The Complete Procedure Coding Book

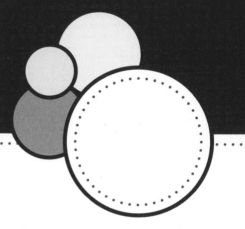

Shelley C. Safian, MAOM/HSM, CCS-P, CPC-H, CHA

Herzing College
Orlando, Florida

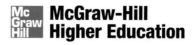

McGraw-Hill Higher Education

Boston   Burr Ridge, IL   Dubuque, IA   New York   San Francisco   St. Louis
Bangkok   Bogotá   Caracas   Kuala Lumpur   Lisbon   London   Madrid   Mexico City
Milan   Montreal   New Delhi   Santiago   Seoul   Singapore   Sydney   Taipei   Toronto

Mc Graw Hill **McGraw-Hill
Higher Education**

THE COMPLETE PROCEDURE CODING BOOK

Published by McGraw-Hill, a business unit of The McGraw-Hill Companies, Inc., 1221 Avenue of the Americas, New York, NY, 10020. Copyright © 2009 by The McGraw-Hill Companies, Inc. All rights reserved. No part of this publication may be reproduced or distributed in any form or by any means, or stored in a database or retrieval system, without the prior written consent of The McGraw-Hill Companies, Inc., including, but not limited to, in any network or other electronic storage or transmission, or broadcast for distance learning. Some ancillaries, including electronic and print components, may not be available to customers outside the United States.
This book is printed on acid-free paper.

Printed in China

3 4 5 6 7 8 9 0 CTP/CTP 10

ISBN   978-0-07-340187-4
MHID   0-07-340187-0

Vice President/Editor in Chief: *Elizabeth Haefele*
Vice President/Director of Marketing: *John E. Biernat*
Senior sponsoring editor: *Deborah Fitzgerald*
Managing developmental editor: *Patricia Hesse*
Marketing manager: *Roxan Kinsey*
Lead media producer: *Damian Moshak*
Director, Editing/Design/Production: *Jess Ann Kosic*
Senior project manager: *Rick Hecker*
Production supervisor: *Janean A. Utley*
Designer: *Marianna Kinigakis*
Senior photo research coordinator: *Carrie K. Burger*
Media project manager: *Mark A. S. Dierker*
Cover design: *Pam Verros, pv design*
Interior design: *Marianna Kinigakis*
Typeface: *10.5/13 Melior*
Compositor: *Lachina Publishing Services*
Printer: *CTPS*
Cover credit: *Photos 1 and 3: Chassenet by BSIP/PhototakeUSA.com; Photo 2: C Sovereign by ISM/PhototakeUSA.com; Photo 4: C Beranger by BSIP/PhototakeUSA.com; Photo 5: C Microworks Color/PhototakeUSA.com*
Credits: The credits section for this book begins on page 483 and is considered an extension of the copyright page.

The names of the facilities, health care professionals, and patients have all been changed to protect the privacy and confidentiality of all concerned in these patient records. Any similarities to actual persons or places are purely coincidental. These cases are to be used for educational purposes only.

Library of Congress Cataloging-in-Publication Data
Safian, Shelley C.
    The complete procedure coding book / Shelley C. Safian.
        p. ; cm.
    Includes index.
    ISBN-13: 978-0-07-340187-4 (alk. paper)
    ISBN-10: 0-07-340187-0 (alk. paper)
    1. Medicine—Terminology—Code numbers. I. Title.
    [DNLM: 1. Forms and Records Control—methods. 2. Medical Records. W 80 S128c 2009]
R123.S18 2009
610.1'4—dc22
        2007039568

The Internet addresses listed in the text were accurate at the time of publication. The inclusion of a web site does not indicate an endorsement by the authors or McGraw-Hill, and McGraw-Hill does not guarantee the accuracy of the information presented at these sites.

www.mhhe.com

About the Author

Shelley C. Safian, Chair of the Allied Health Department at Herzing College, is also the Senior Assistant Professor for the Medical Billing and Insurance Coding program. She is currently teaching coding and medical office administration at both Herzing College–Winter Park (Orlando), Florida, and Herzing College Online.

Safian is a Certified Coding Specialist–Physician-based (CCS-P) from the American Health Information Management Association (AHIMA) and a Certified Professional Coder–Hospital (CPC-H) from the American Academy of Professional Coders (AAPC). She also holds a National Certified Insurance Coding Specialist (NCICS) designation, as well as that of Certified HIPAA Administrator (CHA).

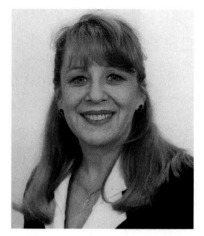

Shelley C. Safian

Safian completed her Graduate Certificate in Health Care Management in June 2005 at Keller Graduate School of Management. The University of Phoenix awarded her Master of Arts/Organizational Management degree in 2002.

Herzing College–Winter Park honored Safian by naming her 2007 Teacher of the Year, and she was awarded the Faculty Scholarship Award–First Runner Up for the Herzing College System.

Safian is a volunteer AHIMA mentor, working with health information management students from all across the country, and sits on the AHIMA Classification Practice Council. She attends local chapter meetings of the Central Florida Health Information Management Association (CFHIMA) whenever her schedule permits, and encourages her students to join her at the Florida Health Information Management Association (FHIMA) Annual Convention every year.

McGraw-Hill Higher Education published *Insurance Coding & Electronic Claims for the Medical Office* by Safian in July 2005. Her second, third, and fourth books, *The Complete Procedure Coding Book, The Complete Diagnosis Coding Book,* and *You Code It! A Case Studies Workbook* were published simultaneously in February 2008.

Brief Contents

Contents

CHAPTER 14 Coding Medical Supplies, Durable Medical Equipment, Pharmaceutical, and Ambulance and Other Transportation Services 338

CHAPTER 15 HCPCS Level II Modifiers 367

Preface

A rather unique aspect of working in the health care industry is the fact that everyone who works in it will at some point become one of its customers. As a larger portion of the population of the United States moves into their older stage of life, the number of customers (patients) will continue to increase. The longer the human body lives, the more maintenance and repair it needs—the services of both preventive and therapeutic health care.

Every time a patient and a health care professional meet, the details of this meeting, known as an encounter, must be documented. Certain details must be reported to government agencies for statistical purposes, such as determining which type of research should be funded and prioritized, which preventive measures should be promoted to the public, or which type of care should be paid for by certain programs. Coders and health information managers are the professionals who interpret the information from the physicians, therapists, radiologists, and so forth, and report the data, in code, so that the agencies can process and work with it.

In addition, the same codes are used to gain payment—reimbursement from insurance carriers and other third party payers—to cover the expense of health care received by patients from their providers. Of course, all the professionals working in health care (physicians, nurses, medical assistants, health information managers) want to—deserve to—get paid for their expertise and hard work.

Coders are in high demand. According to the Bureau of Labor Statistics, the demand for health information management professionals will increase 40 to 50% by the year 2012. Every type of health care facility needs coders: hospitals, doctors' offices, nursing homes, assisted living facilities, clinics, laboratories, radiology centers, and more.

This textbook has been created to begin the journey of learning how to code.

THE AUDIENCE

This book is written to speak directly to the reader and encourage him or her to understand the critical thinking, as well as the technical processes involved in health care coding.

WHAT MAKES THIS BOOK SPECIAL?

The author is a classroom instructor who wants to see her students succeed in their chosen health information management careers. This textbook has been created from her experiences, interacting with students learning coding and watching and evaluating their challenges in learning this demanding skill.

Responding to the comments and recommendations of these students, as well as classroom instructors, the author has created a student-friendly text presenting the step-by-step processes involved with abstracting health care professionals' documentation and accurately translating the facts into the best, most accurate codes.

OVERVIEW

Chapter Structure

This textbook is written on the basis of layered learning—segmented into three stratums.

Layer 1. Preparation

Each chapter begins with a list of **Learning Outcomes** and **Key Terms** to get the reader ready to become educated about the topic of that chapter. **Employment Opportunities** are also listed at the opening of each chapter to help the reader identify a link between the topics they are about to learn and where they can work once they complete their studies.

Layer 2. Knowledge Acquisition

The elements of each chapter's subject matter are presented along with **Key Term Definitions**. **Coding Tips** include helpful memory triggers, as well as ways to avoid common errors. **Examples** are included to help the reader establish a connection between the concepts and real life. Then the unique feature, **Let's Code It! Case Scenarios,** present the reader with a step-by-step guide through the coding process from abstracting physician's notes to choosing key words, finding those key words in the alphabetic index, and then confirming the code or codes in the tabular (numeric) listing. These scenarios are used to reinforce key competencies.

Layer 3. Confirmation of Knowledge Acquisition

Once the reader has gained the knowledge cluster for the chapter, the textbook provides opportunities for testing what has actually been learned. With the concept of layered learning, it is important that the reader confirms that knowledge has been acquired before moving on to the next concept. Testing is provided using several methodologies: **You Code It! Case Studies** enable readers to test themselves several times within each chapter. A short case study is provided with the challenge to the reader to find the most accurate code or codes. Then the answer(s) are presented for comparison. The end of each chapter continues to test the acquisition of knowledge presented in three ways:

> **Chapter Review** is a short, multiple-choice quiz on chapter theory.
> **You Code It! Practice** gives the reader 15 short scenarios to practice coding.
> **You Code It! Simulation** presents five actual case studies for the reader to practice abstracting and going through the entire coding process, as learned in the chapter.

Chapter Review, You Code It! Practice, and **You Code It! Simulation** answers are not included in the textbook, but in the separate Instructor's Manual.

FEATURES

- **Learning Outcomes**

  Each chapter begins with a bulleted list of **Learning Outcomes** to preview the knowledge concepts that will be covered within that particular chapter.

- **Key Terms**

  Each chapter also begins with a list of 10 **Key Terms** to highlight important terminology elements.

- **Employment Opportunities**

  Chapter openers also identify the specific types of health care facilities in which the chapter knowledge concepts are used.

- **Coding Tips**

  Every chapter includes tips for understanding and remembering particular knowledge concepts or coding guidelines. These tips also illuminate strategies for avoiding errors.

- **Examples**

  As each knowledge cluster is presented, examples are provided to establish a connection in the reader's mind between the concept and its use in reality.

- **Let's Code It! Scenario**

  Once the textbook has completed the explanation of a knowledge cluster, the readers are taken, step by step, through a case scenario. It is the literary equivalent to holding their hand and walking them through abstracting the physician's notes and performing the coding process to find the most accurate code or codes.

- **You Code It! Case Study**

  Periodically, each chapter will then provide readers with a case study to practice both the knowledge cluster and the coding process on their own. The answer is then provided so concepts can be reviewed until they are completely understood.

- **Chapter Summary**

  At the end of each chapter, a summary provides a recap of the main concepts covered.

- **Chapter Review**

  A short, multiple-choice quiz tests the reader's knowledge of chapter concepts.

- **You Code It! Practice**

  Readers can test their coding skills with these 15 short case scenarios.

- **You Code It! Simulation**

  Five actual case studies are presented for readers to test their ability to abstract physician's notes and find the most accurate code or codes.

TEACHING AND LEARNING SUPPLEMENTS

Instructor's Manual includes the answers to the end-of-chapter exercises, chapter outlines and overviews, discussion activities, and additional resources.

Instructor Productivity Center CD-ROM contains PowerPoint® presentations for each chapter, exam questions using the EZ-Test format, and the Instructor's Manual.

Online Learning Center at www.mhhe.com/ SafianProcedure offers an extensive array of learning and teaching tools. The site includes quizzes for each chapter, links to websites, crossword puzzles, concentration games and flashcards for vocabulary reinforcement. Instructor resources on the site include PowerPoint® slides, links to professional associations, and the Instructor's Manual.

ACKNOWLEDGMENTS

Every textbook is created by a team, and I, as the author, am only a small part. I wish to thank every member of my team.

Thank you to the students of Herzing College, for without them I would not have the input, the direction, or the motivation to write this book. As if that weren't enough, they also served as testers, using the manuscript for this book as their text to ensure this book works to help students learn in the best possible manner.

Thank you to the administration of Herzing College, especially Tammy Files and Drew Warren, who encouraged me, supported me, and gave me the opportunities to teach and share with my students.

Thank you to my team at McGraw-Hill Higher Education. The professionals in the editorial, marketing, production, and media departments are a pleasure to work with. You all have really helped make this the best book it can be, especially Roxan, Pat, Wendy, Rick, and certainly Ben, who started it all.

And thank you to April Waye, without whom I would not even know what coding was!

REVIEWERS

I would like to thank the many instructors who provided detailed recommendations for improving chapter content throughout the review process.

Bobette Anderson, CPC
MedVance Institute
Lauderdale Lakes, FL

Darlene Boschert, CPC, CPC-H
Career Institute of Florida
St. Petersburg, FL

Gerry Brasin, AS
Premier Education Group
Springfield, MA

Lisa G. Bynoe, BS, MBA
ASA Institute
New York, NY

Christine M. Cole, CCA
Williston State College
Williston, ND

Rosalind Collazo, BS, MS
ASA Institute
Brooklyn, NY

Christine M. Enz, BA, MEd
Rochester Business Institute
Rochester, NY

Theresa Errante-Parrino, AS, BS
Indian River Community College
Port St. Lucie, FL

Kristina Ferry, MAED
Heritage College
Las Vegas, NV

Janet Hunter, MBA, MS,
Northland Pioneer College
Holbrook, AZ

Judy Hurtt
East Central Community College
Decatur, MS

Carol Lee Jarrell, MLT, AHI
Brown Mackie College
Merrillville, IN

Jennifer Lame, MPH, BS, RHIT
Southwest Wisconsin Technical College
Fennimore, WI

Martha Luebke, AA, BA
High Tech Institute
Las Vegas, NV

Pat Moeck, PhD, MBA, BA
El Centro College
Dallas, TX

Della Moon, AA
San Jacinto College
Houston, TX

John E. Nurge, MEd
CCI Training Center, Inc.
Dallas, TX

Sheba Schlailger, BA, RHIT
Colorado Tech University
Sioux Falls, SD

Shirely Eittrein Shaw, MA
Northland Pioneer College
Holbrook, AZ

Anna M. Slaski, JD
International Institute of the Americas
Tucson, AZ

Jim Wallace, MHSA
Maric College
Los Angeles, CA

Teach Me...Show Me...Let Me Try

This text takes a unique approach to the learning process by presenting content to the student in a format the author calls *layered learning*.

Teach Me

Learning Outcomes

Key Terms

Employment Opportunities

Coding Tips

Provides expectations, definitions, goals, and coding process hints.

Show Me

Examples

Let's Code It! Scenario

Establishes a connection between concepts and real life.

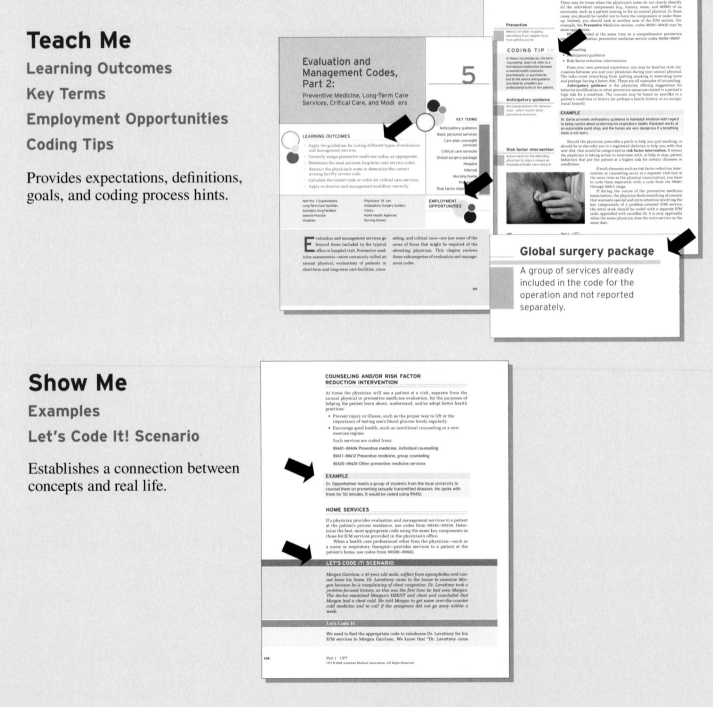

Let Me Try

You Code It! Case Study

Promotes student coding practice using real life cases.

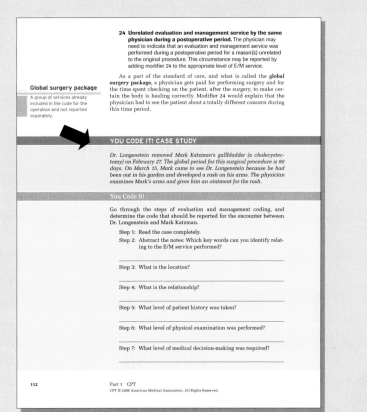

Review

Chapter Review Quizzes
You Code It! Practice
You Code It! Simulation

Reinforces chapter content.

To the Student

YOUR CAREER

This class introduces you to skills you will need in order to work in the health information management profession. A fundamental part of an insurance coding and medical billing specialist's job is to work with the insurance companies that will reimburse your health care facility for the services and treatments you provide to your patients. You may be employed by a hospital, clinic, doctor's office, health maintenance organization, mental health care facility, insurance company, government agency, or long-term care facility. This career is challenging, interesting, and one of the 10 fastest growing allied health occupations.

HOW CAN I SUCCEED IN THIS CLASS?

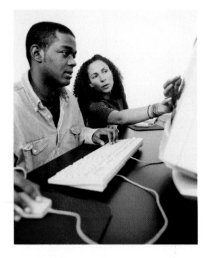

If you're reading this, you're on the right track.

> *"You are the same today that you are going to be five years from now except for two things: the people with whom you associate and the books you read."* Charles Jones

Right now, you're probably leafing through this book feeling just a little overwhelmed. You're trying to juggle several other classes (which probably are equally as intimidating), possibly a job, and on top of it all, a life.

These helpful hints have been designed specifically to help you focus. They're here to help you learn how to manage your time and your studies to succeed.

START HERE

It's true—you are what you put into your studies. You have a lot of time and money invested in your education. Don't blow it now by putting in only half of the effort this class requires. Succeeding in this class (and life) requires

- Making a commitment—of time and perseverance
- Knowing and motivating yourself
- Getting organized
- Managing your time

This text will help you learn how to be effective in these areas, as well as offer guidance in

- Getting the most out of your lecture
- Thinking through—and applying—the material

- Getting the most out of your textbook
- Finding extra help when you need it

Making a Commitment—of Time and Perseverance

Learning—and mastering—takes time, and patience. Nothing worthwhile comes easily. Be committed to your studies and you will reap the benefits in the long run.

Consider this: Your college education is building the foundation for your future—a future in your chosen profession. Sloppy and hurried craftsmanship now will only lead to ruin later.

Side note: A good rule of thumb is to allow two hours of study time for every hour you spend in lecture.

For instance, a three-hour lecture deserves six hours of study time. If you commit time for this course daily, you're investing a little less than one hour per day, including the weekend. Study time includes writing reports, completing practice problems, reading textual material, and reviewing notes.

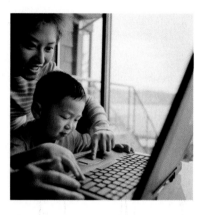

Knowing and Motivating Yourself

What type of a learner are you? When are you most productive? Know yourself and your limits and work within them. Know how to motivate yourself to give your all to your studies and achieve your goals. Quite bluntly, you are the one who benefits most from your success. If you lack self-motivation and drive, you are the first person that suffers.

Knowing yourself—there are many types of learners and no right or wrong way of learning. Which category do you fall into?

Visual learner—you respond best to "seeing" processes and information. Particularly focus on text illustrations and charts and course handouts, and check to see if there are animations on the course or text website to help you. Also, consider drawing diagrams in your notes to illustrate concepts.

Auditory learner—you work best by listening to—and possibly tape recording—the lecture and by talking through information with a study partner.

Tactile/kinesthetic learner—you learn best by being "hands on." You'll benefit by applying what you've learned during lab time. Think of ways to apply your critical thinking skills in application ways.

Identify your personal preferences for learning and seek out the resources that will best help you with your studies. Also, learn by recognizing your weaknesses and try to compensate/work to improve them.

Getting Organized

It's simple, yet it's fundamental. It seems, the more organized you are, the easier things come. Take the time before your course begins to look around and analyze your life and your study habits. Get organized now and you'll find you have a little more time—and a lot less stress.

- **Find a calendar system that works for you.** The best kind is one that you can take with you everywhere. To be truly organized, you

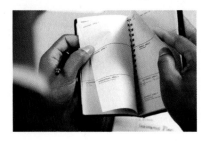

should integrate all aspects of your life into this one calendar—school, work, leisure. Some people also find it helpful to have an additional monthly calendar posted by their desk for "at a glance" dates and to have a visual of what's to come. If you do this, be sure you are consistently synchronizing both calendars so as not to miss anything. *More tips for organizing your calendar can be found in the time management discussion.*

- By the same token, **keep everything for your course or courses in one place**—and at your fingertips. A three-ring binder works well because it allows you to add or organize handouts and notes from class in any order you prefer. Incorporating your own custom tabs helps you flip to exactly what you need at a moments notice.

- **Find your space.** Find a place that helps you be organized and focused. If it's your desk in your dorm room or in your home, keep it clean. Clutter adds confusion and stress and wastes time. Or perhaps your "space" is at the library. If that's the case, keep a backpack or bag that's fully stocked with what you might need—your text, binder or notes, pens, highlighters, Post-its, phone numbers of study partners (a good place to keep phone numbers is in your "one place for everything calendar").

A helpful hint—add extra "padding" into your deadlines for yourself. If you have a report due on Friday, set a goal for yourself to have it done on Wednesday. Then, take time on Thursday to look over your project again, with a fresh eye. Make any corrections or enhancements and have it ready to turn in on Friday.

Managing Your Time

Managing your time is the single most important thing you can do to help yourself. And it's probably one of the most difficult tasks to master.

You are in college taking this course because you want to succeed in life. You are preparing for a career. In college, you are expected to work much harder and to learn much more than you ever have before. To be successful, you need to invest in your education with a commitment of time.

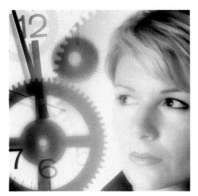

We all lead busy lives. But we all make choices as to how we spend our time. Choose wisely and make the most of every minute you have by implementing these tips:

- **Know yourself and when you'll be able to study most efficiently.** When are you most productive? Are you a late nighter? Or an early bird? Plan to study when you are most alert and can have uninterrupted segments. This could include a quick, five-minute review before class or a one-hour problem-solving study session with a friend.

- **Create a set study time for yourself daily.** Having a set schedule for yourself helps you commit to studying and helps you plan instead of cram. Find—and use—a planner that is small enough that you can take it with you—everywhere. This can be a $2.50 paper calendar or a more expensive electronic version. They all work on the same premise—**organize all of your activities in one place.**

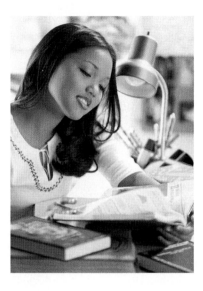

- Less is more. **Schedule study time using shorter, focused blocks with small breaks.** Doing this offers two benefits:
  1. You will be less fatigued and gain more from your effort.
  2. Studying will seem less overwhelming and you will be less likely to procrastinate.

- **Plan time for leisure, friends, exercise, and sleep.** Studying should be your main focus, but you need to balance your time—and your life.

- Make sure you **log your projects and homework deadlines** in your personal calendar.

- **"Plot" your assignments on your calendar or task list.** If you have a large report, for instance, break down the assignment into smaller targets. Set a goal for a first draft, second draft, and final copy.

- Try to **complete tasks ahead of schedule.** This will give you a chance to review your work carefully before you hand it in (instead of at 1 A.M., when you are half awake). You'll feel less stressed in the end.

- **Prioritize!** In your calendar or planner, highlight or number key projects; do them first, and then cross them off when you've completed them. Give yourself a pat on the back for getting them done!

- **Review your calendar and reprioritize daily.**

- Try to **resist distractions by setting and sticking to a designated study time** (remember your commitment and perseverance!). Distractions include friends and surfing the Internet.

- **Multitask when possible.** You may find a lot of extra time you didn't think you had. Review material or organize your term paper in your head while walking to class or doing laundry.

Side note: Plan to study and plan for leisure. Being well balanced will help you focus when it is time to study.

Tip: Try combining social time with studying or social time with mealtime or exercise. Being a good student doesn't mean you have to be a hermit. It does mean you need to know how to budget your time smartly.

- **Learn to manage or avoid time wasters.**

Don't

- **Let friends manage your time.**

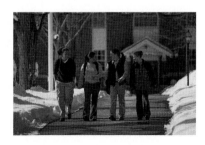

Tip: Kindly ask, "Can we talk later?" when you are trying to study; this will keep you in control of your time without alienating your friends.

- **Get sucked into the Internet.**

  It's easy to lose hours in front of the computer surfing the web. Set a time limit for yourself and stick to it.

Do

- **Use small bits of time to your advantage.**

  Example: Arrive to class five minutes early and review notes. Review your personal calendar for upcoming due dates and events while eating meals or waiting for appointments.

- **Balance your life.**

  Sleep, study, and leisure are all important. Keep each in balance.

Getting the Most Out of Lectures

Believe it or not, instructors want you to succeed. They put a lot of effort into helping you learn and preparing their lectures. Attending class is one of the simplest, most valuable things you can do to help yourself. But it doesn't end there—getting the most out of your lectures means being organized. Here's how:

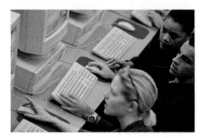

Prepare Before You Go to Class

You'll be amazed at how much more comprehensible the material will be when you preview the chapter before you go to class. Don't feel overwhelmed by this already. One tip that may help you is to plan to arrive to class 5–15 minutes before the lecture. Take your text with you and skim the chapter before lecture begins. At the very least, this will give you an overview of what may be discussed.

Be a Good Listener

Most people think they are good listeners, but few really are. Are you? Following are obvious but important points to remember:

- You can't listen if you're talking.
- You aren't listening if you're daydreaming.
- Listening and comprehending are two different things. If you don't understand something your instructor is saying, ask a question or jot a note and visit the instructor after hours. Don't feel dumb or intimidated; you probably aren't the only person who "doesn't get it."

Take Good Notes

- Use a standard-size notebook or, better yet, a three-ring binder with loose-leaf notepaper. The binder will allow you to organize and integrate your notes and handouts, integrate easy-to-reference tabs, and so on.
- Use a standard black or blue ink pen to take your initial notes. You can annotate later using a pencil, which can be erased if need be.
- Start a new page with each lecture or note-taking session (yes—you can and should also take notes from your textbook).
- Label each page with the date and a heading for each day.
- Focus on main points and try to use an outline format to take notes to capture key ideas and organize subpoints.

- Review and edit your notes shortly after class—at least within 24 hours—to make sure they make sense and that you've recorded core thoughts. You may also want to compare your notes with a study partner's later to make sure neither of you has missed anything.

Get a Study Partner

Having a study partner has so many benefits. First, he or she can help you keep your commitment to this class. By having set study dates, you can combine study and social time, and maybe even make it fun! In addition, you now have two sets of eyes and ears and two minds to help digest the information from the lecture and the text. Talk through concepts, compare notes, and quiz each other.

An obvious note: Don't take advantage of your study partner by skipping class or skipping study dates. You obviously won't have a study partner—or a friend—very long if it's not a mutually beneficial arrangement!

Helpful hint: Take your text to lecture, and keep it open to the topics being discussed. You can take brief notes in your textbook margin or reference textbook pages in your notebook to help you study later.

How to Study for an Exam

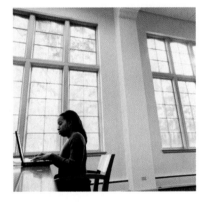

- Study, don't simply reread material.
- Be an active learner.
- Finish reading all material—text, notes, handouts—at least three days prior to the exam.
- Be an active participant in class; ask questions.
- Apply what you've learned; think through scenarios rather than memorize your notes.
- Three days prior to the exam, set aside time each day to do self-testing, to practice problems, and to review notes.
- Create an "I don't know this yet" list. Focus on strengthening these areas and narrow your list as your study.
- Create your own study tools, such as index card flash cards and checklists, and practice writing short essays if this is how your instructor tests.
- Very important: Be sure to sleep and eat well before the exam.

Getting the Most Out of Your Textbook

McGraw-Hill and the author of this book have invested their time, research, and talents to help you succeed, as well. The goal is to make learning—for you—easier. Here's how:

- Use the chapter objectives to guide you through the material presented.
- Review the key terms and definitions, and make certain you understand them.
- Read and jot down the important notes.
- Use the memory tips.
- Practice critical thinking skills.

- Practice coding using the sample cases and examples.
- Read chapter summaries.
- Complete You Code It! Reviews.
- Explore the online learning center activities.

PART ONE

CPT

1

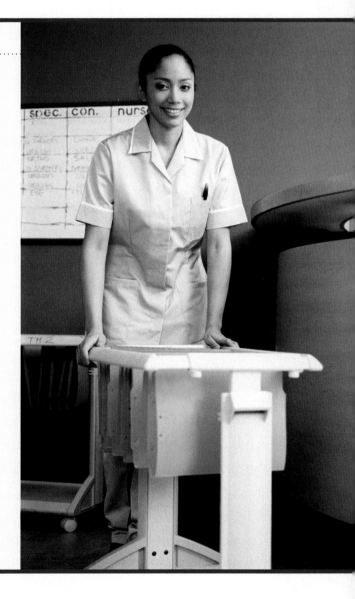

1

Legal and Ethical Issues

LEARNING OUTCOMES

- Identify your responsibilities under HIPAA's Privacy Rule to protect a patient's information.
- Detect signs of health care fraud and abuse.
- Apply the rules of ethical and legal coding.
- Detect ethical danger zones that might exist in the workplace.
- Use the guidelines to determine the legally correct code.
- Outline a compliance program.
- Identify the points within AHIMA Code of Ethics, AHIMA's Standards of Ethical Coding, and the AAPC's Code of Ethics that will direct your conduct as a professional coder.

EMPLOYMENT OPPORTUNITIES

Physicians' offices
Hospitals
Clinics
Nursing homes

Family practice
General practice
Assisted living facilities
Pharmacies

As health care professionals, you will have special legal and ethical responsibilities that others, working in a standard business office, do not have. You will have the privilege to work with other health care professionals to help their patients and clients. In order to do this properly, you will have access to very personal and private information about that individual. In addition, as an insurance coding specialist, you will be working with data that also directly relate to how much your facility will be paid for its services—this is called reimbursement. As you can imagine, working with these two categories of information—personal information about an individual's health and how much professionals are being paid for their services—requires confidentiality, honesty, and accuracy.

Legal and ethical issues can be very complicated. Some working professionals are misinformed. Others never had the opportunity to learn the proper way to handle certain situations. This chapter helps you establish a firm foundation for your future career.

HEALTH INSURANCE PORTABILITY AND ACCOUNTABILITY ACT

The Health Insurance Portability and Accountability Act of 1996, known as HIPAA (pronounced *hip-aah*), was enacted by the federal government, and directly applies to you as a coding professional.

Like most federal laws, HIPAA covers many different issues and concerns. The Privacy Rule, one part of this law, is the section that you are obligated to know and understand.

HIPAA's Privacy Rule was written to protect an individual's privacy with regard to personal health information, without getting in the way of the flow of data that is necessary to provide appropriate care for that patient. Essentially, the lawmakers tried to make certain that *a patient's information is easily accessible to those who should have access to it* (such as the physician, insurance coder and biller, and therapist), *and still keep it secured against unauthorized people* (such as potential employers, co-workers, or neighborhood gossips) so that they do not see things they have no business seeing.

HIPAA's Privacy Rule

A portion of HIPAA that ensures the availability of patient information for those who should see it while protecting that information from those who should not.

Who Is Responsible for Obeying This Law

HIPAA went into effect on April 14, 2003, and concerns every physician's office, clinic, hospital, health insurance carrier—every type of business that is directly involved in the delivery of and/or payment for health care services, no matter how big or small. The largest of corporations owning hundreds of hospitals around the country and an office with one physician working alone are all included. HIPAA calls these businesses **covered entities**, and they all must comply with the terms of the law.

Covered entities are divided into three categories:

Covered entities

Health care providers, health plans, and health care clearinghouses—businesses that have access to the personal health information of patients.

- Health care providers
- Health plans
- Health care clearinghouses

You probably already know the definition of a health care provider: any person or organization that gives health care services as the primary business purpose.

EXAMPLE

Health care providers as defined by HIPAA: physicians, dentists, hospitals, clinics, pharmacies, and laboratories.

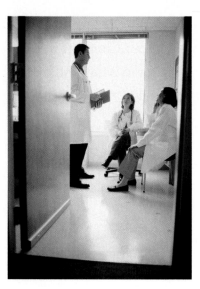

Health plans are described as organizations that provide and/or pay for health care services as their main reason for being in business. They include health insurance carriers, HMOs, employee welfare benefit plans, government health plans (such as TriCare, Medicare, and Medicaid), and group health plans provided through employers and associations. It doesn't matter whether the plan is offered to an individual or a group—all companies offering this coverage are included.

EXAMPLE

Health care plans as defined by HIPAA: Medicare, Medicaid, TriCare, BlueCross/Blue Shield, and Prudential.

In addition, technology has created another type of organization involved in this process, called health care clearinghouses. These companies help process electronic health insurance claim forms. Medical billing services, medical review services, and health information management system companies are included in this definition.

EXAMPLE

Health care clearinghouses as defined by HIPAA: National Clearinghouse, NDC Electronic Claims, and WebMD Network Services.

The workforces of covered entities are also included under HIPAA. A covered entity's workforce consists of every single person who is involved with the company—full time, part time, volunteer, intern, extern, physician, nurse, assistant—and this has nothing to do with whether they are paid. Everyone must comply with the terms of this law.

EXAMPLE

A covered entity's workforce as defined by HIPAA: Full-time staff members, part-time staff members, volunteers, interns, externs, and janitorial staff members.

What This Law Covers

You are certainly familiar with the topic of doctor-patient confidentiality. It means that anything a patient tells his or her doctor must be kept private. The doctor is not allowed, under most circumstances, to reveal to anyone what was said. The exclusion includes family members, parents (in many cases), and friends. This is important so that an individual will feel comfortable being open and honest and tell the physician things that are very, very personal, possibly even embarrassing or private facts that this person has never told anyone else. However, in order for the physician to properly treat this individual, the physician must know everything.

In order for you to do your job properly, you have access to all this confidential information. You need to know very personal and private facts about each and every one of your patients in order to accurately

CODING TIP »»

HIPAA's Privacy Rule is mostly about protecting your patient's privacy.

Part 1 CPT

report the data. You know what is wrong with them (their diagnoses) now and in the past; you know why they came to see this health care provider and why they saw others before they came to your facility; and you know what the health care provider thinks (observations and impressions) about these patients, as well as what has been done, is being done, and will be done to treat them. You know all these things because you have access to patients' health care records including all the physician's notes. HIPAA calls this personal health care information (past, present, and future conditions) individually identifiable health information. In other words, it is information that anyone could look at and know exactly which individual is being discussed—one specific person. Specific pieces of data, called **protected health information (PHI)**, are pieces of information related to an individual that must be kept confidential. The grouping of facts that might have someone say, "Oh, I know him! Oh, and he has that!"

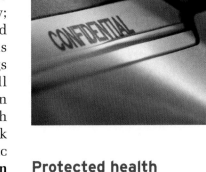

Protected health information (PHI)

Any patient identifiable health information regardless of the form in which it is stored (paper, computer file, etc.).

EXAMPLE

Evan Montgomery is a patient of Dr. Cowell, and the pieces of paper inside his chart contain his records, charts, lab reports, and physician's notes documenting everything Evan has ever discussed with his physician. Donna needs all this information to do her job as the office's coding specialist. At this moment, Donna has stepped away from her desk. Evan Montgomery's file is sitting on Donna's desk, lying open.

From the color of the folder, even from a distance, it is obvious that this is a patient of Dr. Cowell's. The top piece of paper indicates that his patient has been diagnosed with a sexually transmitted disease. *At this point, you couldn't really know whose chart this is because Dr. Cowell has hundreds of patients.*

Right above the diagnosis you can see that this patient is a male. *While this will eliminate some of Dr. Cowell's patients, there are still too many to know for certain.*

Upon closer examination of the paperwork in the folder, anyone could see that this male patient with the sexually transmitted disease lives on Main Street in Our Town, Florida. *The list of Dr. Cowell's patients that is being referred to is getting very short now.*

In the upper right corner, you can see Dr. Cowell's male patient, of Main Street, Our Town, Florida, who has a sexually transmitted disease, was born on June 13, 1985. *Oh my, did you know Evan Montgomery lives on Main Street in Our Town, and his birthday is June 13th! It must be Evan that has that terrible disease!*

Did Donna fulfill her responsibility to protect Evan Montgomery's privacy? What could she have done differently to ensure that this patient's PHI was protected?

Evan Montgomery's private health record is no longer private. His diagnosis of a sexually transmitted disease is health information. After discovering his gender, address, and birth date, you connected this diagnosis directly to one particular person. All these details, and any other pieces of information, are protected to be private under the law. This means that all this information is confidential, and it is against the law for you to reveal any of it with only a few exceptions:

1. You can tell other health care professionals who are directly involved in the course of doing your job.
2. You can tell someone when given written permission from the patient to do so.
3. You can tell in situations, as outlined in the law, based on "best professional judgment."

The Use and Disclosure of PHI

HIPAA's Privacy Rule is very specific as to how you can handle the PHI that you work with every day. The guidelines offer two terms to describe how you might deal with this data.

The term **use** (with regard to HIPAA) means that the information is being shared between people who work together in the same office and need to exchange PHI in order to better serve the patient.

Use

The sharing of information between people working in the same health care facility for purposes of caring for the patient.

EXAMPLE

You are getting ready to code the diagnosis for Jayne Hite's recent visit and need additional information. You speak with the attending physician, Dr. Samson, to discuss Jayne's PHI, so you can make certain you find the best, most appropriate diagnosis code. You are using that patient's PHI because the information is being shared between you and the physician in the same office for the benefit of the patient.

Disclosure

The sharing of information between health care professionals working in separate entities, or facilities, in the course of caring for the patient.

The second term is **disclosure.** HIPAA defines the term disclosure to mean that PHI is being revealed to someone outside of the health care office or facility. For example, you prepare a health insurance claim form to send to the patient's insurance company so it will pay your office for the procedures provided. On that claim form, you must put the patient's full name and address, birth date, diagnosis codes, and procedure codes. As you learned earlier in this chapter, each piece of data is not necessarily confidential. When you put all this information together in one place, it becomes PHI because this health information (diagnosis codes) is now connected to a specific person (identified by the name, address, birth date, etc.) on one piece of paper. However, you must disclose this information to the insurance carrier in order to get paid. You are disclosing the information because the insurance company personnel who will read this claim form do not work for your health care facility—they are an outside company.

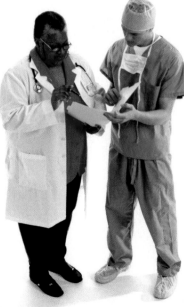

EXAMPLE

Dr. Morton indicates that his patient, John Smith, needs some lab work. Dr. Morton will use Mr. Smith's PHI in his orders for which tests should be performed. Then you need to call the laboratory and *disclose* Mr. Smith's PHI (his name and diagnosis) along with what specific tests should be performed by the lab.

Remember that everyone in your office and everyone at the insurance carrier and the lab are all members of a covered entity's workforce. You are all bound by the same terms of the HIPAA law, and cannot reveal any patient's PHI, except under particular circumstances (such as *use* and *disclosure*), unless you have the patient's written permission.

Getting Written Approval

In all situations, other than those already mentioned, the health care provider must get a patient's written permission to disclose the PHI. While there are many preprinted forms that your office or facility may purchase, the Privacy Rule of HIPAA insists that all these documents have the following characteristics:

1. Are written in plain language (not legalese), so that the average person can understand what he or she is signing.

2. Are very specific as to exactly what information will be disclosed or used.

3. Specifically identify the person or organization that will be disclosing the information.

4. Specifically identify the person(s) who will be receiving the information.

5. Have a definite expiration date.

6. Clearly explain that the person signing this release may retract this authorization in writing at any time.

Figure 1-1 is an example of a form that your facility might use for this purpose.

Permitted Uses and Disclosures

The Privacy Rule outlines six particular circumstances in which health care professionals are permitted, with or without written patient permission, to use their best professional judgment as to whether or not they should use and/or disclose a patient's PHI.

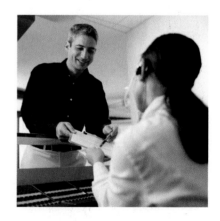

1. **To the individual.** Health care professionals can *use their best professional judgment to decide whether or not a patient should be told* certain things contained in their health care record. Questions come up especially when mental health issues and terminal conditions (when a patient is almost certain to die in the near future) might be concerned and there is doubt if the patient can deal with the medical facts. In almost all cases, providing patients with their own PHI is allowed.

2. **Treatment, payment, and/or operations.** This means that health care professionals are free to use and/or disclose PHI when it comes to making decisions, coordinating, and managing the *treatment* of a patient's condition.

EXAMPLE

A physician needs to be able to discuss PHI details with a therapist so that they can establish a proper course of treatment for the patient.

CIPHER, VICTORS, & ASSOCIATES
A Complete Health Care Facility
234 MAIN STREET • ANYTOWN, FL 32711 • 407-555-1234

AUTHORIZATION FOR RELEASE OF CONFIDENTIAL HEALTH INFORMATION

REGARDING:

_____   _____   _____   _____
PATIENT'S NAME   DATE OF BIRTH   SOCIAL SECURITY #   TELEPHONE NUMBER

I AUTHORIZE   _____

ADDRESS   _____

CITY, STATE, ZIP _____

TO DISCLOSE   _____
                  (EXACTLY WHAT INFORMATION HAS YOUR PERMISSION TO BE DISCLOSED.)

                  _____

TO RECEIVING PARTY _____

ADDRESS   _____

CITY, STATE, ZIP _____

NOTE TO RECEIVING PARTY: THIS INFORMATION IS DISCLOSED TO YOU FROM RECORDS WHOSE CONFIDENTIALITY IS PROTECTED BY LAW. ANY REDISCLOSURE IS STRICTLY PROHIBITED WITHOUT THE WRITTEN PERMISSION OF THE PATIENT/CLIENT/LEGAL REPRESENTATIVE IDENTIFIED BELOW.

THIS AUTHORIZATION FOR RELEASE OF CONFIDENTIAL HEALTH INFORMATION EXPIRES ON _____, AND MAY BE REVOKED AT ANY TIME WITH WRITTEN NOTIFICATION OF REVOCATION TO THE NAMED PARTY ABOVE.

_____   _____   _____
PATIENT/LEGAL REPRESENTATIVE'S SIGNATURE   RELATIONSHIP TO PATIENT   DATE

_____   _____   _____
WITNESS SIGNATURE   TITLE   DATE

Figure 1-1   Example of Authorization Form to Release Health Information.

In addition, PHI can be disclosed for *payment* activities, such as billing and claims processing as mentioned earlier in this chapter. In this description, the term *operations* refers to the health care facility's own management of case coordination and quality evaluations.

3. **Opportunity to agree or object.** This relates to a more informal situation where the patient is present and alert and has the ability to give verbal permission, or not, with regard to a specific disclosure.

One important point to remember: While it is much easier to simply ask someone and get their oral approval than to go get a form and make the patient sign first, it is in your best interest to get written approval whenever possible. People's memories may fail, or they may change their mind later about what they really did tell you. If there is nothing on paper, you cannot prove what was said. For your own protection, get it in writing whenever possible!

4. **Incidental use and disclosure.** As long as reasonable safeguards are in place, this portion of the rule addresses the fact that information might accidentally be used or disclosed during the regular course of business.

This is called incidental use and is understandable within a working environment; therefore, it is not considered a violation of the law.

However, it is important for conversations like this to include only the *minimum necessary* PHI to accomplish the goal. Minimum necessary refers to the caution that should be used to release only the smallest amount of information required to accomplish the task and no more.

Not only is it unnecessary, it is unprofessional.

5. **Public Interest.** There are times when, in the public's best interest, you should disclose what you know about a patient. Very often, this is mandated by state laws, which would then take priority over the federal HIPAA law. In other words, if the federal law says you

≪≪ CODING TIP

Incidental is close to the word *accidental*—if someone accidentally overhears what you say.

are allowed to tell, and your state's law says you must tell—then, you must! These situations may include the reporting of suspected abuse (child abuse, elder abuse, or domestic violence) or the reporting of sexually transmitted and other contagious diseases. You are included in the health care team and must think about the community, which must be warned if someone is walking around with a contagious (communicable) disease. Most states require notification to the police in cases where the patient has been shot or stabbed. It is your responsibility to find out what the laws are in your state and how to correctly file a report.

If the physician does not report suspected child abuse of one of your patients, it is your obligation to pick up the phone and call.

6. **Limited data set.** For research, public health statistics, or other health care operations, PHI can be revealed but only after it has been depersonalized. In other words, if the data that connects this information to one specific individual are removed or blacked out, the information is no longer individually identifiable health information, so it does not need to be protected any longer.

EXAMPLE

You can release a health record that has no name, address, telephone number, e-mail address, Social Security number, or photographs attached to it. Even certain physician's notes can be released, after they have been stripped of that personal data. Following is a sample portion of a record that can be shown without fear of violating anyone's privacy:

"____ is 25 years old. Back in December, ____ was in a motor vehicle accident on the job. ____ is complaining about some neck pain. ____ has tingling into the right hand."

The example above is a direct quote from the medical record of an actual patient after the specified direct identifiers have been removed. You cannot connect this health information to any one particular person. Therefore, the information is no longer protected, and can be used for research and in other ways that may help the community.

Privacy Notices

HIPAA instructs all its covered entities to create policies and procedures with regard to the use and disclosure of PHI. In addition, the law actually states that once policies and procedures are developed, the facilities must follow these policies. Copies of the written policy must be given to every individual patient and posted in a general area where it can be seen by all patients.

Privacy practices notices written in compliance with HIPAA's Privacy Rule must contain the following points:

1. A full description of how the covered entity may use and/or disclose a patient's PHI.

2. A statement about the covered entity's responsibility to protect a patient's privacy.

3. Complete information about the patient's rights, including contact information for the Department of Health and Human Services (HHS) should the patient wish to lodge a complaint that his or her privacy was violated.

4. A specific employee of the covered entity must be named as *privacy officer*. This person's name, as well as contact information, must be included in the written notice to handle patient's questions and complaints.

5. The covered entity must receive written acknowledgment from each patient stating that he or she received the written privacy practices notice. This is usually one of the papers that a patient has to sign when going to a health care facility for the first time.

One of the most important aspects of this portion of the Privacy Rule is that the law specifically says that the covered entity not only has to create these policies and procedures but also has to abide by them. If it doesn't, it is considered to be in violation of federal law and punishable by fines and/or imprisonment.

While some health care staff members feel that HIPAA and its Privacy Rule are a pain in the neck, think about what this law actually means: respecting your patients' privacy and dignity.

Isn't that what you expect from your health care professionals when you go for help? It is not enough that only the doctor be bound to protect the patient's information as confidential, because the doctor is no longer the only person who has access. Your health care facility is no place for gossip or telling tales. You might find this person's hemorrhoids funny or that person's rash gross. As a professional, you should not be concerned with entertaining your friends with your patients' private circumstances. How would you feel if it were *your* personal problem that your health care team members were giggling about with their friends? Or you might consider telling your brother his girlfriend came in with a sexually transmitted disease. You cannot! Everyone is entitled to privacy. As difficult as it may be, you must remain a professional.

««« CODING TIP

This law simply assures each and every person coming to your health care facility that his or her personal and private information will be protected and treated with respect.

Violating HIPAA's Privacy Rule

Any individual who discovers that his or her privacy has been misused or disclosed without permission can file a complaint with the HHS that the health care provider, health plan, or clearinghouse has not followed HIPAA's regulations. When writing this law, Congress included specifications for both civil and criminal penalties to be applied against any covered entity that fails to protect its patients' PHI. These penalties include fines—up to $250,000—and up to 10 years in prison.

A covered entity is responsible for any violation of HIPAA requirements by any of its employees, business associates or any other members of its workforce, such as interns and volunteers. Generally, the senior officials of the covered entity may be punished for the lack of compliance; however, middle managers and staff members are not exempt.

Civil Penalties

1. $100 with no prison for each single violation of a HIPAA regulation with a maximum of $25,000 for multiple violations of the same portion of the regulation during the same calendar year.

> **EXAMPLE**
>
> You tell your best friend that Alan Olin, who you both went to school with, came into your physician's office and tested positive for a sexually transmitted disease. You, of course, swear her to secrecy. Later that day, she bumps into Alan's fiancée and feels obligated to tell her about Alan's condition. Alan puts two and two together, after his fiancée breaks up with him, and he files a complaint that you disclosed his PHI without permission. You and/or your physician are fined $100.

Criminal Penalties

2. Up to $50,000 *and* up to one year in jail for the unauthorized or inappropriate disclosure of individually identifiable health information.

> **EXAMPLE**
>
> After you are fined the $100 civil penalty for the above inappropriate disclosure of Alan Olin's PHI, you and/or your physician are charged with criminal penalties for this same disclosure, including a fine of $50,000 and a year in jail.

3. Up to $100,000 *and* up to five years in prison for the unauthorized or inappropriate disclosure of individually identifiable health information through deception.

> **EXAMPLE**
>
> Your best friend since high school, Roxanne Rogers, just got a great new job as a pharmaceutical representative. To help her, you give her a list of all the patients from your facility who have been diagnosed with diabetes so she can advertise her company's new drug to them. You and she both know this is illegal, so you tell Roxanne that you got permission from each of the patients to release the information (and that is a lie). After a patient complains to the HHS, the investigation discovers your relationship with Roxanne. You and your physician are fined $100,000 per occurrence (that's for each person on the list), as well as sentenced to five years in prison.

4. Up to $250,000 *and* up to 10 years in prison for the unauthorized or inappropriate disclosure of individually identifiable health information through deception with intent to sell or use for business-related benefit, personal gain, or hateful detriment.

> **EXAMPLE**
>
> A famous television star is a patient of the physician's office down the hall from yours. You get a call from a tabloid newspaper offering you a lot of money for any information on the celebrity's health. So

you call the manager of the pathology lab and tell him you are filling in at the other physician's office and need test results for Mr. TV. Then you call the tabloid reporter and tell him what you found out. You used deception (you lied about working in the other physician's office) to gain PHI that you then sold for personal financial gain. You (and possibly your physician) are fined a quarter of a million dollars and sentenced to 10 years in prison. Definitely not worth it!

HEALTH CARE FRAUD AND ABUSE CONTROL PROGRAM

HIPAA also created the *Health Care Fraud and Abuse Control Program.* This program, under the direction of the Attorney General and the secretary of the HHS, acts in association with the Office of the Inspector General (OIG) and coordinates with federal, state, and local law enforcement agencies to discover those who attempt to defraud or abuse the health care system, including Medicare and Medicaid patients and programs.

In 2003, approximately $723 million was returned to the Medicare Trust Fund and another $151.6 million was reimbursed to the Centers for Medicare and Medicaid Services (CMS). Since this program was created in 1997, over $5.69 billion has been returned to the Medicare Trust Fund.

Also, in 2003, 362 criminal indictments were filed in health care fraud cases, and 437 defendants were convicted for health care fraud–related crimes. Another 231 civil cases were filed, and 1,277 more civil matters were pending during this year. This program also prohibited 3,275 individuals and organizations from working with any federally sponsored programs (such as Medicare and Medicaid). Most of these were as a result of convictions for Medicare- or Medicaid-related crimes, including patient abuse and patient neglect, or as a result of providers' licenses having been revoked.

RULES FOR ETHICAL AND LEGAL CODING

As a coder, you have a very important responsibility—to yourself, your patients, and your facility. The work you do results in the creation of health claim forms, which are legal documents. Your responsibilities can help your facility stay healthy (businesswise) or contribute to the business's being fined and shut down by the Office of the Inspector General and your state's attorney general. It is important that you clearly understand the ethical and legal aspects of your new position. Following are some issues, with regard to the ethics and legalities of coding, with which you should become very familiar.

1. It is very important that the codes indicated on the health claim form represent the services actually performed and are supported by notes and other documentation in the patient's health record. Don't use a code on a claim form without having **supporting documentation** in the file.

Supporting documentation

The paperwork in the patient's file that corroborates the codes presented on the claim form for a particular encounter.

Code for coverage

To choose a code by the insurance company's rules of what it will pay for, rather than a code that accurately reflects the truth about the encounter.

Upcoding

Using a code on a claim form that indicates a higher level of service than that which was actually performed.

Unbundling

Coding individual parts of a specific procedure rather than one combination, or bundle, that includes all the components.

Mutually exclusive codes

Codes that are identified as those that are not permitted to be used on the same claim form with other codes.

2. Some health care providers instruct their coders to **code for coverage.** This means that codes (both diagnostic and procedural) are not chosen for the best, most accurate code available but, rather, with regard to the procedures the insurance company will pay for, or "cover." This is dishonest and is considered fraud. Some providers will rationalize this process by saying they are doing it so the patient can get the treatment he or she really needs to be paid for by the insurance company. Altruism aside, it is still illegal.

3. If you find yourself in an office or a facility that insists that you include codes for procedures that you know, or believe, were never performed, this might be a case of fraud. It might be that you just didn't know. However, sometimes this is done out in the open, even though it is illegal. Your participation in the process of getting money on false pretenses is serious. If you are found guilty of fraud, you might have to pay a fine and/or go to jail. This is not something to take lightly.

4. **Upcoding,** another illegal process, is using a code that reports a higher level of service than that which was actually performed. Upcoding is considered falsifying records. Even if all you do is fill out the claim form, it is still an unethical and illegal act.

> ### EXAMPLE
>
> Using a code for a colonoscopy when a sigmoidoscopy was actually done is an example of upcoding. A colonoscopy is a more complex procedure that requires patient preparation as well as a sedative. It also takes more time to perform. Therefore, the physician would be paid more to perform a colonoscopy than a sigmoidoscopy. You can see that it would be wrong to get paid for providing a more involved procedure when a simpler procedure was actually done.

5. If you resubmit a claim that has been lost, identify it as a "tracer" or "second submission." If you don't, you might be found guilty of double billing: billing the insurance company twice for a service provided only once. This also constitutes fraud.

6. It is not permissible to code and bill for individual (also known as component) services when a comprehensive or combination (bundle) code is available. This is referred to as **unbundling,** and it is illegal. For Medicare billing, refer to the Medicare National Correct Coding Initiative (CCI), which lists standardized bundled codes. The CCI is used to find coding conflicts, such as unbundling, the use of **mutually exclusive codes,** and other unacceptable reporting of CPT codes. When these errors are discovered, those claims are pulled for review and may be subject to possible suspension or rejection.

> ### EXAMPLE
>
> Dr. Federman's notes indicate that Ellen Thompson, a 5-year-old female, received an MMR vaccine. Reporting 90704 Mumps virus vaccine, 90705 Measles virus vaccine, and 90706 Rubella virus vaccine separately—instead of the combination code of 90707 Measles, mumps, and rubella virus vaccine—would be considered unbundling and is unethical.

7. Separating the codes relating to one encounter and placing them on several claim forms over the course of several days is neither legal nor ethical. This not only indicates a lack of organization in the office but also can cause suspicion of duplicating service claims. Even if you are reporting procedures that were done for diagnoses that actually exist, remember that the claim form is a legal document. All data on that claim form, including dates of service, must be accurate. Do not submit the claim form until you are certain it is complete, with all diagnoses and procedures listed.

If, after you submit a claim, an additional service provided comes to light (such as a lab report with an extra charge), then you must file an amended claim. While not illegal because you are identifying that this claim contains an adjustment, most third-party payers dislike amended claims. You can expect an amended claim to be scrutinized.

《《 CODING TIP

Always remember to read the complete descriptions in the provider's notes in addition to referencing the encounter form, and then, carefully, find the best available code, according to the documentation.

CODES OF ETHICS

There are two premier trade organizations for professional coding specialists. Each has published a code of ethics to guide members of our industry on the best professional way to conduct themselves.

American Health Information Management Association Code of Ethics

The American Health Information Management Association (AHIMA) is the preeminent professional organization for health information workers, including insurance coding specialists. The AHIMA House of Delegates designated the elements in Box 1-1 as being critical to the highest level of honorable behavior for its members.

In this era of reimbursements based on diagnostic and procedural coding, the professional ethics of health information coding professionals continue to be challenged. Standards of ethical coding practices—developed by AHIMA's Coding Policy and Strategy Committee and approved by AHIMA's board of directors—for coding professionals are shown in Box 1-2.

American Academy of Professional Coders Code of Ethical Standards

American Academy of Professional Coders (AAPC) is an influential organization in the health information management industry. Their members, and their certifications, are well respected throughout the United States and the world. Its Code of Ethical Standards, shown in

BOX 1-1 AHIMA Code of Ethics

This Code of Ethics sets forth ethical principles for the health information management profession. Members of this profession are responsible for maintaining and promoting ethical practices. This Code of Ethics, adopted by the American Health Information Management Association, shall be binding on health information management professionals who are members of the Association and all individuals who hold an AHIMA certification.

The following ethical principles are based on the core values of the American Health Information Management Association and apply to all health information management professionals. Health information management professionals must

1. Advocate, uphold, and defend the individual's right to privacy and the doctrine of confidentiality in the use and disclosure of information.

2. Put service and the health and welfare of persons before self-interest and conduct themselves in the practice of the profession so as to bring honor to themselves, their peers, and the health information management profession.

3. Preserve, protect, and secure personal health information in any form or medium and hold in the highest regard the contents of the records and other information of a confidential nature, taking into account the applicable statutes and regulations.

4. Refuse to participate in or conceal unethical practices or procedures.

5. Advance health information management knowledge and practice through continuing education, research, publications, and presentations.

6. Recruit and mentor students, peers, and colleagues to develop and strengthen a professional workforce.

7. Represent the profession accurately to the public.

8. Perform honorably health information management association responsibilities, either appointed or elected, and preserve the confidentiality of any privileged information made known in any official capacity.

9. State truthfully and accurately their credentials, professional education, and experiences.

10. Facilitate interdisciplinary collaboration in situations supporting health information practice.

11. Respect the inherent dignity and worth of every person.

Box 1-3, also illuminates the importance of an insurance coding and billing specialist exhibiting the most ethical and moral conduct.

COMPLIANCE PROGRAMS

A formal compliance program is strongly recommended by the Office of the Inspector General (OIG) of the Department of Health and Human Services (HHS) to help all health care facilities establish their organization's respect for the laws and their agreement to follow the direction from those laws. A compliance program will officially create policies and procedures; establish the structure to adhere to those policies; set up a monitoring system to ensure that it works; and correct conduct that does not comply.

BOX 1-2 AHIMA Standards of Ethical Coding

1. Coding professionals are expected to support the importance of accurate, complete, and consistent coding practices for the production of quality health care data.

2. Coding professionals in all health care settings should adhere to the ICD-9-CM (International Classification of Diseases, 9th revision, Clinical Modification) coding conventions, official coding guidelines approved by the Cooperating Parties,* the CPT (Current Procedural Terminology) rules established by the American Medical Association, and any other official coding rules and guidelines established for use with mandated standard code sets. Selection and sequencing of diagnoses and procedures must meet the definitions of required data sets for applicable health care settings.

3. Coding professionals should use their skills, their knowledge of currently mandated coding and classification systems, and official resources to select the appropriate diagnostic and procedural codes.

4. Coding professionals should only assign and report codes that are clearly and consistently supported by physician documentation in the health record.

5. Coding professionals should consult physicians for clarification and additional documentation prior to code assignment when there is conflicting or ambiguous data in the health record.

6. Coding professionals should not change codes or the narratives of codes on the billing abstract so that meanings are misrepresented. Diagnoses or procedures should not be inappropriately included or excluded because payment or insurance policy coverage requirements will be affected. When individual payer policies conflict with official coding rules and guidelines, these policies should be obtained in writing whenever possible. Reasonable efforts should be made to educate the payer on proper coding practices in order to influence a change in the payer's policy.

7. Coding professionals, as members of the health care team, should assist and educate physicians and other clinicians by advocating proper credentialing documentation practices, further specificity, and re-sequencing or inclusion of diagnoses or procedures when needed to more accurately reflect the acuity, severity, and occurrence of events.

8. Coding professionals should participate in the development of institutional coding policies and should ensure that coding policies complement, not conflict with, official coding rules and guidelines.

9. Coding professionals should maintain and continually enhance their coding skills, as they have a professional responsibility to stay abreast of changes in codes, coding guidelines, and regulations.

10. Coding professionals should strive for optimal payment to which the facility is legally entitled, remembering that it is unethical and illegal to maximize payment by means that contradict regulatory guidelines.

*The Cooperating Parties are the American Health Information Management Association, American Hospital Association, Health Care Financing Administration, and National Center for Health Statistics.

Source: Copyright © 2007 American Health Information Management Association. All rights reserved.

CHAPTER SUMMARY

Knowing your legal and ethical responsibilities as a health care professional will give you a strong foundation for a healthy career. HIPAA's Privacy Rule, along with the codes of ethics from both AHIMA and AAPC, should help guide you through any challenges. Confidentiality, honesty, and accuracy are three watchwords that all health information management professionals should live by.

BOX 1-3 Code of Ethical Standards

This Code of Ethical Standards for members of the American Academy of Professional Coders strives to promote and maintain the highest standard of professional service and conduct among its members. Adherence to these standards assures public confidence in the integrity and service of professional coders who are members of the American Academy of Professional Coders. Failure to adhere to these standards may result in the loss of credentials and membership with the American Academy of Professional Coders.

Members of the American Academy of Professional Coders shall be dedicated to providing the highest standard of professional coding and billing services to employers, clients and patients. Behavior of the American Academy of Professional Coders members must be exemplary.

American Academy of Professional Coders members shall maintain the highest standard of personal and professional conduct. Members shall respect the rights of patients, clients, employers and all other colleagues.

Members shall use only legal and ethical means in all professional dealings, and shall refuse to cooperate with or condone by silence, the actions of those who engage in fraudulent, deceptive or illegal acts.

Members shall respect the laws and regulations of the land, and uphold the mission statement of the American Academy of Professional Coders.

Members shall pursue excellence through continuing education in all areas applicable to their profession.

Members shall strive to maintain and enhance the dignity, status, competence and standards of coding for professional services.

Members shall not exploit professional relationships with patients, employees, clients or employers for personal gain.

Above all else, we will commit to recognizing the intrinsic worth of each member.

Chapter 1 Review
Legal and Ethical Issues

1. According to HIPAA, covered entities include all *except*

   a. Health care providers.

   b. Health plans.

   c. Health care computer software manufacturers.

   d. Health care clearinghouses.

2. HIPAA's Privacy Rule is all about the

   a. Training of medical assistants.

   b. Use and disclosure of protected health information.

   c. Security of health records.

   d. Insurance billing and coding issues.

3. An example of protected health information is

   a. Patient's Social Security number.

   b. Patient's next of kin.

   c. All codes in the CPT book.

   d. Patient's state of residence.

4. HIPAA states that all covered entities must comply with the Privacy Rule as of

   a. October 16, 2003.

   b. April 14, 2003.

   c. September 15, 2003.

   d. March 1, 2004.

5. A patient calls your office and asks for the results of her recent blood tests. You

   a. Get her file and answer her questions honestly.

   b. Tell her to hold on so that she can speak with the doctor.

   c. Offer to make an appointment for her to come in to get the results.

   d. Tell her she is breaking the law and hang up.

6. Most state laws mandate that when a health care professional suspects abuse of any kind he or she *must*

   a. Call the appropriate authorities.

   b. Talk to the patient about the suspicions.

   c. Wait until he or she is absolutely certain.

   d. Talk to the patient's family.

7. The intent of HIPAA's Privacy Rule is to properly

   a. Protect an individual's privacy.

   b. Not interfere with the flow of information necessary for care.

   c. Restrict health care professionals from doing their jobs.

   d. (*a*) and (*b*).

8. All covered entities must create and implement written

   a. PHI information flow charts.

   b. Customer service rules.

   c. Privacy practices notices.

   d. Coding guidelines.

9. Protected health information (PHI) is

   a. Any health information that can be connected to a specific individual.

   b. A listing of diagnosis codes.

   c. Current procedural terminology.

   d. Covered entity employee files.

10. Taking authorization for the release of protected health information over the phone from an individual is

    a. Acceptable, as long as you recognize their voice.

    b. Never acceptable.

    c. Acceptable, as long as someone else gets on the phone to vouch for the caller.

    d. Acceptable under emergency situations.

11. The term *use* per HIPAA's Privacy Rule refers to the exchange of information between health care personnel

    a. And health care personnel in other health care facilities.

    b. And family members.

    c. Within the same office.

    d. And the pharmacist.

12. The term *disclosure* per HIPAA's Privacy Rule refers to the exchange of information between health care personnel

    a. And health care personnel in other covered entities.

    b. And family members.

    c. Within the same office.

    d. And the patient.

13. Ensuring that patients' privacy is protected is the responsibility of

    a. The clinical staff.

    b. The attending physician.

    c. The registered nurse.

    d. All staff members.

14. HIPAA is a _____ law.

    a. local

    b. county

    c. state

    d. federal

15. Which of the following is *not* a covered entity under HIPAA

    a. County Hospital.

    b. Blue Cross Blue Shield.

    c. Physician Associates medical practice.

    d. MediSoft technical support.

16. A woman comes into the hospital emergency room. The attending physician suspects that her husband has been physically abusing her. The Privacy Rule says the physician is permitted, but not mandated, to disclose this information to the police. The state says the physician must report this to the police or lose his or her license. The physician should:

    a. Call his or her attorney.

    b. Get the patient to sign a release form before telling anyone.

    c. Call the police immediately.

    d. Say nothing.

17. A new Walgreen's store opens two blocks away from the office where you work. The manager of the store calls your medical practice and offers to pay for a copy of the names and addresses of your patients who have been taking prescribed medication on a regular basis. Do you

    a. Meet with the doctor to determine how much to charge?

    b. Explain that this would be against the law under HIPAA's Privacy Rule?

    c. Provide the list for free to be a good neighbor?

    d. Get the money for the list upfront?

18. According to HIPAA's rules and regulations, a covered entity's workforce includes

    a. Only paid, full-time employees.

    b. Only licensed personnel working in the office.

    c. Volunteers, trainees, and employees, part time and full time.

    d. Business associates' employees.

19. HIPAA's Privacy Rule has been carefully crafted to

    a. Protect a patient's health care history.

    b. Protect a patient's current medical issues.

    c. Protect a patient's future health considerations.

    d. All of the above.

20. A written form to release PHI should include all except
    a. Specific identification of the person who will be receiving the information.
    b. The specific information to be released.
    c. Legal terminology so it will stand up in court.
    d. An expiration date.

21. There can be _____ penalties for any violation of HIPAA's rules.
    a. civil
    b. criminal
    c. both civil and criminal
    d. no

22. Those who are permitted to file an official complaint with HHS are
    a. Health care providers.
    b. Any individual.
    c. Health plans.
    d. Clearinghouses.

23. Penalties for violating any portion of HIPAA apply to
    a. Patients.
    b. Patients' families.
    c. All covered entities.
    d. Health care office managers.

24. If you disclose PHI improperly and under false pretenses, you can
    a. Be fined $100 for each occurrence.
    b. Be fined $50,000 and get up to one year in jail.
    c. Be fined $10,000 and get up to five years in prison.
    d. Be fined $100,000 and get up to three years in prison.

25. HHS stands for
    a. Department of Home and Health Services.
    b. Division of Health and Health Care Sciences.
    c. Department of Health and Human Services.
    d. District of Health and HIPAA Systems.

26. Changing a code from one that is most accurate to one you know the insurance company will pay for is called
    a. Coding for coverage.
    b. Coding for packaging.
    c. Unbundling.
    d. Double billing.

27. Unbundling is an illegal practice in which coders
    a. Bill for services never provided.
    b. Bill for services with no documentation.
    c. Bill using several individual codes instead of one combination code.
    d. Bill using a code for a higher level of service than what was actually provided.

28. Upcoding is an illegal practice in which coders
    a. Bill for services never provided.
    b. Bill for services with no documentation.
    c. Bill using several individual codes instead of one combination code.
    d. Bill using a code for a higher level of service than what was actually provided.

29. Medicare's Correct Coding Initiative (CCI) looks for
    a. Unbundling.
    b. The improper use of mutually exclusive codes.
    c. Unacceptable reporting of CPT codes.
    d. All of the above.

30. Coding improperly on a claim form can cause that claim to be
    a. Rejected.
    b. Reviewed.
    c. Suspended.
    d. All of the above.

Below and on the following pages are health care scenarios. Determine the best course of action that you, as the health information management professional for the facility, should take. Identify and explain how you would deal with any legal and/or ethical issues that you find.

CIPHER, VICTORS, & ASSOCIATES
A Complete Health Care Facility
234 MAIN STREET • ANYTOWN, FL 32711 • 407-555-1234

PATIENT: SUSQUEHANNA, MARION
MRN: SUSQMA001
Date: 17 September 2008

Attending Physician: Valerie R. Victors, MD

This 25-year-old female is 21 weeks pregnant. She presents today in tears. She is suffering from hemorrhoids and cannot stand it anymore. The pain and itching are making life difficult for her, as it hurts to sit for any length of time, and she cannot sleep. As it is difficult for her to lie on her stomach, due to the pregnancy, she can only find some comfort by either walking around or lying on her side. She is asking (more like begging) for a hemorrhoidectomy—a simple surgical procedure that can be done in the office and will almost immediately provide her with complete relief.

The correct ICD-9-CM diagnosis code for Marion's condition is

455.3 External hemorrhoids without mention of complication

However, Marion's insurance carrier will not pay for a hemorrhoidectomy with a diagnosis that indicates there are no complications. According to the insurance customer service representative, it will pay in full for the procedure, but only with a diagnosis of

455.5 External hemorrhoids with mention of complication

Marion's husband, David, is a civilian who works for a defense contractor and is currently in Iraq supporting the troops. Money is tight for the family because David's paycheck has been delayed due to a mix-up in paperwork when he was transferred to the Middle East. There is no way they can afford to pay for the hemorrhoidectomy.

All you need to do is change the one number of the code, and Marion can have the relief she so desperately needs. What should you do?

_____

_____

_____

Part 1 CPT

CIPHER, VICTORS, & ASSOCIATES
A Complete Health Care Facility
234 MAIN STREET • ANYTOWN, FL 32711 • 407-555-1234

PATIENT: MARINOSCI, CHRISTOPHER
MRN: MARICH001
Date: 5 October 2008

Attending Physician: James I. Cipher, MD

As the coding specialist for this facility, you are given the chart for this patient, after his recent encounter with Dr. Cipher. On the face sheet you notice that Dr. Cipher has indicated the diagnosis for this patient to be:

Gram-negative pneumonia

However, there is nothing at all in the rest of the documentation, including the encounter notes and lab reports, to support this diagnosis.

What should you do?

_____

_____

_____

CIPHER, VICTORS, & ASSOCIATES
A Complete Health Care Facility
234 MAIN STREET • ANYTOWN, FL 32711 • 407-555-1234

PATIENT: KELLOGG, JOAN
MRN: KELLJO001
Date: 15 October 2008

Attending Physician: James I. Cipher, MD

Today, Felicia Masterson comes into your office. She states that she is Joan Kellogg's sister and that she has been asked by her sister to collect a copy of her complete medical record. Ms. Masterson tells you that her sister has moved to another town and needs the records for an upcoming medical appointment with her new doctor. She hands you a printout of an e-mail, supposedly from Ms. Kellogg, to serve as documentation that she should have the records.

What should you do?

_____

_____

_____

CIPHER, VICTORS, & ASSOCIATES
A Complete Health Care Facility
234 MAIN STREET • ANYTOWN, FL 32711 • 407-555-1234

PATIENT: BORNER, EMILY
MRN: BORNEM001
Date: 25 September 2008

Attending Physician: James I. Cipher, MD

The patient is a 16-year-old female who came in for counseling on birth control.

Today, Glenda Borner came into the office. She stated that she is Emily's mother and found an appointment card for this facility in her daughter's jeans. She demands to know why her daughter came to see the physician. She is angry and frustrated and states that she will not leave until she is told why her daughter saw the doctor.

What should you do?

_____

_____

_____

CIPHER, VICTORS, & ASSOCIATES
A Complete Health Care Facility
234 MAIN STREET • ANYTOWN, FL 32711 • 407-555-1234

PATIENT: GRANGER, ALLEN
MRN: GRANAL001
Date: 1 December 2008

Attending Physician: Ronald Jones, DPM

The patient came to see the physician because of problems with his feet. He is diagnosed with stress fractures of the metatarsals. In reality, this condition is due to the patient's morbid obesity. The physician's notes document the patient's weight is 435 pounds, and his height as 5 ft. 9 in.

However, you have been told not to code the morbid obesity and only to code the stress fractures, because the insurance carrier will not pay for any procedures for conditions related to the patient's weight.

What should you do?

_____

_____

_____

Part 1   CPT

Introduction to Coding and CPT

2

KEY TERMS

KEY TERMS

Abstracting

Diagnosis

Durable medical equipment (DME)

Inpatient

Medical necessity

Outpatient

Procedure

Query

Superbill

Supporting documentation

LEARNING OUTCOMES

- Explain the purpose of diagnosis coding.
- Relate diagnosis coding to procedure coding.
- Apply correctly the steps to accurate coding.
- Use official guidelines provided to apply the best, most accurate code.
- Abstract documentation thoroughly.
- Interpret notations and symbols to code accurately.

EMPLOYMENT OPPORTUNITIES

Family practice	Physicians' offices
Chiropractor office	Hospitals
Non-profit organizations	Clinics
General practice	Nursing homes

The purpose of coding is to make every effort to ensure clear and concise communication about health care issues among all parties involved. These parties include health care providers, the insurance companies (third-party payers), and government agencies.

The processing of health care information is an important part of our country's health care system. As you are probably aware, insurance carriers use this data to determine how much they should pay health care profession-als for the attention they provide to a patient. This is called the reimbursement process. The codes make it easier for the organizations involved to evaluate and manage all the data. In addition, these codes are used in the study of diseases and conditions that affect our population. Foundations and government agencies use statistical information to develop programs and policies that will best address the health of our residents. For example, they can only know that a disease such as Alzheimer's needs diagnostic tests, treatment, and possibly a vaccine or a cure by studying statistics to see what individuals are being diagnosed with around the country and the world.

Coding is simply interpreting health care terms and definitions into numbers or number-letter combinations (alphanumeric codes) that specifically relate to diagnoses and procedures.

DIAGNOSIS CODES AND MEDICAL NECESSITY

Diagnosis

Physician's determination of a patient's condition, illness, or injury.

Medical necessity

The assessment that the provider was acting according to standard practices in providing a procedure or service for an individual with a specific diagnosis.

The International Classification of Diseases, 9th revision, Clinical Modification (ICD-9-CM) is a directory of every **diagnosis,** or reason, that a health care provider would spend time and/or provide a service to a patient. Diagnosis codes are very important because they give the information about why the physician provided a particular service or treatment. These codes establish **medical necessity,** and every procedure code reported must be accompanied by a diagnosis code that justifies that specific procedure. Some examples of diagnoses are a broken ankle, diabetes, or the flu.

ICD-9-CM diagnosis codes can be all numbers (three, four, or five digits) or a combination of numbers and letters.

EXAMPLE

ICD-9-CM Diagnosis Codes

486	Pneumonia
002.0	Typhoid fever
596.51	Hypertonicity of bladder
V11.0	Personal history of schizophrenia

EXAMPLE

Diagnosis Codes Supporting Procedures Performed

Jerri Cavanaugh, a 13-year-old female, is brought to the Emergency Department by her mother after Jerri fell off her skateboard and hurt her ankle. Dr. Roberts orders x-rays that confirm Jerri's ankle is broken, and he applies a short leg (knee-to-toe) cast.

The diagnosis of a broken ankle makes the application of the lower leg cast a good medical decision. Dr. Roberts had a documented medical reason to provide this treatment. This diagnosis explains the medical necessity for the application of the cast.

Morris Cruz, a 65-year-old male, went to see his physician, Dr. Bridges. Morris was complaining of pain upon urination. Dr. Bridges orders an urinalysis. The results of the test showed that Morris had a urinary tract infection (UTI). Dr. Bridges was in a hurry and scribbled in his notes what looked like "URI."

The problem here is that URI stands for upper respiratory infection (chest congestion). You can see that the diagnosis of an upper respiratory infection does not justify the lab test that was ordered. This will be looked at as either an error or very poor medical judgment. In either case, the claim will be denied for lack of medical necessity.

PROCEDURES (SERVICES AND TREATMENTS)

This and the following chapters in this text take you through three directories that you will use in the process of health care translating **procedures** (services and treatments) into codes. These three directories are Current Procedural Terminology (CPT), Healthcare Common Procedure Coding System (HCPCS) Level II, and ICD-9-CM Volume 3.

Current Procedural Terminology, fourth edition, is similar to the ICD-9-CM, except that, instead of listing codes for diagnoses, the CPT catalogs codes for procedures, treatments, and services provided to patients, such as an x-ray, a vaccination, or the removal of a cyst. Technically, CPT codes are HCPCS Level I codes. However, professionals in the health care industry refer to these procedure codes simply as CPT codes.

CPT codes are chiefly five numbers, all in a row. Some CPT codes can have four numbers followed by a letter.

Procedure

A treatment or service provided by a health care professional.

EXAMPLE

CPT Codes

31750 Tracheoplasty; cervical

0058 T Cryopreservation; reproductive tissue, ovarian

The Healthcare Common Procedure Coding System, Level II, lists codes used to identify **durable medical equipment (DME),** dental procedures, medications, and certain other services not listed in the CPT book. Items coded from HCPCS (pronounced *hick-picks*) might include a wheelchair, crutches, or a unit of blood for a transfusion. HCPCS Level II codes have one letter followed by four numbers.

Durable medical equipment (DME)

Items that are used in the care and treatment of a patient that can either last a long time, or can be used again and again.

EXAMPLE

HCPCS Codes

E0607 Home blood glucose monitor

D0120 Periodic oral examination

J0128 Injection, abarelix, 10 mg

When a hospital provides services and treatments to an individual who has been admitted into the hospital as an **inpatient,** codes will be used from the third volume of ICD-9-CM. Unlike the first two volumes of ICD-9-CM that lists diagnosis codes, this volume lists codes for procedures.

ICD-9-CM Volume 3 procedure codes use two, three, or four numbers.

Inpatient

A patient staying overnight in a hospital.

ICD-9-CM Volume 3 Procedure Code

32.1   Other excision of bronchus

07.22 Unilateral adrenalectomy

SPECIFIC CODE DEFINITIONS

Each set of numbers or numbers/letters means something so specific that a code just one digit off could mean something totally unrelated. Transposing two numbers is a typical error, for example, when jotting down a phone number. You think one-seven-one but write down 711. However, instead of having a wrong phone number, an incorrect code could cause a claim to be rejected, denied, or pulled for investigation, resulting in your office having to deal with delayed payment or no payment at all. This is why it is critical to be careful and accurate when coding and *always* double-check your codes.

Specific Definitions: The Difference between 305 and 503

30520 Septoplasty or submucous resection, with or without cartilage scoring, contouring or replacement with graft . . . *nose surgery.*

50320 Donor nephrectomy (including cold preservation); open, from living donor . . . *the removal of a kidney from a live person to be transplanted into another.*

CODING TIP »»»

Documentation is your watchword. You must have the information *in writing*. If it is not written down (or in a computer document), then, as far as you are concerned, it never happened and, therefore, you cannot code it.

Superbill

A form preprinted with the diagnosis codes and procedure codes most frequently used in a particular facility.

Abstracting

The process of identifying the relevant words or phrases in health care documentation in order to determine the best, most appropriate code(s).

SEVEN STEPS TO ACCURATE CODING

There is a seven-step process for coding a health care encounter in the approved manner. As you gain experience, coding a patient encounter will take less time. However, remember that time is not the number one consideration—no matter what anyone says—accuracy is the most important factor.

The steps are as follows:

1. *Read* the **superbill** and the physician's notes for this encounter completely, from beginning to end. Make a copy of the pages relating to this visit, so that you can write on these pages without marking the originals.

2. *Reread* the physician's notes, and *highlight key words* regarding diagnoses and procedures directly relating to this encounter. Pulling out the key words is also called **abstracting** physician's notes.

3. *Make a list* of any questions you have regarding unclear or missing information necessary to code this encounter. **Query** the health care provider who treated the patient and, if necessary, ask the provider to update the chart. Never assume. Code only what you know from actual documentation. As you read in Chap. 1, Box 1-2, "AHIMA Standards of Ethical Coding," the fourth standard directs

you to have the **supporting documentation** to back up every code you submit on a claim form.

EXAMPLE

The Importance of Querying the Physician

The documentation indicates that the physician performed a posterior vestibuloplasty on Marion Jones. You pull out the key words: vestibuloplasty; posterior. However, when you look up this procedure in the CPT book, you see that there are two codes to choose from:

> 40842 Vestibuloplasty; posterior, unilateral
>
> 40843 Vestibuloplasty; posterior, bilateral

You must query the physician to find out whether the procedure was done unilaterally (one side) or bilaterally (both sides). Make certain the physician answers your question *and* writes the answer down in the chart—and initials and dates it. Now, you know which code is the best, most appropriate code.

4. *Code the diagnosis or diagnoses* as stated by the physician. In the absence of a definitive diagnosis, code the identified signs and symptoms describing why the patient came to see the health care provider for this encounter. Use the best, most accurate code available based on the documentation. In the ICD-9-CM, you will:

   a. Look up the key terms regarding the diagnosis abstracted from the notes in the alphabetic index (ICD-9-CM, volume 2).

   b. Verify the correct code in the tabular listings (ICD-9-CM, volume 1).

   c. Double-check your codes to ensure accuracy, specificity, and adherence to guidelines.

5. *Code the procedure or procedures* as stated in the notes describing what the provider did for the patient. Use the best, most appropriate codes available based on the documentation. In the ICD-9-CM, volume 3, for inpatient procedures, or CPT for physician services and outpatient services, you will:

   a. Look up the key terms regarding the procedures and services abstracted from the notes in the alphabetic index.

   b. Verify the correct code in the numerical listings.

   c. Double-check your codes to ensure accuracy, specificity, and adherence to guidelines.

6. *Link every procedure code to at least one diagnosis code* shown on the same claim form to document medical necessity. Not only is this required, but also it is an excellent way to confirm that all your procedure codes are justified by a diagnosis code.

7. *Double-check your work* by *back coding* to ensure that you did not accidentally transpose any numbers, copy the wrong code, or misread a description.

Following these steps will help you code precisely, resulting in a greater number of your claims getting paid quickly, at the highest earned reimbursement rate.

Query

To ask.

Supporting documentation

The written reports that provide evidence of what was provided to the patient and why.

《《《 **CODING TIP**

Never, never, never code directly from the alphabetic index. Always verify the suggested code in the numerical listing before using a code.

《《《 **CODING TIP**

Patient = *who* came to see the provider for health care

Diagnosis = *why* the individual came to see the provider for this visit

Procedure = *what* the provider did for the individual

LuAnne Cannellis, a 55-year-old female, has a family history of colon cancer, so she came in today for a screening colonoscopy. Dr. Cousins removed a polyp by snare during the examination.

Let's Code It!

Go through the steps of coding, and determine the codes that should be reported for this encounter between Dr. Cousins and LuAnne Cannellis.

First, read the case completely. These notes are nice and short (whereas some notes can go on for many pages). Second, let's abstract the notes together. What key words identify the procedures performed? *screening colonoscopy, removed a polyp by snare*

Do you need to query the provider? I think that, for right now, we seem to have all the information we need. Sometimes, you may not know if information is missing until you get to the code descriptions.

Because our lessons here are all about coding the procedures, I will tell you that the diagnosis is clearly stated in the notes: *family history of colon cancer.*

Now, we have to code the procedure or procedures. Turn to the alphabetic index in the CPT book, and find *Colonoscopy.* Below the subheading, read down the list of words, and find a word that was used in the description of the procedure. Do you see *Removal*? Indented underneath *Removal*, you will see the same term that Dr. Cousins wrote in his notes regarding what he removed: *Polyp.* The index suggests codes 45384–45385.

Turn to the page within the numeric listing of the CPT book, so we can look at the complete code descriptions.

45384 Colonoscopy, flexible, proximal to splenic flexure; with removal of tumor(s), polyp(s), or other lesion(s) by hot biopsy forceps or bipolar cautery

45385 Colonoscopy, flexible, proximal to splenic flexure; with removal of tumor(s), polyp(s), or other lesion(s) by snare technique

The difference between these two codes is the technique by which the physician removed the polyp. Which technique does the notes indicate? The notes state *by snare.* This means that the code description for 45385 matches the notes perfectly!

Next, you must link the procedure codes to at least one diagnosis code. This step is pretty easy. We only have one diagnosis code, and they go together very well. The diagnosis of a family history of colon cancer establishes medical necessity for a colonoscopy.

The last step is to *always* double-check your answers. Just as you looked in the alphabetic index first, by the terms, and then found the numeric code, double-check your work by doing this process backward. I call this *back coding.* Look at the number and see if the code description matches your physician's notes. It does! Excellent.

CODING FROM SUPERBILLS INSTEAD OF PHYSICIAN'S NOTES

Health information management administrators are the staff members responsible for choosing the system that their health care facilities use to handle coding diagnoses and procedures. Some organizations outsource this very important job to an independent company. Large facilities, such as hospitals and some physician groups, typically establish a separate department. Smaller practices may opt to have one or two people in their office handle this process.

Health care facilities differ in more ways than simply the logistics of where coding occurs. Some have their coders use only the superbill to create the first health claim form and refer to the physician's notes only if that claim is rejected, denied, or questioned by the third-party payer. (Figure 2.1 shows a sample Superbill.) This may happen because the staff believes that it is the quickest way to process claim forms. When an office is dealing with 60 or 100 patients a day, this seems to make sense: "Get those claim forms coded and sent as soon as possible, and we will deal with the rejected ones later! We don't have time for people to sit around, reading physician's notes." On the surface, it may appear that coding from superbills saves time and, therefore, money (fewer hours for coders equals lower payroll).

The reality is that coding only from superbills is not efficient with regard to either time or money. The policy of coding from superbills can result in a higher number of rejected or underpaid claims. When this happens, the facility loses money in several ways:

1. Extra time is needed for the coder to go back over a rejected claim.

2. A rejected claim means lost money, because it will take longer for the money to get from the third-party payer to your health care office.

3. There may be a more accurate code not included on the superbill. This means the office is not getting paid as much as it is entitled for its legitimate work.

In addition, the ICD-9-CM Official Guidelines for Coding and Reporting, effective April 1, 2005, state, *"The entire record should be reviewed to determine the specific reason for the encounter and the conditions treated."* While these are the guidelines regarding the process of coding diagnoses, you can see that this level of accuracy is beneficial for coding procedures and services, as well.

LET'S CODE IT! SCENARIO

Jake Mathers, a 23-year-old male, came to see his regular physician, Dr. Patterson. Jake has twenty-two common warts and is very self-conscious of them. Dr. Patterson removes the warts. Because his office uses superbills, Dr. Patterson checked off the only code available on the sheet, "17110 Destruct wart."

Family Doctors Associates
123 Main Street • Anytown, FL 32711
(407) 555-1200

Date: September 16, 2005   Attending Physician: J. Healer, MD

Patient Name: Sasha White

CPT DESCRIPTION	CPT DESCRIPTION	CPT DESCRIPTION
OFFICE/HOSPITAL	**PATHOLOGY/LAB/RADIOLOGY**	**PROCEDURES/TESTS**
☐ 99201 OFFICE-NEW; FOCUSED	☒ 71020 X-RAY CHEST TWO VIEWS	☐ 12011 SIMPLE SUTURE, FACE
☒ 99202 OFFICE-NEW; EXPANDED	☒ 72040 X-RAY SPINE-C, TWO VIEWS	☐ 29125 SPLINT-SHORT ARM
☐ 99203 OFFICE-NEW; DETAILED	☒ 73030 X-RAY SHOULDER COMP	☐ 29355 WALKER CAST-LONG LEG
☐ 99204 OFFICE-NEW; COMPREHEN	☐ 76085 MAMMOGRAM-COMP DET	☐ 29540 STRAPPING-ANKLE
☐ 99205 OFFICE-NEW; COMPREHEN	☐ 76092 MAMMOGRAM SCREENING	☐ 45378 COLONOSCOPY-DIAGNOSTIC
☐ 99211 OFFICE-ESTB; MINIMAL	☐ 80050 BLOOD TEST-GEN HEALTH	☐ 45385 COLONOSCOPY-POLYP REM.
☐ 99212 OFFICE-ESTB; FOCUSED	☐ 80061 BLOOD TEST-LIPID PANEL	☐ 50390 ASPIRATION, RENAL CYST
☐ 99213 OFFICE-ESTB; EXPANDED	☐ 82947 BLOOD TEST-GLUCOSE	☐ 90703 TETANUS INJECTION
☐ 99214 OFFICE-ESTB; DETAILED	☐ 83718 BLOOD TEST-HDL	☐ 92081 VISUAL FIELD EXAM
☐ 99215 OFFICE-ESTB; COMPREHEN	☐ 85025 BLOOD TEST-CBC	☐ 93000 ECG, 12 LEADS, W/RPT
☐ 99281 EMER DEPT; FOCUSED	☐ 86403 STREP TEST, QUICK	☐ 93015 TREADMILL STRESS TEST
☐ 90844 COUNSELING – 50 MIN.	☐ 87430 ENZY IMMUNOASSAY-STREP	☐ 99173 VISUAL ACUITY SCREEN

ICD DESCRIPTION	ICD DESCRIPTION	ICD DESCRIPTION
☐ 034.0 STREP THROAT	☐ 511.0 PLEURISY	☐ V01.5 RABIES EXPOSURE
☐ 042 HUMAN IMMUNO VIRUS	☐ 538 STOMACH ULCER	☐ V16.0 FAMILY HISTORY-COLON
☐ 250.51 DIABETES W/VISION	☐ 643.00 HYPEREMESIS/PREGNANCY	☐ V16.3 FAMILY HISTORY- BREAST
☐ 250.80 DIABETES, W/OTHER	☐ 707.14 ULCER OF HEEL/MID FOOT	☐ V20.2 WELL CHILD
☐ 307.51 BULIMIA NON-ORGANIC	☐ 788.30 ENURESIS	☐ V22.0 PREGNANCY-FIRST NORM
☐ 354.0 CARPEL TUNNEL SYNDROME	☐ 815.00 FRACTURE, HAND	☐ V22.1 PREGNANCY-NORMAL
☐ 362.01 RETINOPATHY (DIABETIC)	☐ 823.20 FRACTURE, TIBIA	☐ E816.2 MOTORCYCLE ACCT
☐ 486 HYPERTENSION, UNSPEC	☐ 831.00 DISLOCATION, SHOULDER	☐ E826.1 FALL FROM BICYCLE
☐ 482.30 PNEUMONIA	☐ 845.00 SPRAINED ANKLE	☐ E849.0 PLACE OF OCCUR-HOME
☐ 490 BRONCHITIS, UNSPECIFIED	☐ 880.03 OPEN WOUND UPPER ARM	☐ E881.0 FALL FROM LADDER
☐ 493.92 ASTHMA, UNSPECIFIED	☒ 912.0 ABRASION, SHOULDER	☐ E906.0 DOG BITE

FOLLOW-UP

PRN _____

WEEKS _____

NXT APPT. _____

TIME _____

Figure 2-1   An Example of a Superbill.

If you only work from the superbill, then all you know is what is checked off. Let's look up this code in the CPT book. The full description is:

17110 Destruction (e.g., laser surgery, electrosurgery, cryosurgery, chemosurgery, surgical curettement), of benign lesions other than skin tags or cutaneous vascular proliferative lesions; up to 14 lesions

It is the only procedure code related to warts offered on the office's preprinted form. Let's read this code description, along with others near it in the CPT book. You will note a few facts:

- 17110 is used if the physician destroyed 14 lesions or fewer. It is the next code that is actually more accurate for this encounter:

- 17111 Destruction (e.g., laser surgery, electrosurgery, cryosurgery, chemosurgery, surgical curettement), of benign lesions other than skin tags or cutaneous vascular proliferative lesions; 15 or more lesions

- If 15 or more lesions (warts) were destroyed, the physician would have done more work, entitling him or her to be paid more. The only way to report this would be to use code 17111.

If all you have is the check mark on the superbill, next to 17110 Destruct wart, you won't know which code is the most specific and the most accurate. You will have to refer to the complete physician's notes of the encounter to answer these questions.

With a policy of creating claim forms only from superbills, the office would have received less payment than it actually deserved.

CPT PROCEDURE CODING BOOK

The CPT book lists services, procedures, and treatments, provided by all types of health care professionals. These codes may be used to report services provided in either inpatient facilities or **outpatient** facilities. Services such as counseling, treatments such as the application of a cast, or procedures such as the surgical removal of a mole are each assigned a special code to simplify reporting for purposes of reimbursement and statistical analysis. In addition, ancillary services, such as imaging (x-rays, CT scans, magnetic resonance imaging) and pathology and laboratory (biopsy analysis, blood tests, cultures), are also reported using CPT codes.

Outpatient

A patient treated without being hospitalized.

EXAMPLE

Facilities

Inpatient facilities: Acute care facility, a hospital.

Outpatient facilities: A physician's office, clinic, ambulatory care center, or emergency department.

The Organization of the CPT Book

The CPT book has two parts, which have many sections.

1. The main body of the CPT book has six sections, presented in numerical order by code number:
   - Evaluation and Management: 99201–99499
   - Anesthesia: 00100–01999 and 99100–99140
   - Surgery: 10021–69990
   - Radiology: 70010–79999
   - Pathology and Laboratory: 80048–89356
   - Medicine: 90281–99199, 99500–99602

   You may notice that while each section within itself is in numerical order, the sections are not in numerical order; for example, the Evaluation and Management (E/M) section is presented first.

2. The second part of the CPT book contains several sections, including:
   - Category II codes: For supplemental tracking of performance measurement.
   - Category III codes: Temporary codes for emerging technological procedures.
   - Appendixes A–M: Modifiers and other relevant additional information.
   - Alphabetic index: All the CPT codes in alphabetical order by code description, presented in four classes of entries:
     a. Procedures or services, such as removal, implantation, or debridement.
     b. Anatomical site or organ, such as heart, mouth, or pharynx.
     c. Condition, such as miscarriage, cystitis, or abscess.
     d. Eponyms, synonyms, or abbreviations, such as Baker's cyst or EKG.

Guidelines, Formats, and Notations

Official Guidelines

The official guidelines you will use to ensure that you are coding procedures correctly are presented right in your CPT. Notice the pages in front of each of the six sections of the main part of the book.

The Layout of the CPT Book

- Evaluation and Management Guidelines
- Evaluation and Management Numerical Listings
- Anesthesia Guidelines
- Anesthesia Numerical Listings
- Surgery Guidelines
- Surgery Numerical Listings
- Radiology Guidelines
- Radiology Numerical Listings
- Pathology and Laboratory Guidelines

- Pathology and Laboratory Numerical Listings
- Medicine Guidelines
- Medicine Numerical Listings

The guidelines identify important rules and directives that coders must follow when assigning codes from each section. For example:

- Evaluation and management services guidelines include the definitions of commonly used terms.
- Surgery guidelines include a listing of services that are bundled into the surgical package definition.
- Medicine guidelines include instructions on how to code multiple procedures and the proper use of add-on codes.

Also, there are additional guidelines and instructions throughout each section, shown in paragraphs under various subheadings. These instructional notations, ranging from a short sentence to several paragraphs, provide specific information regarding the proper coding appropriate to that anatomic site or type of procedure.

EXAMPLE

Instructional Notations in a Subsection

Repair–Intermediate
Sum of lengths of repairs for each group of anatomic sites.

Echocardiography
Echocardiography includes obtaining ultrasonic signals from the heart and great arteries, with two-dimensional image and/or Doppler ultrasonic signal documentation, and interpretation and report. When interpretation is performed separately, use modifier 26.

Formats

The Formats of the Codes

As reviewed earlier in this chapter, the codes listed in the CPT book are structured as follows:

CPT codes (category I codes) are five-digit codes: numbers with no punctuation; for example, 51100 Aspiration of bladder; by needle.

Category II codes are five-character codes: four numbers followed by the letter F; for example, 2001F Weight recorded.

Category III codes are five-character codes: four numbers followed by the letter T; for example, 0031T Speculoscopy.

Modifiers: There are special circumstances when a 2-digit modifier must be appended to a CPT code. When this is required, the modifier will be added, after a hyphen, after the main CPT code; for example, 47600-54 Cholecystectomy, surgical care only.

The Format of the Book

As you look through the CPT book, both the numeric listings and the alphabetic index show their data in columns. Notice that some information is indented under other descriptions or terms. An indented description or term attaches to the description or term that appears at the margin of the column above, or before, the indented words.

Notice that this description is set at the inner margin of the column. The positioning indicates that it is the complete description of this code.

Now, let's look right below this code, at the next code listed.

35501   Bypass graft, with vein; common carotid-ipsilateral internal carotid

35506   carotid-subclavian or subclavian-carotid

You can see that the description next to code 35506 is indented, not at the inner margin of the column. This means you must not only read 35506's description but also attach it to the description above. But before you do that, look at the punctuation of the first code:

35501   Bypass graft, with vein; carotid

Notice the semicolon (the dot over the comma) after the word *vein*. The semicolon is very important. When you read the description for a code that has an indented term or phrase, attach it to the description of the code above, but only *up to the semicolon*.

Read it as shown by the underlines:

35501   <u>Bypass graft, with vein</u>; common carotid-ipsilateral internal carotid

35506   <u>carotid-subclavian</u> or subclavian-carotid

Putting both lines together means that the actual complete description of code 35506 is:

35506   Bypass graft, with vein; carotid-subclavian or subclavian-carotid

Again, the rule is to read the part of the code above *up to the semicolon* and then attach the indented description to it. The CPT book does this to save space.

Let's look at an example from the alphabetic index.

Let's look at the words at the margin and those indented.

The heading of this part of the index is identified as *Excision*, a type of procedure. This heading is at the margin of the column. Underneath this, also at the margin of the column, is the word *Abscess*. Underneath this, indented, is the word *Brain*, followed by two suggested codes. Read backward, and you have *Brain, Abscess, Excision*. The physician's notes are more likely to read:

<u>Excision</u> of an <u>Abscess</u> in the <u>Brain</u>

Part 1   CPT

Just like with the descriptions in the numeric listing, you must be careful as you read and connect the indented words and phrases. Using a ruler or other straight edge may make it easier to see which words are indented and which are at the margins.

Notations and Symbols

Throughout the CPT book, you will see notations and symbols. Let's review them together.

See

A "see" reference is found under a heading in the alphabetic index. Let's return to an earlier example.

EXAMPLE

Find "excision" in the alphabetic index.

> Excision
>
> *See* Debridement; Destruction

In our example, under the heading "Excision," the notation "*See* Debridement; Destruction" provides two alternate terms that the physician may have used in his or her notes. The CPT book is suggesting that if you cannot find a match to the documentation under "Excision," you might find it under one of these other terms.

+

The plus symbol (+) identifies an *add-on code*. An add-on procedure is most often performed with a main procedure. These services or treatments are additional to, and associated with, that main procedure, and are never performed or reported alone (without the main procedure). Due to this relationship with the main procedure, add-on codes never use the modifier *51 Multiple Procedures*. (You will learn all about modifiers later in this book.) All the add-on codes are grouped and listed in Appendix D for additional reference.

> **+ 22328**   each additional fractured vertebrae or dislocated segment (List separately in addition to code for primary procedure)

(List separately in addition to code for primary procedure)

Seen at the end of the description of an add-on code, this notation reminds you that the code represents a procedure that is done as a part of another procedure, reported separately. Again, this should also remind you that this code cannot be used by itself.

EXAMPLE

Add-On Code Listing

> 22630 Arthrodesis, posterior interbody technique, including laminectomy and/or diskectomy to prepare interspace (other than for decompression), single interspace, lumbar
>
> + 22632   each additional interspace (List separately in addition to code for primary procedure.)
>
> (Use 22632 in conjunction with 22630.)

(Use . . . in conjunction with . . .)

The notation "Use . . . in conjunction with . . ." is found below the description of an add-on code. Here, the CPT book is going one step further. In addition to the + symbol and the notation "List separately," the book states the primary procedure code or codes with which the add-on code may be reported.

•

The bullet symbol (•) identifies a new code, one that is in the CPT book for the first time. During the annual update of the CPT book, various codes and guidelines are added, deleted, or revised. The new updated printed version of CPT is effective every January 1.

▲

The triangle symbol (▲) distinguishes a code whose description has been changed since the last edition of CPT.

►◄

The double sideways triangles (►◄) mark the beginning and end of text that has been revised or is being shown for the first time in this year's CPT book. This symbol may highlight code descriptions, guidelines, and/or instructional paragraphs throughout the CPT book.

⊙

The bull's-eye symbol (⊙), a circle with a dot in the center, indicates that the code includes the administration of conscious sedation along with the procedure shown. The bull's-eye symbol tells you that you should not include a separate code when conscious sedation is provided during this treatment. All codes that include conscious sedation are grouped together and listed in Appendix G.

⦸

The symbol of a circle with a slash through it (⦸) identifies codes that are not permitted to be appended with modifier *51 Multiple Procedures*. These codes are procedures that are sometimes done at the same time as another procedure (like an add-on code) but can also be performed alone (unlike an add-on code). Consequently, when such a procedure is performed along with other procedures, you are not allowed to attach the multiple procedure modifier. All codes that are modifier 51 exempt are grouped and listed in Appendix E. There will be a lot more about modifiers as you go through this text.

Some versions of the CPT book may also include the following symbol:

⮌

The circle with the arrow symbol (⮌) points you toward an AMA published reference that may be of additional guidance. The notation may direct you toward a particular edition of either the *CPT Assistant* newsletter or the book *CPT Changes: An Insider's View.*

Part 1   CPT

Melanie Terlington, a 23-year-old female, and her husband, Matthew, have been trying to have a baby. Melanie comes in so Dr. Petard can perform a pregnancy test (urine, by visual comparison).

You Code It!

Go through the steps of coding, and determine the codes that should be reported for this encounter between Dr. Petard and Melanie Terlington.

Step 1: Read the case completely

Step 2: Abstract the notes: Which key words can you identify relating to the procedure performed?

_____

Step 3: Query the provider, if necessary.

Step 4: Diagnosis: Pregnancy test.

Step 5: Code the procedure(s).

_____

Step 6: Link the procedure code(s) to at least one diagnosis code.

Step 7: Back code to double-check your choices.

Answer

Did you find the correct code to be:

81025 Urine pregnancy test, by visual color comparison methods

Excellent work!

CHAPTER SUMMARY

In this chapter you learned about the important role that coding plays in our health care system. As coding specialists, you must strive to accurately report the services and procedures provided to each and every patient. Health care professionals are responsible for ensuring that the supporting documentation is complete, so that the coding specialist has the information necessary to find the best, most accurate code.

The seven steps to accurate coding may help you establish an effective sequence for reviewing the documentation and interpreting the information.

The Current Procedural Terminology (CPT), fourth edition, contains thousands of codes for reporting services, treatments, and procedures. The book includes guidelines for each section, as well as additional notations, symbols, and references to assist you in your quest for the correct code or codes.

1. The seven steps to accurate coding are

    1. _____

    2. _____

    3. _____

    4. _____

    5. _____

    6. _____

    7. _____

2. The most important factor in coding is

    a. Speed of coding process.
    b. Accuracy of codes.
    c. Quantity of codes.
    d. Level of codes.

3. When you find unclear or missing information in the physician's notes, you should

    a. Ask a co-worker.
    b. Figure out the information yourself; you should know what the doctor is thinking.
    c. Query the physician.
    d. Place the file at the bottom of the pile.

4. Diagnosis codes identify

    a. What the provider did for the patient.
    b. Who the policyholder is.
    c. At which facility the patient was seen by the provider.
    d. Why the patient saw the provider.

5. Procedure codes identify

    a. What the provider did for the patient.
    b. Who the policyholder is.
    c. At which facility the patient was seen by the provider.
    d. Why the patient saw the provider.

6. Coding from superbills instead of physician's notes can cause the facility to

    a. Lose time.
    b. Lose money by undercoding.
    c. Lose money by delaying payments received.
    d. All of the above.

7. CPT guidelines

    a. Must be memorized by professional coders.
    b. Can be found in the front of every CPT section.
    c. Can be found in a separate guidelines book.
    d. Change every two months.

8. An example of a CPT guideline is

    a. The proper way to read a superbill.
    b. The way to determine the principle diagnosis.
    c. The alphabetical listing of procedures and services.
    d. The proper use of add-on codes.

9. A CPT code has

    a. Five numbers.
    b. Five letters.
    c. Three numbers followed by three letters.
    d. The letter *P* followed by four numbers.

10. HCPCS Level II codes may be used to report

   a. Evaluation services.

   b. Blood tests.

   c. Durable medical equipment.

   d. Diagnoses.

11. ICD stands for

   a. International Classification of Diseases.

   b. International Classification of Diagnoses.

   c. International Categories of Drugs.

   d. Internal Classifications of Diseases.

12. CPT stands for

   a. Current Procedural Trailers.

   b. Classification of Procedural Techniques.

   c. Current Procedural Terminology.

   d. Classification of Procedural Terms.

13. ICD-9-CM Volume 3 procedure codes are used to report

   a. Procedures done for inpatients.

   b. Procedures done in a physician's office.

   c. Diagnoses for inpatients.

   d. Diagnoses of patients seen in an ambulatory care center.

14. A superbill is

   a. A claim form for a major surgical procedure.

   b. A form preprinted with the most often used codes in a facility.

   c. A claim form for more than $5,000.

   d. A claim form issued from a hospital with more than 200 beds.

15. The plus symbol (+) identifies

   a. A new code.

   b. An add-on code.

   c. A revised code.

   d. A code that includes conscious sedation.

16. The ⊙ symbol identifies

   a. A new code.

   b. An add-on code.

   c. A revised code.

   d. A code that includes conscious sedation.

17. An outpatient can be treated at a facility including but *not*

   a. A doctor's office.

   b. Emergency room.

   c. Admitted into a hospital.

   d. Same-day surgery center.

18. CPT codes are used for

   a. Reimbursement from third-party payers.

   b. Government agencies for funding allotment.

   c. Foundations for research directions.

   d. All of the above.

19. The term "procedure" can also mean

   a. Treatment.

   b. Counseling.

   c. Surgery.

   d. All of the above.

20. The CPT book is revised and in effect beginning each year on

   a. October 1.

   b. November 1.

   c. December 1.

   d. January 1.

1. Anna Samuels was taken to the OR for an anterior cervical discectomy with decompression of a single interspace of the spinal cord and nerve roots and including osteophytectomy. She is a healthy, 37-year-old female.

   _____

2. Robert Mourning, a 25-year-old male, was taken to the OR for a corneal transplant, lamellar, to the left eye.

   _____

3. Stuart Pencil, an 87-year-old male, has been taken to the OR for a single lung transplant with a cardiopulmonary bypass. Dr. Labelle is concerned because Stuart was not expected to survive without the transplant.

   _____

4. Marlene Stapleton, an otherwise healthy 16-year-old female, was taken to the OR for a total thyroidectomy to remove a left thyroid mass.

   _____

5. Dr. Shoun inserted a nontunneled centrally inserted central venous catheter into Ted Thomas, a four-year-old male. Ted was given conscious sedation so he could more easily withstand the procedure.

   _____

6. Barbara Dunedun, a 17-year-old female who is an amateur gymnast, was brought to the OR for the insertion of a plate with screws to assist the healing of the malunion of a humeral shaft fracture. An open procedure began.

   _____

7. Elaine Avalino, a 31-year-old female, was brought to the OR for a c-section. Anesthesia was administered. She has type 1 diabetes that is currently under control. Dr. Benito came to perform the cesarean delivery only.

   _____

Part 1   CPT

8. John Johnson, a 39-year-old male, was rushed to the hospital by ambulance and taken directly to the OR for an appendectomy for a ruptured appendix and generalized peritonitis. Patient is otherwise healthy.

   _____

9. Dr. Cordoba performed a spigelian hernia repair in the lower abdomen on Michael Dollern, an 8-month-old male.

   _____

10. Viviana Markum, a 13-year-old female, came to see her physician, Dr. Lovern. She had something in her eye, and it was irritating her. Nothing she did could get it out. Dr. Lovern took a problem-focused history and examined the area. He then applied a topical anesthetic and removed the foreign body from the conjunctiva of her eye.

    _____

11. Drew Hansen, a 73-year-old male, was seen by his physician at an ambulatory surgical center for the insertion of a temporary transvenous single-chamber cardiac electrode. Conscious sedation was administered. The patient tolerated the procedure well. Code the procedure only.

    _____

12. Nancy Carrington, a 5-month-old female, was taken to the OR for an excision of a 1.3 cm malignant neoplasm on her left cheek right below her eye. It is expected that the carcinoma was caught before any spread. The patient is in otherwise healthy condition.

    _____

13. Sunshine Cannin, an otherwise healthy 41-year-old female, was admitted to the same-day surgery center after having an abnormal shoulder x-ray in the clinic the week before. Dr. Provan decided to do a diagnostic arthroscopy.

    _____

14. Jason Munsey, a 15-year-old male, had severe pain in his right thumb. His mother believes it is from too much Playstation. Dr. Wienert took an x-ray, two views, of Jason's finger.

    _____

15. Lorraine Osage, a 5-year-old female, saw Dr. Blander for a screening audiologic function test, pure tone, air only, to check her hearing.

On the following pages, you will see physician notes documenting encounters with patients at our textbook's health care facility, Cipher, Victors, & Associates. Carefully read through the notes, and find the best code or codes for each case.

Part 1   CPT

CIPHER, VICTORS, & ASSOCIATES
A Complete Health Care Facility
234 MAIN STREET • ANYTOWN, FL 32711 • 407-555-1234

PATIENT: STARKER, SHARON
MRN: STARSH001
Date: 08/11/08

Attending Physician: Willard B. Reader, MD

S: This new patient is a 41-year-old female, who comes in with a complaint of severe neck pain and difficulty turning her head. She states she was in a car accident two days ago, her car was struck from behind when she was driving home from work.

O: PE reveals tightness upon palpitation of ligaments in neck and shoulders, most pronounced C3 to C5. X-rays are taken of the cervical vertebrae, three views (AP, Lat, and PA). Radiological review denies any fracture.

A: Anterior longitudinal cervical sprain

P: 1. Prescribed cervical collar to be worn during all waking hours.
     2. Rx Vicodin (hydrocodone) 500 mg po prn
     3. 1,000 mg aspirin qid
     4. Pt to return in 2 weeks for follow-up

Willard B. Reader, MD

DRC/pw   D: 08/11/08 09:50:16   T: 08/13/08 12:55:01

Find the best, most appropriate CPT code or codes.

_____

_____

_____

CIPHER, VICTORS, & ASSOCIATES
A Complete Health Care Facility
234 MAIN STREET • ANYTOWN, FL 32711 • 407-555-1234

PATIENT: WESTERBY, ELMO
ACCOUNT/EHR #:   WESTEL001
Date: 09/16/08

Attending Physician: Suzanne R. Taylor, MD

PREOPERATIVE DX: Orbital mass, OD

POSTOPERATIVE DX: Herniated orbital fat pad, OD

PROCEDURE: Excision of lesion and repair, right superior conjunctiva

SURGEON: Raul Sanchez, MD

ANESTHESIA: Local

PROCEDURE: After Proparacaine was instilled in the eye, it was prepped and draped in the usual sterile manner and 2 percent Lidocaine with 1:200,000 epinephrine was injected into the superior aspect of the right orbit. A corneal protective shield was placed in the eye. The eye was placed in down-gaze.

   The upper lid was everted and the fornix examined. The herniating mass was viewed and measured at 0.75 cm in diameter. Westcott scissors were used to incise the fornix conjunctivae. The herniating mass was then clamped, excised, and cauterized. It appeared to contain mostly fat tissue, which was sent to pathology.

   The superior fornix was repaired using running suture of 6-0 plain gut. Bacitracin ointment was applied to the eye followed by an eye pad. The patient tolerated the procedure well and left the operating room in good condition.

_____

Suzanne R. Taylor, MD

SRT/pw   D: 9/16/08 09:50:16   T: 9/18/08 12:55:01

Find the best, most appropriate CPT code or codes.

_____

_____

_____

CIPHER, VICTORS, & ASSOCIATES
A Complete Health Care Facility
234 MAIN STREET • ANYTOWN, FL 32711 • 407-555-1234

PATIENT: GAYLORD, NITA
ACCOUNT/EHR #:   GAYLNI001
Date: 09/16/08

Attending Physician: Suzanne R. Taylor, MD

The patient is a 61-year-old female with a very long history of schizoaffective disorder with numerous hospitalizations who was brought in by ambulance from the YMCA where she resides for increasing paranoia, increasing arguments with other people, and in general an exacerbation of her psychotic symptoms which had been worsening over the previous two weeks.

I am here to provide psychoanalysis.

Initially, the patient was very agitated and uncooperative. She refused medications. She wanted to leave the hospital. A 2PC* was done and the patient had a court hearing that results in retention. Eventually the patient agreed to a trial of a Risperdal, and then she fairly rapidly improved once she was started on Risperdal 2 mg twice daily. At the time of discharge compared to admission, the patient is much improved. She is usually pleasant and cooperative with occasional difficult moments, some continuing mild paranoia. She has no hallucinations. She has no thoughts of harming herself or anyone else. She is compliant with her medication until the recently refused hydrochlorothiazide. She is irritable at times, but overall she is redirectable and is considered to be at or close to her best baseline. She is considered no imminent danger to herself nor to others at this time.

Final DX: Schizoaffective disorder; hypothyroidism; hypercholesterolemia; borderline hypertension.

Prescriptions for 30-day supplies were given:

Ativan 2 mg po tid; Celexa 40 mg po daily; Risperdal 2 mg po bid; Synthroid 0.088 mg po qam; Zocor 40 mg po qhs

---

Suzanne R. Taylor, MD

SRT/pw   D: 9/16/08 09:50:16   T: 9/18/08 12:55:01

*2PC stands for "two physicians certify"—a medical certification testifying that an individual requires involuntary treatment at a psychiatric facility.

Find the best, most appropriate CPT code or codes.

_____

_____

_____

CIPHER, VICTORS, & ASSOCIATES
A Complete Health Care Facility
234 MAIN STREET • ANYTOWN, FL 32711 • 407-555-1234

PATIENT: KELLO, JOAN
ACCOUNT/EHR #:   KELLOJO001
Date: 09/16/08

Attending Physician: Suzanne R. Taylor, MD

S: This patient is a 25-year-old female who I have not seen in ten months. She has a history of recurrent sinus infections was well until five days ago. She presents with fever, severe frontal headache, facial pain, and runny nose. Patient states she has been having difficulty concentrating.

O: T 101.5° HEENT: Tenderness over frontal and left maxillary sinuses. Nasal congestions visible. CT scan of the maxillofacial area, without contrast, reveals opacification of both frontal and left maxillary, sphenoid sinuses and a possible large nonenhanced lesion in the brain.

A: Epidural abscess with frontal lobe lesions caused by significant compression on frontal lobe.

P: Recommendation for surgery to evacuate the abscess. Patient will think about it and call in a day or two.
Rx antibiotics and pseudoephedrine

Suzanne R. Taylor, MD

SRT/pw   D: 9/16/08 09:50:16   T: 9/18/08 12:55:01

Find the best, most appropriate CPT code or codes.

_____

_____

_____

Part 1   CPT

CIPHER, VICTORS, & ASSOCIATES
A Complete Health Care Facility
234 MAIN STREET • ANYTOWN, FL 32711 • 407-555-1234

PATIENT: KLACKSON, KEVIN
MRN: KLACKE01
Date: 15 September 2008

Diagnosis: Primary cardiomyopathy with chest pain

Procedure: Arterial catherization

Physician: Frank Vincent, MD

Anesthesia: Local

Procedure: The patient was placed on the table in supine position. Local anesthesia was administered. Once we were assured that the patient had achieved no nervous stimuli, the incision was made and the catheter was introduced percutaneously. The incision was sutured with a simple repair. The patient tolerated the procedure well and was transferred to the recovery room.

_____

Frank Vincent, MD

FV/mg   D: 9/15/08 09:50:16   T: 9/15/08 12:55:01

Find the best, most appropriate CPT code or codes.

_____

_____

_____

3

Introduction to CPT Modifiers

LEARNING OUTCOMES

- Determine when a modifier is required.
- Apply the guidelines to determine the best, most appropriate modifier.
- Append multiple modifiers in the proper sequence.
- Correctly use anesthesia physical status modifiers.
- Identify circumstances that require a supplemental report.
- Distinguish between CPT modifiers and HCPCS modifiers.

In addition to the code for the specific procedure or service provided to the patient, there may be times when you will have to apply a **modifier**. Modifiers are two-character codes that add clarification and additional details to the procedure code's original description, as listed in the main portion of the CPT book. At times, the modifier provides necessary explanation that directly relates to the reimbursement that the facility or physician will receive.

PROCEDURE CODE MODIFIERS

Modifiers clarify a report, or claim form, in regard to the following:

- A service or procedure had both a professional component and a technical component.
- A service or procedure was performed by more than one physician.
- A service or procedure was performed in more than one location.
- A service or procedure was not performed in total (only part of it was done).
- An adjunctive service was performed.
- A bilateral procedure was performed.
- A service or procedure was performed more than once.
- Unusual events arose.

The CPT book lists all modifiers in Appendix A, found directly after the category III codes. Each modifier is shown in numerical order by category, accompanied by an explanation of when and how you would use that particular modifier.

There are four categories of modifiers:

- **CPT code modifiers** are two-digit codes that can be attached to regular codes from the main portion of the CPT book.

EXAMPLE

CPT Modifiers

-23 Unusual anesthesia

-66 Surgical Team

- Anesthesia **physical status modifiers** are two-character **alphanumeric** codes, used only with CPT codes reporting anesthesia services.

EXAMPLE

Physical Status Modifiers

P1 A normal healthy patient

P3 A patient with severe systemic disease

- **Ambulatory surgery center (ASC)** *hospital outpatient use modifiers* are two-digit codes used only when reporting services provided at this type of outpatient facility.

EXAMPLE

ASC Modifiers

27 Multiple outpatient hospital E/M encounters

73 Discontinued outpatient procedure

- **HCPCS Level II modifiers** are two-character alphabetic or alphanumeric codes that are used to provide additional information about services provided to patients covered by a third-party payer that

Modifier

A two-character code that affects the meaning of another code; a code addendum that provides more meaning to the original code.

CPT code modifier

A two-character code that may be appended to a code from the main portion of the CPT book to provide additional information.

Physical status modifier

A two-character alphanumeric code used to describe the condition of the patient at the time anesthesia services are administered.

Alphanumeric

Containing both letters and numbers.

Ambulatory surgery center (ASC)

A facility specially designed to provide surgical treatments without an overnight stay; also known as a *same-day surgery center*.

HCPCS Level II modifier

A two-character alphabetic or alphanumeric code that may be appended to a code from the main portion of the CPT book or a code from the HCPCS Level II book.

accepts HCPCS Level II codes. (Lots more about this later in this chapter and the text.)

CPT CODE MODIFIERS

Using modifiers is often a judgment that you, the coding specialist, will have to make as you review the details of each case. As you are analyzing the descriptions of the procedures performed, written by the physician, and comparing them to the descriptions of the codes in the CPT book, you may find that there is more to the story.

On occasion, the CPT book will remind you of a special circumstance that requires a modifier.

Modifier 50 is used to identify that a health care professional has provided a service or performed a procedure bilaterally (both sides).

In some locations of the CPT book, you will find the directions regarding modifier use in the instructional paragraph at the beginning of a subheading.

Modifier 52 indicates that the service or procedure, as described, was not completed in full. If both ears are included in the code description but only one ear is tested, then a reduced service was provided.

Personnel modifiers

A modifier providing additional information about the professionals attending to the treatment of the patient.

PERSONNEL MODIFIERS

As you read through the descriptions of each of the modifiers, most of them will seem very straightforward. **Personnel modifiers** explain special circumstances relating to the health care professionals involved in the treatment of the patient.

Personnel Modifier

62 Two surgeons

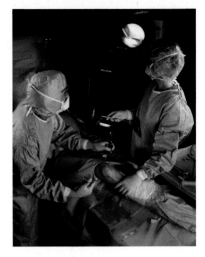

Modifier 62, clearly, is used when the operative notes indicate that two surgeons worked side by side, both as primary surgeons, during a procedure. If the modifier is not there to explain that there *were* two primary surgeons involved, how else could the insurance carrier know that receiving two separate claim forms for the same patient on the same day is legitimate? The insurance carrier would certainly think that one of the physicians is fraudulently billing it for work done by another. The second claim filed, and possibly even the first one, might be denied or set aside for further investigation, and the carrier may even initiate a fraud investigation. This little two-digit code tells the insurance carrier that no one is cheating and both surgeons actually did provide for the patient.

The same scenario works for other personnel modifiers:

- 66 Surgical team
- 80 Assistant surgeon
- 81 Minimum assistant surgeon
- 82 Assistant surgeon (when qualified resident surgeon not available)

Using any of these modifiers provides an explanation, very directly and simply, why more than one health care professional is claiming reimbursement for providing service to the same patient on the same date.

YOU CODE IT! CASE STUDY

Reina Gold, a 39-year-old female, has been diagnosed with endometriosis and is admitted to Barton Hospital to have Dr. Thomas perform a vaginal, radical hysterectomy. While Reina is in the OR and under anesthesia, Dr. Peters is going to perform an open sling operation for stress incontinence on her bladder. She tolerates both procedures well and is taken back to her room.

You Code It!

Go through the steps of coding and determine the codes that should be reported for this encounter between Reina Gold, Dr. Thomas, and Dr. Peters.

Step 1: Read the case completely.

Step 2: Abstract the notes: Which key words can you identify relating to the procedures performed?

Step 3: Query the provider, if necessary.

Step 4: Diagnosis: Endometriosis, stress incontinence.

Step 5: Code the procedure(s).

Step 6: Link the procedure codes to at least one diagnosis code.

Step 7: Back code to double-check your choices.

Answer

Did you find the correct codes to be:

58285-62 Vaginal hysterectomy, radical (Schauta type operation); two surgeons

57288-62 Sling operation for stress incontinence; two surgeons

MULTIPLE MODIFIERS

There may be circumstances where one case is so complex, unusual, or special that you need more than one modifier to explain the whole scenario.

LET'S CODE IT! SCENARIO

Dr. Lazenby performed a bilateral osteotomy on the shaft of Jack Banyon's femur. Another surgeon performed the same procedure on Jack two weeks ago, but was unsuccessful, so Dr. Lazenby repeated the procedure. As an expert in this procedure, he was brought in to perform the surgery only, and will not be involved in any preoperative or postoperative care of the patient.

Let's Code It!

To accurately report Dr. Lazenby's surgical services to Jack Banyon, you would need:

27448 Osteotomy, femur, shaft or supracondylar; without fixation
  -50 Modifier to report that it was a bilateral procedure
  -54 Modifier to report Dr. Lazenby was providing surgical care only
  -77 Modifier to report that this is a repeat procedure by another physician

Therefore, box 24D on the claim form CMS-1500 (find a sample of this form in Appendix A of this text) would look like this: 27448-50-54-77.

The CMS-1500 claim form, upon which you will record your chosen codes and other information to request reimbursement from the third-party payer, has a limited amount of space to place the necessary information, particularly when it comes to the inclusion of modifiers. Some third-party payers do not permit multiple modifiers to be listed on the same line as the CPT code. Therefore, should your case require two or more modifiers to completely explain all of the circumstances involved, you can use modifier 99.

99 Multiple Modifiers: *Under certain circumstances two or more modifiers may be necessary to completely delineate a service. In such situations modifier 99 should be added to the basic procedure, and other applicable modifiers may be listed as part of the description of the service.*

ANESTHESIA PHYSICAL STATUS MODIFIERS

Anesthesia physical status modifiers are two-character alphanumeric codes: the letter *P* followed by a number. These modifiers identify the condition of the patient at the time anesthesia services are provided and highlight health circumstances that might dramatically impact the anesthesiologist's ability to successfully care for the patient. By explaining the level of the patient's health at the time the anesthesiologist administers the service, the third-party payer can better understand how hard this physician had to work. For example, if a patient has uncontrolled hypertension at the time anesthesia is administered, the anesthesiologist must monitor the patient more carefully, perhaps use a different type of anesthetic, and watch for possible complications that would not be an issue with an otherwise healthy patient. This status modifier, for the most part, does not relate to the reason the patient is having the anesthesia administered, but is in relation to the patient's entire health. You can see that without understanding the difference between treatment issue and overall health, it might be hard for you to identify a patient as "P1 A normal healthy patient" when the person is in your facility to have a diseased gallbladder removed. However, if the patient is *otherwise healthy*, P1 would be the correct status modifier.

The physical status modifiers, P1 through P6, may only be appended to codes from the Anesthesia section of the CPT book, codes 00100 through 01999.

EXAMPLE

Use of a Physical Status Modifier
Anesthesia for a diagnostic arthroscopy of the knee on a professional basketball player who is otherwise healthy.

   01382-P1

There may be a case when a CPT modifier must also be used with an anesthesia code. When this is done, the physical status modifier is to be placed closest to the procedure code.

EXAMPLE

Using a Physical Status Modifier with a CPT Modifier
Anesthesia for a third-degree burn excision, 5% of total body surface area, for patient with uncontrolled diabetes and essential hypertension. The procedure was discontinued due to sudden onset of arrhythmia.

   01952-P3-53

You will read more about the anesthesia physical status modifiers in Chap. 6, "Anesthesia Coding."

««« **CODING TIP**

All anesthesia codes and *only* anesthesia codes are appended with a physical status modifier, immediately following the anesthesia code.

Like the CPT modifiers, ambulatory surgery center (ASC) hospital outpatient facilities use modifiers that are two-digit codes.

Many of the modifiers in this subheading are the same as the CPT modifiers. However, there are three additional modifiers specifically for ASC coders:

> **27 Multiple Outpatient Hospital E/M Encounters on the Same Date:** *For hospital outpatient reporting purposes, utilization of hospital resources related to separate and distinct E/M encounters performed in multiple outpatient hospital settings on the same date may be reported by adding modifier 27 to each appropriate level outpatient and/ or emergency department E/M code(s). This modifier provides a means of reporting circumstances involving evaluation and management services provided by physician(s) in more than one (multiple) outpatient hospital setting(s) (e.g., hospital emergency department, clinic).*

EXAMPLE

Using Modifier 27

Patricia Anatoly, a 35-year-old female, cut her hand and went to the Barton Hospital clinic. After Dr. Aden evaluated her hand, he sent her to the emergency department because the cut was so deep it needed more intense care. Dr. Knight saw and treated Patricia's laceration in the ED.

As the coding specialist for the hospital, you would be responsible for coding the services provided in all your facilities, including the clinic as well as the emergency department (ED). Patricia Anatoly was seen in two different facilities on the same day for the same injury. First, you would code the services that Dr. Aden did—the evaluation and management of Patricia's injury and his decision to send her to the ED for a higher level of care. Second, you would report the services that Patricia received in the ED, which certainly included additional evaluation and then the repair of her wound.

Without the use of modifier 27, you would have difficulty in getting the claim paid, because the third-party payer is liable to think that this is a case of duplicate billing or an error.

Occasionally, a planned surgical event is not performed due to circumstances that might put the patient in jeopardy. In such cases, all the preparation has been done, the team was ready, and your facility needs to be reimbursed, even though you have not performed the service or treatment. Modifiers 73 and 74 will identify these unusual circumstances.

> **73 Discontinued Outpatient Hospital/Ambulatory Surgery Center (ASC) Procedure prior to the Administration of Anesthesia:** *Due to extenuating circumstances or those that threaten the well-being of the patient, the*

physician may cancel a surgical or diagnostic procedure subsequent to the patient's surgical preparation (including sedation when provided, and being taken to the room where the procedure is to be performed), but prior to the administration of anesthesia (local, regional block(s) or general). Under these circumstances, the intended service that is prepared for but canceled can be reported by its usual procedure number and the addition of modifier 73.

74   Discontinued Outpatient Hospital/Ambulatory Surgery Center (ASC) Procedure after Administration of Anesthesia: *Due to extenuating circumstances or those that threaten the well-being of the patient, the physician may terminate a surgical or diagnostic procedure after the administration of anesthesia (local, regional block(s) or general), or after the procedure was started (incision made, intubation started, scope inserted, etc.). Under these circumstances, the procedure started, but terminated can be reported by its usual procedure number and the addition of modifier 74.*

LET'S CODE IT! SCENARIO

Kenneth Bonner, a 61-year-old male, was brought into Room 9 to be prepared for a bunionectomy. He changed into a gown, got into bed, and the nurse took his vital signs. Kenneth's temperature was 38.9°C (102°F). Dr. Richter ordered a complete CBC, the results of which proved that Kenneth had an active infection in his system. The bunionectomy was canceled, and Kenneth was sent home.

Let's Code It!

Dr. Richter and her team were prepared and ready to perform a bunionectomy. However, it is not wise to operate on a patient with an active infection, so the procedure had to be canceled in the best interest of the patient. The facility still deserves to be reimbursed for its time, materials and supplies, and efforts. Therefore, the facility will submit a claim form to Kenneth's insurance carrier with the code for the bunionectomy and the modifier 73 to indicate that the procedure was canceled *prior to the administration of anesthesia:* 28290-73.

HCPCS/NATIONAL LEVEL II MODIFIERS

The Healthcare Common Procedure Coding System (HCPCS) has two parts. The first (Level I) is the Current Procedural Terminology (CPT). Even though all the codes come from HCPCS, only Level II codes are referred to as HCPCS, and they have their own modifiers. Part Two of this text (Chaps. 13–15) go into complete detail on HCPCS Level II codes and modifiers.

Laterality

Relating to the side or sides of the body, *unilateral* meaning one side and *bilateral* meaning both sides.

A short list of HCPCS (Level II) modifiers is included in Appendix A of the CPT book. The modifiers are two-character codes, either one letter and one number or two letters. You'll notice that most of the HCPCS modifiers included in Appendix A specify **laterality**.

- E1 through E4 identify right/left/upper/lower eyelids.
- F1 through FA identify each of the 10 fingers.
- T1 through TA identify each of the 10 toes.
- LC through LD identify portions of the left coronary artery.
- RC identifies the right coronary artery.
- LT = left.
- RT = right.

There are two modifiers shown that have nothing to do with anatomical sites: QM and QN are related to the use of ambulance services.

It is very important that you know when you may or may not use HCPCS modifiers. Essentially, the insurance carrier you are billing will either accept these codes and modifiers or not accept them. Medicare uses HCPCS codes and modifiers, along with CPT. This is true nationwide. However, it is your responsibility to find out whether other third-party payers with which you work want you to use them.

YOU CODE IT! CASE STUDY

Yamile Tourhy, a 67-year-old female, came to the Barton Ambulatory Surgery Center so that Dr. Bhmiami could excise a benign tumor from her right foot's big toe. She tolerated the procedure well, and was discharged.

You Code It!

Go through the steps of coding and determine the codes that should be reported for this encounter between Dr. Bhmiami and Yamile Tourhy.

Step 1: Read the case completely.

Step 2: Abstract the notes: Which key words can you identify relating to the procedures performed?

_____

Step 3: Query the provider, if necessary.

Step 4: Diagnosis: Benign neoplasm, great toe.

Step 5: Code the procedure(s).

_____

Step 6: Link the procedure codes to at least one diagnosis code.

Step 7: Back code to double-check your choices.

Answer

Did you find the correct codes to be:

28108-T5 Excision or curettage of bone cyst or benign tumor, phalanges of foot; right foot, great toe

Part 1   CPT

SEQUENCING MULTIPLE MODIFIERS

Should a particular case require the use of several different types of modifiers, it is important that you place them in the correct order.

A CPT modifier should be placed closest to the procedure code.

EXAMPLE

24201-53 Removal of foreign body, upper arm or elbow area; deep, discontinued procedure

When more than one CPT modifier is required, place the **service-related modifier** closest to the procedure code, followed by the personnel modifier.

EXAMPLE

24201-22-80 Removal of foreign body, upper arm or elbow area; deep, unusual procedural service, assistant surgeon

When a HCPCS Level II modifier is used in addition to a CPT modifier, the CPT modifier is placed closest to the procedure code and the HCPCS Level II modifier follows.

EXAMPLE

24201-76-LT Removal of foreign body, upper arm or elbow area; deep, repeat procedure by same physician, left side

SUPPLEMENTAL REPORTS

Remember: Documentation is your watchword. It is the backbone of the health information management industry. In many situations when a modifier is used, a **supplemental report** is needed for additional clarification.

Generally, while the modifier itself provides a certain amount of explanation, the insurance carrier wants more. You can be efficient and send the details along with the claim, or you can wait until the carrier requests additional information. Either way, you will have to supply all the facts. However, if you wait to be asked, you will be delaying payment to your facility.

Service-related modifier

A modifier relating to a change or adjustment of a procedure or service provided.

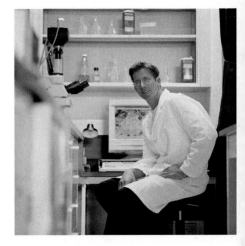

Supplemental report

A letter or report written by the attending physician or other health care professional to provide additional clarification or explanation.

LET'S CODE IT! SCENARIO

Leland Alexander, an 11-year-old boy, had a superficial cut, about 3.3 cm, on his left cheek, after being in a car accident and hit by broken glass. Dr. Chandra is ready to perform a simple repair of the wound, but she is very concerned. Leland has Tourette's syndrome that causes him to jerk or move abruptly, especially when nervous. Although anesthesia is not typically used for a simple repair of a superficial wound, Dr. Chandra administers general anesthesia. Jacob Haverty, a CRNA, assists Dr. Chandra with monitoring Leland during the procedure.

Dr. Chandra performed a *simple repair* of Leland's *superficial wound* on his *face*. Go to the alphabetic index and look up *Repair*. As you look down the list of anatomical sites, you do not see face or cheek listed. You know that the repair was simple, and when you look at that listing, you note the direction, "*See* Integumentary System, Repair, Simple." Once you go to that listing, you find the suggested codes 12001–12021. Let's take a look at the complete description in the numeric listing.

12011 Simple repair of superficial wounds of face, ears, eyelids, nose, lips and/or mucous membranes; 2.5 cm or less

The basic description matches the notes exactly. However, several choices are determined by the size of the wound. The notes state that Leland's wound was 3.3 cm. This brings you to the correct code:

12013 Simple repair of superficial wounds of face, ears, eyelids, nose, lips and/or mucous membranes; 2.6 cm to 5.0 cm

Great! Now, you have to address the fact that Dr. Chandra gave Leland *general anesthesia*. This was done for a very valid medical reason, and Dr. Chandra (and her facility) should be properly reimbursed for the service. Anesthesia is not included with code 12013 because it is not normally required. Leland's case is unusual. Unusual circumstances often require modifiers, so let's look at Appendix A to see if there is an applicable modifier. Modifier 23 seems to fit:

> **23 Unusual Anesthesia:** *Occasionally, a procedure, which usually requires either no anesthesia or local anesthesia, because of unusual circumstances must be done under general anesthesia. This circumstance may be reported by adding modifier 23 to the procedure code of the basic service.*

So modifier 23 should be appended, or attached, to the procedure code.

12013-23

You also know that you have to code the anesthesia service as well.

00300 Anesthesia for all procedures on the integumentary system, muscles and nerves of head, neck, and posterior trunk, not otherwise specified

Now, let's look at Appendix A to see if there is an applicable modifier to explain that an anesthesiologist was not involved. Modifier 47 seems to fit.

> **47 Anesthesia by surgeon:** *Regional or general anesthesia provided by the surgeon may be reported by adding modifier 47 to the basic service. (This does not include local anesthesia.) NOTE: Modifier 47 would not be used as a modifier for the anesthesia procedures.*

Well, the *note* in the description of modifier 47 tells you that this modifier is necessary, but not with code 00300. You have to attach the modifier to the procedure code. Therefore, you submit the claim with one CPT code and two modifiers: 12013-23-47. In addition, it is smart to include a supplemental report with the claim to explain the use of general anesthesia. You are aware that the insurance company wants to know the details before paying the claim.

CHAPTER SUMMARY

Modifiers provide additional explanation to the third-party payer so they can fully appreciate any special circumstances that affected the procedures and services provided to the patient. In health care, as well as in so many other instances of our lives, most things do not fit neatly into predetermined descriptions. By using modifiers correctly, you provide an additional explanation and promote the efficient and more accurate reimbursement of your facility.

The following chapters in this text review, in detail, the proper use of all the modifiers listed in Appendix A of the CPT book, with reference to the specific type of procedure code each affects.

1. A modifier explains

   a. The reason why a procedure was performed.

   b. An unusual circumstance.

   c. The date of service.

   d. The level of education of the physician.

2. Modifiers are attached to

   a. Policy numbers.

   b. Diagnosis codes.

   c. Procedure codes.

   d. Pharmaceutical codes.

3. A modifier is a code made up of

   a. Two numbers.

   b. Two letters.

   c. One number and one letter.

   d. All of the above.

4. A physical status modifier may only be attached to

   a. Anesthesia codes.

   b. Surgical codes.

   c. Radiology codes.

   d. Evaluation and Management codes.

5. An example of a HCPCS Level II modifier is

   a. 23.

   b. P4.

   c. E2.

   d. 99.

6. An example of a personnel modifier is

   a. 81.

   b. 47.

   c. LC.

   d. 57.

7. If a third-party payer limits your use of multiple modifiers, you should use

   a. No modifiers.

   b. 91.

   c. 51.

   d. 99.

8. P5 is an example of a

   a. HCPCS Level II modifier.

   b. CPT modifier.

   c. Physical status modifier.

   d. Personnel modifier.

9. When appending both a CPT modifier and a HCPCS modifier to a procedure code,

   a. The HCPCS modifier comes first.

   b. The CPT modifier comes first.

   c. It doesn't matter which comes first.

   d. Use neither, they cancel each other out.

10. A supplemental report is _____ when using a modifier.

   a. sometimes required

   b. always required

   c. never required

   d. given upon request of the third-party payer only

Find the best modifier for each of the following scenarios.

1. Dr. White removed Vanetta Johns' gallbladder 10 days ago. Today, she comes to see Dr. White because of a problem in her knee. Which modifier should be appended to the encounter's E/M code?

   _____

2. Dr. Regis performed an appendectomy on Wilfred Maxell. However, the operation took twice as long as usual because Wilfred weighs 432 pounds. Which modifier should be appended to the code for the surgical procedure?

   _____

3. Dr. Calhoun performed a biopsy on the left external ear of Janise Smith, a 71-year-old female. Which HCPCS modifier will Medicare require you to append to the procedure code?

   _____

4. Adrian Matthews, a 15-year-old male, was brought into the operating room in the Barton ASC to have a programmable pump inserted into his spine for pain control. After the anesthesia was administered and Adrian was fully unconscious, Dr. Clayton made the first incision. Adrian began to hemorrhage. The bleeding was stopped, the incision was closed, and the procedure was discontinued. Which modifier should be appended to the code for the insertion of the pump?

   _____

5. Elizabeth Julienne, a 53-year-old female, goes to see Dr. Rodriquez at the referral of her family physician, Dr. Roth, for his opinion as to whether or not she should have surgery. After the evaluation and Elizabeth's agreement, Dr. Rodriquez schedules surgery for Thursday. Which modifier should be appended to Dr. Rodriquez's consultation code for today's evaluation?

   _____

6. Sophia Alvera, a 71-year-old female, is having Dr. Young remove a cyst from her left ring finger. Which modifier does Medicare require you to append to the procedure code for the removal of the cyst?

   _____

7. John Jung, a 2-week-old male, was rushed into surgery for repair of a septal defect. If the repair is not completed successfully, he may not survive. What is the correct anesthesia physical status modifier?

_____

8. Dr. Kidman is preparing to perform open-heart surgery on Frank Wenami. Dr. Fortner is asked to assist because a surgical resident is not available. Which modifier should be appended to the procedure code on Dr. Fortner's claim for services?

_____

9. Nancy Nemeir, a 41-year-old female, comes to see Dr. Parker for a complete physical examination, required by her insurance carrier. Which modifier should be appended to the code for the physical?

_____

10. Earl Hillier, a 5-week-old male, was born prematurely and weighs 3.8 kg. Dr. Volkesberg performs a cardiac catheterization on Earl. Which modifier should be appended to the procedure code?

_____

11. Dr. Koenig excised an abscess on Harold Crenshaw's great toe, right foot. Which modifier does Medicare require you to append to the procedure code?

_____

12. Debra Dumont, a 9-year-old female, has been complaining of hearing a constant ringing in her right ear. Dr. Lowell performs an assessment for tinnitus in the one ear only. Which modifier should be appended to the procedure code?

_____

13. Dr. Nevradi performed a percutaneous transluminal coronary atherectomy, by mechanical method, on Maxine Burwell's left circumflex artery. Which modifier does Medicare require you to append to the procedure code?

_____

14. Ronald Aswan, a 15-year-old male, came to Dr. Pollard to have corrective surgery on both of his eyes. Which modifier is appended to the procedure code?

_____

15. Carlo Yawya, a 19-year-old male, hurt his shoulder while camping. The clinic in the area took an x-ray but did not have a radiologist, so Carlo brought the films to Dr. Ellerton for interpretation and evaluation. Which modifier should Dr. Ellerton's coder append to the code for the x-rays?

_____

You Code It! Simulation
Chapter 3. Introduction to CPT Modifiers

On the following pages, you will see physician notes documenting encounters with patients at our textbook's health care facility, Cipher, Victors, & Associates. Carefully read through the notes, and find the best code or codes, and modifiers when applicable, for each case.

CIPHER, VICTORS, & ASSOCIATES
A Complete Health Care Facility
234 MAIN STREET • ANYTOWN, FL 32711 • 407-555-1234

PATIENT: MORRISON, GARRET

ACCOUNT/EHR #:   MORRGA001

Date: 11/13/08

Diagnosis: Morbid obesity

Procedure: Gastric bypass, secondary to skin infection—CANCELED

Physician: Marion M. March, MD

Anesthesiologist: George Harland, MD

Anesthesia: General endotracheal anesthesia

Location: AMBULATORY SURGICAL CENTER–EAST

Procedure: Pt is a 30-year-old male with a long history of morbid obesity, recently underwent silastic gastric banding, and, due to reflux disease, subsequently required a procedure to loosen the band. Most recently, he has experienced significant reflux disease, and presents for removal of his band and to have short limb Roux-en-Y gastric bypass.

    The patient is brought into the OR and placed in the supine position. General endotracheal anesthesia was administered. The patient's gown was removed for prepping, at which point clinicians noticed there were small, acnelike lesions over the anterior surface of his abdomen, his inguinal areas, and on his legs. Several of the lesions fell on the incision line.

    Additionally, there was a large midline abdominal wall defect, which was assumed to represent an abdominal wall hernia, and most likely will require a mesh repair. For these two reasons the case was canceled after general anesthesia was administered. The patient was awakened from anesthesia and taken to the recovery room. There were no immediate complications evident.

_____

Marion M. March, MD

MMM/mg   D: 11/13/08 09:50:16   T: 11/13/08 12:55:01

Find the best, most accurate codes, and modifiers, as appropriate.

_____

_____

_____

CIPHER, VICTORS, & ASSOCIATES
A Complete Health Care Facility
234 MAIN STREET • ANYTOWN, FL 32711 • 407-555-1234

PATIENT: ATWELL, SARAH

ACCOUNT/EHR #:   ATWESA001

Date: 10/3/08

Diagnosis: Fecal incontinence, diarrhea, constipation

Procedure: Total colonoscopy with hot biopsy destruction of sessile 3 mm mid-sigmoid
                                   colon polyp and multiple cold biopsies taken randomly throughout the colon

Physician: Marion M. March, MD

Anesthesia: Demerol 50 mg and Versed 3 mg both given IV

Procedure: Pt is a 43-year-old female. Patient was placed into position. Digital examination revealed no masses. The pediatric variable flexion Olympus colonoscope was introduced into the rectum and advanced to the cecum. A picture was taken of the appendiceal orifice and the ileocecal valve.

The scope was then carefully extubated. The mucosa looked normal. Random biopsies were taken from the ascending colon, the transverse colon, the descending colon, sigmoid colon, and rectum. There was a 3 mm sessile polyp in the mid-sigmoid colon that a hot biopsy destroyed.

Impression: Sigmoid colon polyp destroyed by hot biopsy
Recommendations: The physician asked the patient to call the office in a week to get the results
                                   of the pathology. At a later time, take cold biopsies because of history of
                                   diarrhea.

___

Marion M. March, MD

MMM/mg   D: 10/3/08 09:50:16   T: 10/5/08 12:55:01

Find the best, most accurate codes, and modifiers, as appropriate.

___

___

___

CIPHER, VICTORS, & ASSOCIATES
A Complete Health Care Facility
234 MAIN STREET • ANYTOWN, FL 32711 • 407-555-1234

PATIENT: TACOMA, THOMAS

ACCOUNT/EHR #: TACOTH001

Date: 9/13/08

Diagnosis: Family history of colon cancer

Procedure: Colonoscopy

Physician: Marion M. March, MD

Anesthesia: Versed 4 mg, Demerol 75 mg

Procedure: Pt is a 75-year-old male presenting for a colonoscopy. He understands the nature of the procedure, the risks and consequences, and alternative procedures, and consents to the procedure. The patient receives educational materials, information on the risks of the procedure, and answers frequently asked questions.

The patient is placed in the left lateral decubitus position. The rectal exam reveals normal sphincter tone and no masses. A colonoscope is introduced into the rectum and advanced to the distal sigmoid colon. Further advancement is impossible due to the marked fixation and severe angulation of the rectosigmoid colon.

On withdrawal, no masses or polyps are noted, and the mucosa is normal throughout. Rectal vault is unremarkable. The patient tolerates the procedure without difficulty.

Impression: Normal colonoscopy, only to the distal sigmoid colon
Plan: Strong recommendation for a barium enema

Marion M. March, MD

MMM/mg   D: 9/13/08 09:50:16   T: 9/13/08 12:55:01

Find the best, most accurate codes, and modifiers, as appropriate.

Part 1   CPT

CIPHER, VICTORS, & ASSOCIATES
A Complete Health Care Facility
234 MAIN STREET • ANYTOWN, FL 32711 • 407-555-1234

PATIENT:	STERLING, KRISTA
ACCOUNT/EHR #:	STERKR001
Date:	12/1/08
Diagnosis:	Obstructive sleep apnea
Procedure:	Aborted uvulopalatopharyngoplasty
Physician:	Marion M. March, MD
Anesthesia:	Bilateral superior laryngeal nerve blocks
Location:	AMBULATORY SURGICAL CENTER–EAST

Procedure: After obtaining informed consent, the patient was taken to the operating room and placed in a supine position. The patient was properly identified, and Versed 4 mg was injected.

Prior to the anesthesia service being performed, the patient exhibited significant coughing and gagging. After multiple attempts to calm the response, the procedure was aborted. The patient was taken to the recovery room.

Impression: Aborted uvulopalatopharyngoplasty

_____

Marion M. March, MD

MMM/mg   D: 12/1/08 09:50:16   T: 12/7/08 12:55:01

Find the best, most accurate codes, and modifiers, as appropriate.

_____

_____

_____

CIPHER, VICTORS, & ASSOCIATES
A Complete Health Care Facility
234 MAIN STREET • ANYTOWN, FL 32711 • 407-555-1234

PATIENT:	ULVERTON, NATALIE
ACCOUNT/EHR #:	ULVENA001
Date:	11/9/08
Diagnosis:	Chronic obstructive lung disease
Procedure:	Lung transplant, single, with cardiopulmonary bypass
Surgical Team:	Marion M. March, MD, primary; Fredrick Avatar, MD; Gene Lavelle, MD
Anesthesia:	General

Procedure: Pt is a 37-year-old female brought into the OR, placed on the table, and draped in sterile fashion. Anesthesia was administered. At thoracotomy, the left lung was removed by dividing the left main stem bronchus at the level of the left upper lobe. The two pulmonary veins and single pulmonary artery were divided distally. An allograft left lung was inserted. The recipient left main stem bronchus and pulmonary artery were re-resected to accommodate the transplant. The recipient pulmonary veins were opened into the left atrium. An end-to-end anastomosis of the recipient's respective structures (pulmonary artery, main stem bronchus, and left atrial cuffs) was made to the similar donor structures. Two chest tubes were inserted. Bronchoscopy was performed in the operating room. Cardiopulmonary bypass was successfully completed.

   Patient tolerated the procedure well and was taken to the recovery room.

Marion M. March, MD

MMM/mg   D: 11/9/08 09:50:16   T: 11/13/08 12:55:01

Find the best, most accurate codes, and modifiers, as appropriate.

_____

_____

_____

Evaluation and Management Codes, Part 1:

Key Components

LEARNING OUTCOMES

- Apply the guidelines for proper evaluation and management coding.
- Calculate the appropriate level of patient history taken.
- Ascertain the appropriate level of physical exam performed by the physician.
- Determine the appropriate level of medical decision-making provided by the physician.
- Distinguish between the various types of encounters.
- Choose the best, most appropriate code for evaluation and management services.

KEY TERMS

Confirmatory consultation

Consultation

Established patient

Evaluation and management (E/M)

Level of patient history

Level of physical examination

Medical decision-making (MDM)

New patient

PFSH

Relationship

EMPLOYMENT OPPORTUNITIES

Non-profit organizations
Long-term care facilities
Assisted living facilities
General practice
Hospitals

Physicians' offices
Ambulatory surgery centers
Clinics
Home health agencies
Nursing homes

Evaluation and Management (E/M) is the first section in the CPT book and lists codes numbered 99201 to 99499. The codes are used to report and reimburse physicians for their expertise and thought processes involved in diagnosing and treating patients:

- Talking with the patient and their family.

- Reviewing data such as test and examination results.
- Doing research in medical books and journals.
- Consulting with other health care professionals.

All these elements, including the training and education that this health care

73

professional has had, go into the decision of what to do next for the patient—what advice, what prescription, what test, what treatment, what procedure. E/M codes provide a way to reimburse the health care professional for his or her assessment and supervision of the patient's care.

Evaluation and management (E/M)

Specific characteristics of a face-to-face meeting between a health care professional and a patient.

E/M CODES

Evaluation and management codes are used to describe the encounter between provider and patient. The codes are used to compensate the provider for meeting face to face with the patient and his or her family, as well as for evaluating the situation and determining the correct procedures and services to help the patient in the best way. Information that you must have to code the encounter properly includes the following:

1. **Location of the encounter:** Did the provider see the patient in an outpatient location (such as an office), in the hospital, in a skilled nursing facility, or somewhere else?

2. **Relationship:** Is this individual a new patient of the provider, an established patient, or here for a one-time consultation?

3. **Key components:** What type of service was provided? What levels of services were provided?

Location

Let's go to the Evaluation and Management (E/M) section of the CPT book. Look at the first subheading on the first page:

Office or Other Outpatient Services

This, like others throughout the section, identifies the location of the encounter. In other words, where did the physician meet with the patient? Other headings in the E/M section are shown in Box 4-1.

EXAMPLES

Maxwell Edison, a 61-year-old male, was brought into the *emergency department* with sharp pain in his chest, radiating downward into his left arm. The best, most appropriate E/M code will be found in the 99281-99288 range of codes, under *Emergency Department Services.*

Dr. Farber goes to the Suniland Nursing Home *to see his patient, Gail Robbins, a 93-year-old female.* The best, most appropriate E/M code will be found in the 99304-99318 range of codes, under *Nursing Facility Services.*

Amanda Carter, a 21-year-old female, comes to see Dr. Atwater at his office. The best, most appropriate E/M code will be found in the 99201-99215 range of codes, under *Office or Other Outpatient Services.*

Relationship

As you can see in Figure 4-1, throughout the E/M section of the CPT book, subheadings identify the **relationship** between the provider and the individual. Evaluation and management (E/M) codes use three types of relationship for determining the best, most appropriate code. The three relationships are **new patient, established patient,** and **consultation.**

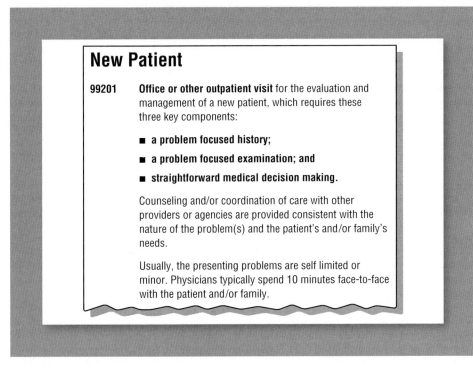

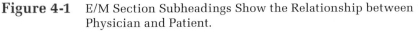

Figure 4-1 E/M Section Subheadings Show the Relationship between Physician and Patient.

Relationship

The level of familiarity between provider and patient.

New patient

A person who has not received any professional services within the past three years from either the provider or another provider of the same specialty who belongs to the same group practice.

Established patient

A person who has received professional services within the last three years from either this provider or another provider of the same specialty belonging to the same group practice.

Consultation

An encounter for purposes of a second physician's opinion or advice, requested by another physician, regarding the management of a patient's specific health concern. A consultation is planned to be a short-term relationship between a health care professional and a patient.

The reason why you must know the relationship between the patient and the provider is so that you can establish an understanding of how familiar the physician is with the patient, his or her personal history, social history, family history, and other elements that may affect the physician's decisions regarding the patient's health. Certainly you can understand that the first time they meet, the physician knows absolutely nothing about the patient at all. He or she must spend time asking questions to help collect the information that will be critical to determining the correct diagnosis and course of treatment. Whereas when the physician sees the patient again, all the doctor will need to do is quickly read through the patient's file to refresh his or her memory of past conditions and issues.

EXAMPLE

Amanda Carter, a 21-year-old female, comes to see Dr. Atwater at his office and complains of severe pain in her right wrist and forearm. She just moved to the area, and this is the *first time* Dr. Atwater has seen her.

The E/M codes applicable for this encounter are now in the smaller range of 99201–99205, Office or Other Outpatient Services, New Patient.

LET'S CODE IT! SCENARIO

Margaret Tanner, an 83-year-old female, broke her hip one month ago. She has been a patient of Dr. Rodriquez for several years. Since her release from the hospital, Margaret has been homebound until her hip completely heals. Therefore, Dr. Rodriquez went to her home to check on her progress.

Let's Code It!

Read the notes again, and look for the key words that tell you the location of the encounter and the relationship between patient and physician.

Margaret has been "a patient of Dr. Rodriquez for several years." Therefore, she is an established patient. Also, the notes state that the doctor went to "her home." That phrase tells us the location of the encounter. As you look through the section of the CPT book, you find the perfect group of E/M codes: 99347–99350, Home Services, Established Patient.

There are times when the relationship between a patient and a health care provider is expected to be temporary. In such cases, a physician will meet and evaluate a patient's condition only to offer his or her own professional opinion about the patient's diagnosis and/or treatment options. This relationship is not defined as new or established, and is coded from the Consultations section. (More details about coding consultations follow in just a few pages.)

Key Components

Once you have found the appropriate subheading with regard to the location and you have determined the relationship between the patient and the physician, there are just a few codes from which to choose.

BOX 4-2 Service Locations Requiring Key Component Levels

Office and Other Outpatient Services

Hospital Observation Services

Hospital Inpatient Services

Consultations

Emergency Department Services

Nursing Facility Services

Domiciliary, Rest Home (e.g., Boarding Home), or Custodial Care Services

Domiciliary, Rest Home (e.g., Assisted Living Facility), or Home Care Plan Oversight Services

Home Services

When evaluation and management services are provided in the locations listed in Box 4-2, you have to determine the level of services that were given.

In the E/M section of the CPT book, look at the key components, identified by bullet points, in the description of each code. Each bullet identifies a different level of work the physician has done, and documented, with regard to:

1. *Patient history* taken.

2. *Physical examination* performed.

3. *Medical decision-making* required.

Let's go back to our first subheading in the E/M section, and use this as an example. There are only five codes under Office or Other Patient Services: New Patient: codes 99201, 99202, 99203, 99204, and 99205. How do you know which is the correct code? How can you tell them apart? You will notice a difference immediately:

99201 is described as *problem-focused*.

99202 is described as *expanded problem-focused*.

99203 is described as *detailed*.

99204 is described as *comprehensive*.

99205 is described as *comprehensive*.

While accurately reporting the level of expertise and knowledge used by the physician during a visit may seem intangible, the coding guidelines give us very specific and tangible measurements to recognize an appropriate level of service.

Level of Patient History

In the E/M section of the CPT book, you will notice that the first key component (bullet) describes the **level of patient history** taken during this encounter by the physician.

There are four levels of patient history. You can measure the level of patient history taken by the physician by reading the notes and matching the documentation to this list.

Level of patient history

The amount of detail involved in the documentation of patient history.

BOX 4-3 **Review of Systems**

1. Constitutional symptoms, such as fever, weight loss, etc.
2. Eyes
3. Ears, mouth, nose, and throat
4. Cardiovascular
5. Respiratory
6. Gastrointestinal
7. Genitourinary
8. Musculoskeletal
9. Integumentary (skin and/or breast)
10. Neurological
11. Psychiatric
12. Endocrine
13. Hematological/lymphatic
14. Allergic/immunologic

1. Problem-focused history:

   a. A brief history of the patient's chief complaint, also known as a presenting problem. This might include a description of the signs and/or symptoms, the timing, severity, location, and any associated elements that might relate to a confirmed diagnosis.

2. Expanded problem-focused history:

   a. A brief history of the patient's chief complaint.

   b. A review of systems (ROS) related to the specific complaint or concern accomplished with a progression of questions that the physician will ask the patient to help him or her identify the problem, shed light on the diagnosis, categorize needed tests, or establish a baseline for possible treatment options. The elements of a system review are listed in the E/M guidelines, and here in Box 4-3.

3. Detailed history:

   a. An extended history of the present health concern.

   b. An extended review of a patient's past problems with the organ system(s) related to the present health concern and any other necessary systems.

   c. A past, family, and/or social history (**PFSH**) with focus only on components related to the present health concern. Overall components of a PFSH are listed in Box 4-4.

4. Comprehensive history:

   a. An extended history of this present health concern.

   b. A complete review of systems (ROS).

   c. A complete PFSH.

Level of Physical Examination

The second key component (bullet) describes the **level of physical examination** that was performed during this encounter by the physician.

There are four levels of physical examination. You can measure the level of examination performed by the physician by reading the notes and matching the documentation to the following list.

CODING TIP »»

The E/M guidelines include an itemized list of the body areas and the organ systems. So you always have a handy list that can be compared to provider's notes.

PFSH

An acronym for *past, family, and social history.*

Level of physical examination

The extent of a physician's clinical assessment and inspection of a patient.

Part 1   CPT

BOX 4-4 **PFSH Components**

Past History (also identified as PMH—Patient's Medical History)

- Prior major illnesses and injuries
- Prior operations
- Prior hospitalizations
- Current medications
- Allergies (e.g., drug, food)
- Age appropriate immunization status
- Age appropriate feeding/dietary status

Family History

- The health status or cause of death of parents, siblings, and children
- Specific diseases related to problems identified in the chief complaint, history of present illness, and/or system review

- Diseases of family members that may be hereditary or place the patient at risk

Social History

- Marital status and/or living arrangements
- Current employment
- Occupational history
- Use of drugs, alcohol, and tobacco
- Level of education
- Sexual history
- Other relevant social factors

---

1. Problem-focused examination:
   a. A limited examination of the body area related to the patient's chief complaint.
2. Expanded problem-focused examination:
   a. A limited examination of the related body area.
   b. Any other indicative or related body area(s) or organ system(s).
3. Detailed examination:
   a. An extended examination of the related body area(s) or organ system(s).
   b. Any other indicative or related body area(s) or organ system(s).
4. Comprehensive examination:
   a. A general, multisystem examination—*or* a complete examination of a single organ system.
   b. An examination of any other indicative or related body area(s) or organ system(s).

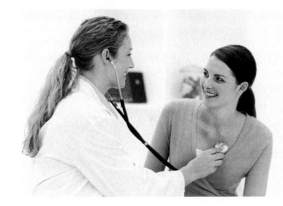

Level of Medical Decision-Making

The third bullet describes the level of **medical decision-making** required by the physician during this encounter.

The four levels of medical decision-making are:

1. Straightforward:
   a. A small number of possible diagnoses.
   b. A small number of treatment or management options.
   c. A low to no risk for complications.
   d. Little to no data or research to be reviewed.

««« CODING TIP

The CPT book categorizes 7 body areas and 11 organ systems in its determination of the best, most appropriate level of physical examination. See Boxes 4-5 and 4-6.

Medical decision-making (MDM)

The level of knowledge and experience needed by the provider to determine the diagnosis or to decide what to do next.

BOX 4-5 Body Areas

1. Head, including the face
2. Neck
3. Chest, including breasts and axilla
4. Abdomen
5. Genitalia, groin, buttocks
6. Back
7. Each extremity (arms and legs)

BOX 4-6 Organ Systems

1. Eyes
2. Ears, mouth, nose, and throat
3. Cardiovascular
4. Respiratory
5. Gastrointestinal
6. Genitourinary
7. Musculoskeletal
8. Skin
9. Neurological
10. Psychiatric
11. Hematological/lymphatic/immunologic

CODING TIP »»

Certain terms in the physician's notes may indicate a more complex process of medical decision-making on the physician's part. Orders for several tests with terms such as *rule out, possible,* and *likely* might indicate the physician is looking for evidence of one of several possible diagnoses.

CODING TIP »»

When the patient history, examination, and the medical decision-making are not performed at the same level to determine one code, the guidelines instruct you to choose the code that identifies key components that have been *met or exceeded* by the physician's documentation.

2. Low complexity:
   a. A limited number of possible diagnoses.
   b. A limited number of treatment or management options.
   c. A limited amount of data to be reviewed.
   d. A low risk for complications.
3. Moderate complexity:
   a. A multiple number of possible diagnoses.
   b. A multiple number of treatment or management options.
   c. A moderate amount of data to be reviewed.
   d. A moderate level of risk for complications, possibly due to other existing diagnoses or medications currently being taken.
4. High complexity:
   a. A large number of possible diagnoses.
   b. A large number of treatment or management options.
   c. A large amount of data and/or research to be reviewed.
   d. A high level of risk for complications, possibly due to other existing diagnoses and/or medications currently being taken.

EXAMPLE

Carter Allison comes in to his physician's office with a large chard of glass in his hand. You can see that the number of potential diagnoses is very small: a foreign body in his hand. There are a small number of treatment options: remove the chard. There are no real health complications, and the physician should not have to research Carter's condition before deciding what to do. This is a straightforward level of medical decision-making.

EXAMPLE

Gina Mulvanney comes to see her family doctor, Dr. Erickson, and complains of malaise and fatigue. She denies any major changes in her diet or lifestyle prior to the onset of her symptoms. This is a complex situation that will take a lot of investigation and knowledge on the part of the physician to determine Gina's underlying condition. There are numerous possible diagnoses and, thereby, a large number of management options. Dr. Erickson may have to perform several diagnostic tests to help him determine the problem. This is a highly complex case.

YOU CODE IT! CASE STUDY

Kenny Wilmington, a 33-year-old male, came to see Dr. Thomas in her office, for the first time, because of a cough, fever, excessive sputum production, and difficulty in breathing. He had been reasonably well until now. Dr. Thomas did an expanded problem-focused exam of the patient's respiratory system and took Kenny's personal, family, and social history in detail. After a chest x-ray was taken to rule out pneumonia, Dr. Thomas's straightforward medical decision-making led her to diagnose him with bronchitis and prescribed an antibiotic and a steroid.

You Code It!

Go through the steps of E/M coding, and determine the evaluation and management code that should be reported for this encounter between Dr. Thomas and Kenny Wilmington.

Step 1: Read the case completely.

Step 2: Abstract the notes: Which key words can you identify relating to the E/M service performed?

_____

Step 3: What is the location?

_____

Step 4: What is the relationship?

_____

Step 5: What level of patient history was taken?

_____

Step 6: What level of physical examination was performed?

_____

Step 7: What level of medical decision-making was required?

_____

Answer

Did you find the correct code to be 99202?

You know, from the notes, that Kenny is a new patient, because Dr. Thomas is seeing him "for the first time." In addition, this first sentence tells us that Kenny saw the doctor "in her office."

You would need to use code 99203 because the physician documented "history in detail." However, the level of physical examination performed would better match code 99202 because she only performed "an expanded problem-focused exam." Code 99202 is also supported by the "straightforward medical decision-making." So when you examine the requirements to meet or exceed the key components of code 99202, you consider the following:

- Expanded problem focused history: *Exceeded.*
- Expanded problem focused exam: *Met.*
- Straightforward decision-making: *Met.*

The correct evaluation and management code for this scenario is 99202.

Time

If the physician spends more than half (51% or more) of the total time *counseling* the patient, the time spent may be used as the key element in determining the best, most appropriate E/M code. In such cases, the time shown in the last paragraph of the E/M code description may override the other key components to determine the appropriate level. In order to use this guideline to choose a code, the documentation must support this fact.

LET'S CODE IT! SCENARIO

Lenore Parker, a 55-year-old female, came to see Dr. Bruce because she had the flu. While she was there, the results of her lab work, ordered by the doctor during her annual physical two weeks earlier, came back. Dr. Bruce examined Lenore's eyes, ears, nose, throat, and chest and quickly determined she had the flu. He advised her to rest and drink hot tea with honey. Then Dr. Bruce spent 30 minutes counseling Lenore on her diet and the changes she needed, due to her extremely high cholesterol level (as shown in the lab results from the physical exam).

Let's Code It

The fact that Lenore "came to see Dr. Bruce" tells us this encounter occurred at Dr. Bruce's office.

The notes document that Lenore had an "annual physical" performed by Dr. Bruce "two weeks earlier." This means that she is an established patient.

Which levels of history, exam, and MDM were met or exceeded? You will note that established patient office E/M codes only require two key

Part 1 CPT

elements to be met. In this case, the physician did not do a history of any kind. However, he did document "examined Lenore's eyes, ears, nose, throat, and chest," a problem-focused examination, and "quickly determined" a straightforward MDM.

All these key elements direct us to the code 99212, *but* the notes also state that Dr. Bruce spent "30 minutes counseling" Lenore on her diet. Code 99212 shows a typical time of 10 minutes. Therefore, using code 99212 would fairly compensate Dr. Bruce for the caring of Lenore's flu, but not her high cholesterol. He deserves to be reimbursed for his counseling. Dr. Bruce spent 10 minutes on Lenore's flu plus 30 minutes on Lenore's cholesterol, totaling 40 minutes. Thirty minutes is more than half of 40 minutes, so the guideline regarding counseling time can be applied, and it is correct to use the E/M code 99215 that indicates 40 minutes face-to-face.

Prolonged Services: 99354–99359

In some cases, patients require greater than the usual amount of attention from a physician; more time than would regularly be spent—either face to face or without direct contact—over the course of one day.

Prolonged service codes report evaluation and management services that are at least 30 minutes longer than the amount of time represented by standard evaluation and management codes. These codes may be reported in addition to standard evaluation and management codes at any level, as appropriate.

To determine the best, most appropriate code from this subcategory, you have to calculate the total number of minutes that the physician spent with, or on behalf of, the patient, during one date of service. Calculate it as follows:

The standard evaluation and management code.

+ 99354 or 99356 for the first 30–74 minutes.

+ 99355 or 99357 for each 30 minutes additionally spent until the total amount of time spent by the physician is represented.

EXAMPLE

Dr. Moro spent a total of 2 hours, in his office, with Gina Fairchild working with her to stabilize her diabetes mellitus.

Report

99213	Office visit, established patient, expanded problem-focused	
+ 99354	Prolonged physician service in the office; first hour	60 min.
+ 99355	additional 30 minutes	30 min.
+ 99355	additional 30 minutes	30 min.
		120 min. = 2 hours

When the health care provider has spent more than the standard time, but less than 30 minutes with the patient, append modifier 21—but only to the highest level of E/M service in that subcategory. Note that typically a report should be submitted with the claim to explain the reasons for the additional service.

Consultations

As mentioned earlier in this chapter, occasionally a patient will only see a physician for a second opinion and not necessarily to establish a health care relationship. Such encounters are typically identified in the physician's notes as a consultation, so usually you will not have to decide. The notes will tell you to code from this section.

First, let's begin with two common terms used and confused: referral and consultation. If one physician *transfers* the care and treatment for a patient (in total or for one particular issue) to another physician, this is a *referral*. The patient is merely being recommended to see another physician and is expected to become a patient of the other physician. If a patient goes to a physician for a *consultation,* it is expected to be a temporary relationship, because the patient is merely seeking a *second opinion* regarding diagnosis and/or treatment.

Within the section of E/M consultation codes 99241–99255, two types of consultation are identified: *Office and Other Outpatient Consultations* and *Initial Inpatient Consultations.*

When a physician requests the advice or opinion of another health care professional regarding the management, care, and/or treatment of a patient with a specific health concern, codes within the range 99241–99255 should be used. This range of codes is divided into two, determined by where the consultation takes place:

- Codes 99241–99245 should be used if the consultation happened in the physician's office or other outpatient location.
- Codes 99251–99255 are used if the consulting physician sees the individual while he or she is an inpatient at a hospital.

CODING TIP »»

If the patient, or a family member, requests the second opinion and not another health care professional, the encounter should be coded as a regular, new patient visit in the applicable location.

CODING TIP »»

If it is decided that after a consulting physician sees a patient, this physician will continue care and/or treatment of the patient, the subsequent encounters will be coded as an *Established Patient.*

EXAMPLE

Loretta Gerbil, a 47-year-old female, was sent to Dr. Harrington, an oncologist, by her family physician, Dr. Catalane, for a consultation. She had been suffering with moderate pelvic pain and a heavy sensation in her lower pelvis. Upon her arrival at Dr. Harrington's office, she was given a pelvic ultrasound. Dr. Harrington evaluated the test results, spoke with Loretta, and sent a report to Dr. Catalane.

This was a *consultation* that was *requested by another physician* and held in the physician's *office,* leading to the code range 99241-99245.

So if Loretta Gerbil's tests are positive for a malignancy and she decides to have Dr. Harrington treat her cancer, she will then become Dr. Harrington's patient, and all future encounters in his office between this doctor and this patient will use E/M codes from 99211-99215 Office or Other Outpatient Services, Established Patient.

YOU CODE IT! CASE STUDY

Dr. Weldon was asked by Dr. Samuels to provide a second opinion on Burton Conner, a 17-year-old male. Burton's pulmonary specialist, Dr. Samuels, wants to perform a lung transplant because of his diagnosis of cystic fibrosis. Dr. Weldon examined Burton's respiratory system in his hospital room, reviewed the x-rays ordered by Dr. Samuels, and wrote a report agreeing that the surgery was medically necessary.

You Code It!

Go through the steps of evaluation and management coding, and determine the code that should be reported for this encounter between Dr. Weldon and Burton Conner.

Step 1: Read the case completely.

Step 2: Abstract the notes: Which key words can you identify relating to the E/M service performed?

_____

Step 3: What is the location?

_____

Step 4: What is the relationship?

_____

Step 5: What level of patient history was taken?

_____

Step 6: What level of physical examination was performed?

_____

Step 7: What level of medical decision-making was required?

_____

Answer

Did you find the correct code to be: 99252 Inpatient consultation for a new or established patient, expanded problem-focused?

The notes indicate that the "consultation" was done in Burton's "hospital" room. Therefore, you turn to the subheading *Consultations, Initial Inpatient Consultations, New or Established Patient,* codes 99251–99255.

When the patient, or a member of the patient's family, requests the consultation because he or she wants a second opinion and this is not requested by a physician, the encounter will be reported using the appropriate codes from another section of the E/M codes, depending upon where the encounter occurred. This is sometimes called a **confirmatory consultation**. For example, if the patient requests a second opinion and the patient is seen by another physician in his or her office, you will use the appropriate code from 99201–99205. If the consulting physician sees the patient while an inpatient at a hospital, you will use the appropriate codes from Initial Hospital Care 99221–99223.

Confirmatory consultation

An encounter for purposes of a second physician's opinion or advice, requested by the patient or a member of the patient's family, regarding the management of a patient's specific health concern.

Harrison Bernardo, a 51-year-old male, was having pain in his lower abdomen, especially when going to the bathroom. His primary care physician, Dr. Mayonni, did a PSA and was not very concerned, so he told Harrison to come back in 6–8 months for a follow-up. Harrison did not feel right about Dr. Mayonni's decision and made his own appointment for a second opinion with Dr. Hamilin, an urologist. Dr. Hamilin did additional tests and diagnosed Harrison with prostate cancer.

Let's Code It!

The notes indicate that it was Harrison, "the patient," who "requested the consultation" with Dr. Hamilin. Therefore, it is coded as a new patient office visit, and you will find the correct code in the 99201–99205 range. In this short version of the physician's notes, we really don't have enough information to determine the exact level. You would need to review the full-length notes or query the physician to narrow it down to one code.

READING THE PHYSICIAN'S NOTES

Sometimes, physicians will actually tell you in their notes with a statement such as "MDM was low complexity."

YOU CODE IT! CASE STUDY

Amanda Carter, a 21-year-old female, comes to see Dr. Atwater at his office with complaints of severe pain in her right wrist and forearm. She just moved to the area, and this is the first time Dr. Atwater will see her. Amanda sees Dr. Atwater for a very specific concern. The doctor asks Amanda about any medical history she may have related to her arm (i.e., diagnosed osteoporosis, previous broken bones, etc.). Next, Dr. Atwater examines Amanda's arm. He suspects that the arm is broken and orders an x-ray to be taken. MDM is straightforward.

You Code It!

Go through the steps of evaluation and management coding, and determine the code that should be reported for this encounter between Dr. Atwater and Amanda Carter.

Step 1: Read the case completely.

Step 2: Abstract the notes: Which key words can you identify relating to the E/M service performed?

_____

Step 3: What is the location?

_____

Step 4: What is the relationship?

_____

Step 5: What level of patient history was taken?

_____

Step 6: What level of physical examination was performed?

_____

Step 7: What level of medical decision-making was required?

_____

Answer

Did you find the correct code to be 99201 Office or other outpatient visit, new patient?

Let's carefully review the physician's notes.

Where did the encounter occur? Amanda went "to see Dr. Atwater at his office." This will lead us to the first subheading in the E/M section, *Office or Other Outpatient Services.*

What is the relationship? The notes state, "She just moved to the area and this is the first time Dr. Atwater will see her." This clearly brings us to the category of *New Patient,* and code range is 99201–99205.

What is the level of history? The notes state, "The doctor asks Amanda about any medical history she may have related to her arm," meaning that all the history he took was *problem-focused.*

What is the level of exam? You will see that "Dr. Atwater examines Amanda's arm." This means only one body area (each extremity) or one organ system (musculoskeletal) was examined. That's *problem-focused.*

What is the level of MDM? In this case, the physician actually wrote in his notes that the medical decision-making was *straightforward.* However, you can see that the documentation supports the definition of this level: There is only one diagnosis; the management options are limited (put a cast on it); there are very few complications; and Dr. Atwater didn't really have to do any research to recommend a course of treatment.

This brings you right to the best, most appropriate E/M code: 99201.

More often, the physicians will not come right out and use this terminology to describe what occurred during the encounter. Let's inspect various statements from patients' charts and identify the key words that lead to the correct E/M code.

1. Arvin Wasserman, a 65-year-old male, was seen for the *first time* by Dr. Frieda in the *office* for a *contusion of his hand*. Dr. Frieda asked questions about the bruise on Arvin's hand and examined his hand thoroughly.

   a. Location: *Office* tells us where the encounter took place.

   b. Relationship: *First time* tells us this is a new patient.

   c. Key Components: *History–problem-focused, physical examination–problem-focused, medical decision-making–straightforward.* Therefore, the correct code is 99201.

2. Dr. Pratt performed an *initial observation at the hospital* of Gerda Illianni, a 27-year-old female. After asking about her personal medical history, including *pertinent history of stomach problems, digestive problems, and pertinent family and social history directly relating to her complaints,* he *examined Gerda's abdomen, chest, neck, and back,* which revealed lower right quadrant pain, accompanied by nausea, vomiting, and a low-grade fever. Dr. Pratt made the *straightforward decision* to admit Gerda *overnight to the hospital* to rule out appendicitis.

   a. Location: *Initial observation at the hospital* tells us this code is in the Hospital Observation Services section.

   b. Relationship: *Observation at the hospital* codes are the same for both new and established patient.

   c. Key Components: *History–detailed, physical examination–detailed, medical decision-making–straightforward, and overnight admission to the hospital* all lead us to the correct code of 99218.

3. Dr. Sierra, a general surgeon, saw Carolina Hommen, a 37-year-old female, *in her office* for a *second opinion requested by Carolina's gynecologist, Dr. Keller,* regarding a lump in her right breast. Dr. Sierra took a *brief history of Carolina's present illness and a personal medical history relating to her hematologic and lymphatic system,* which was positive for breast cancer on her maternal side. After reviewing the existing mammogram and performing a *limited physical examination of her breasts and chest area,* the physician made the *straightforward decision* to advise a lumpectomy.

   a. Location: *In her office* tells us where the encounter took place.

   b. Relationship: *Second opinion requested by a physician* tells us this is a consultation.

   c. Key Components: *History–expanded problem-focused, physical examination–expanded problem-focused, and medical decision-making–straightforward* leads us directly to the correct code of 99242.

4. Matthew Claussen, a 15-year-old male, presented at the *emergency department* with a painful, swollen wrist. Patient stated he was hurt at a softball game. Dr. Alexander took a *brief history and asked some key questions about Matthew's arm/hand.* He then *examined Matthew's wrist and arm, checked his musculoskeletal system,* and x-rays were taken. It was rather *simple to determine* that Matthew's diagnosis is a sprained wrist.

   a. Location: *Emergency department* tells you the location.

   b. Relationship: Codes in the Emergency Department Services section do not differentiate between New and Established Patient.

   c. Key Components: *History–expanded problem-focused, physical examination–expanded problem-focused, and medical decision-making–low complexity* tells you the extent of the encounter. The correct code is 99282.

LET'S CODE IT! SCENARIO

Dr. Abbanni arrived at the Denton Nursing facility to do an annual assessment of her patient, Hannah Swannson, an 80-year-old female. Dr. Abbanni reviewed the latest test results in Hannah's chart, took a comprehensive interval history, and performed a comprehensive physical examination. Decision-making is extremely complex because the patient has senile dementia, hypertension, and hypothyroidism. A new treatment plan is created due to changes in the patient's condition.

Let's Code It!

"Nursing facility" tells us the location, and "her patient" tells us that this is an established patient. Comprehensive interval history, comprehensive physical examination, and highly complex decision-making lead you directly to the correct code of 99310.

CHAPTER SUMMARY

Evaluation and management codes report the energy and knowledge a health care professional puts into gathering information, reviewing data, and determining the best course of treatment for the patient's current condition. Due to the complex formula of such codes, many health information management professionals find these difficult to correctly determine. Don't become overwhelmed. Once you get a job, you will find that one particular portion of this section will become your main focus.

EXAMPLE

- If you work for a provider in a private medical office, most of your E/M codes will be found under the Office heading on the first two pages of the section.

- If you work for a physician who cares for patients at a skilled nursing facility, you will use codes from under the Nursing Facility Services heading.

So in the real world, most of the time, you will be using the same, small set of codes over and over again. But because we don't know where you will be working, you should learn the entire section.

1. Evaluation and management codes enable the physician to be reimbursed for all of these services except

   a. Talking with the patient and their family.
   b. Taking continuing education classes.
   c. Consulting with other health care professionals.
   d. Reviewing data such as test results.

2. Often, finding the correct E/M code begins with knowing

   a. Where the patient met with the physician.
   b. Which credential is held by the provider.
   c. What type of insurance policy is held by the patient.
   d. What the patient does for an occupation.

3. A patient who has not seen a particular physician in the last three years is categorized as

   a. An established patient.
   b. A referral.
   c. A consultation.
   d. A new patient.

4. The three key components of many E/M codes include all of these except

   a. History.
   b. Exam.
   c. Chief complaint.
   d. Medical decision-making.

5. Levels of patient history include all except

   a. Expanded problem-focused.
   b. Comprehensive.
   c. Detailed.
   d. High complexity.

6. Body areas that might be included in a physical examination include

   a. Eyes.
   b. Each extremity.
   c. Respiratory.
   d. Neurological.

7. When services are provided at different levels, the guidelines state you should code to a level of

   a. At least one of three key components achieved.
   b. All must be met or exceeded.
   c. The number of minutes face to face.
   d. The number of diagnosis codes.

8. If _____ of the time with the patient is spent counseling, you should use time rather than key components to determine the level of service code.

   a. 51% or more
   b. 45% or more
   c. 51% or less
   d. 25% or more

9. A consultation is expected to be a(n) _____ relationship with the patient.

   a. extended
   b. transferred
   c. temporary
   d. continuing

10. A patient seen in the office and then admitted to the hospital the same day should be coded with E/M codes from subsection(s)

    a. Office visit only.
    b. Office visit and initial hospital care.
    c. Initial hospital care only.
    d. Emergency department.

YOU CODE IT! Practice
Chapter 4. Evaluation and Management Codes, Part 1

Find the best E/M code for each of these scenarios.

1. Karyn Cassey, a 3-year-old female, sees Dr. Fahey, a pediatrician, for the first time with itchy spots all over her body. After a detailed history and a detailed examination, his MDM is of a low complexity. Dr. Fahey diagnoses her with chicken pox.

   _____

2. Isaac Thomas, a 73-year-old male, collapsed at church during services and was brought to the ED. Dr. Zendar took a comprehensive history, performed a comprehensive examination, and made the decision to admit Isaac into the observation unit of the hospital due to an irregular heartbeat with an unknown cause.

   _____

3. Dr. Maxwell calls in Dr. Frizzola for a consultation on 8-year-old David Harrison to determine if a tonsillectomy should be performed. David is currently in the hospital for treatment of his previously diagnosed leukemia. Dr. Frizzola gathers a comprehensive history, performs a comprehensive examination in his hospital room, and spends time reviewing all prior test results. David's history of allergies and other health concerns makes this a highly complex decision.

   _____

4. Jamie Farmer was admitted into the hospital for lower right quadrant pain, accompanied by nausea, vomiting, and a low-grade fever. Dr. Wadhwa was brought in for a surgical consultation by the attending physician, Dr. Lowen. After a problem-focused history and exam, Dr. Wadhwa recommended that Jamie stay in the hospital overnight to rule out the possibility of a ruptured appendix. Code for Dr. Wadhwa's services.

   _____

5. After five days of antibiotic therapy showed no sign of improvement, Dr. Anderson admitted Randy Taylor, a 2-year-old male, into the hospital with bacterial pneumonia. At Randy's admittance, his vitals showed a temperature of 38.3°C (101°F), with a mild rash on his torso. The following day, Dr. Anderson performed a problem-focused history and examination with MDM of low complexity. Code Dr. Anderson's visit on the second day.

   _____

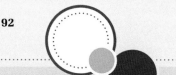

Part 1   CPT

6. Loretta Reubens, a 47-year-old female, was sent by Dr. Porter to Dr. Harrington, an OB-GYN, for an office consultation. She had been suffering with moderate pelvic pain, a heavy sensation in her lower pelvis, and marked discomfort during sexual intercourse. In a detailed history, Dr. Harrington noted the location, severity, and duration of her pelvic pain and related symptoms. In the review of systems, Loretta had positive findings related to her gastrointestinal, genitourinary, and endocrine body systems. Dr. Harrington noted that her past medical history was noncontributory to the present problem. The detailed physical examination centered on her gastrointestinal and genitourinary systems with a complete pelvic exam. Dr. Harrington ordered lab tests and a pelvic ultrasound in order to consider uterine fibroids, endometritis, or other internal gynecological pathology. MDM complexity was moderate.

---

7. Martin Mazzenthorp decided to see Dr. Appleton for a second opinion regarding his own physician's recommendation for surgical repair of a hernia. After a brief problem-focused history of present illness and a problem-focused exam of the affected body area and organ system, Dr. Appleton made a straightforward medical decision to support the original recommendation for surgery.

---

8. Carolina Tanner came into the ED with a wrist sprain that she sustained during a baseball game when she slid into home base. She was in obvious pain, and the wrist was swollen and too painful upon attempts to flex. Dr. Ramada performed an expanded problem-focused history and exam before he ordered radiographs. Reports confirmed a simple fracture of the distal radius. MDM was low.

---

9. Bernard Kristenson, an 82-year-old male, was diagnosed with advanced Alzheimer's disease about one year ago. He was seen by the nursing facility's physician, Dr. Mintz, over concern of the development of urinary and fecal incontinence, as well as a number of other medical problems that have appeared to increase in severity. In addition to the detailed interval history, the physician spoke with family members, the nursing staff, and reviewed the patient's record to create an extended history necessary for an extended review of systems (ROS). Dr. Mintz performed a comprehensive physical exam to assess all body systems. Afterward, he wrote all new orders due to the patient's dramatic change in his physical and mental condition. A new treatment plan was created. The MDM complexity was high.

---

10. Verniece Dantini, a 61-year-old female, sees Dr. Smallerman for the first time for a variety of medical problems. She was diagnosed with insulin-dependent diabetes mellitus with complicating eye and renal problems. In addition, she suffers from hypertensive heart disease with episodes of congestive heart failure. Her peripheral vascular disease has worsened, and she can walk only a block before being crippled with extreme leg pain. The patient reports that a new problem has surfaced: throbbing headaches with radiating neck pain. In order to manage and investigate the multiplicity of problems, Dr. Smallerman performs a comprehensive history and physical exam. A complete ROS is performed, and her complete PFSH is updated. Dr. Smallerman has to take a multitude of factors into consideration, as the patient's problems are highly complex.

_____

11. Maribelle Johannsen, a 75-year-old female, lives in Barton Assisted Living Center where she is seen by Dr. Modesta as a part of her annual assessment. Dr. Modesta completes a detailed interval history with a comprehensive head-to-toe physical exam. He reviews and affirms the medical plan of care developed by the multidisciplinary care team at Barton. Maribelle's condition is stable, her hypertension and diabetes (type II) are in good control, and she has no new problems. There is minimal data for Dr. Modesta to review and several diagnoses to consider. The MDM was moderate.

_____

12. George Carter, a 17-month-old male, is admitted to the hospital by his pediatrician, Dr. Mitchell, after confirming via chest x-ray that the child has pneumonia. The initial hospital care includes a detailed history and detailed physical exam with an extended problem-focused ROS completed with Petula Carter, the child's mother. The course of treatment planned by Dr. Mitchell is straightforward as the child's condition is of low severity. MDM is of low complexity.

_____

13. Tricia Thornwell, a 27-year-old female, is admitted to the hospital for observation after falling from the roof of her carport (approximately 8 feet high). Tricia has complaints of pain in multiple areas, and numerous x-rays are ordered. Dr. Dijohn performs a comprehensive history and physical exam. The possibility of multiple fractures makes the MDM moderately complex.

_____

14. Ellen Onoton, a 45-year-old female, recently diagnosed with asthma, comes to see her family physician, Dr. Pashma with a complaint of severe headaches. He performs a comprehensive history and exam, with highly complex MDM.

_____

15. Raymond Catertell, a 20-year-old male, was admitted into the hospital two days ago for bronchitis. While in the hospital, Raymond requested that his family physician, Dr. Kaminsky, perform a circumcision, so Dr. Kaminsky called in Dr. Longwell, an urologist, for a consultation. Dr. Longwell performs a problem-focused history and problem-focused physical exam and makes the straightforward decision to recommend that Raymond have the surgical procedure done as an outpatient at a later date. Code for Dr. Longwell's services.

_____

YOU CODE IT! Simulation
Chapter 4. Evaluation and Management Codes, Part 1

On the following pages, you will see physicians' notes documenting encounters with patients at our textbook's health care facility, Cipher, Victors, & Associates. Carefully read through the notes and find the best E/M code for each of these cases.

CIPHER, VICTORS, & ASSOCIATES
A Complete Health Care Facility
234 MAIN STREET • ANYTOWN, FL 32711 • 407-555-1234

PATIENT: WHITE, SIERRA
ACCOUNT/EHR #:   WHITSI001
Date: 09/16/08

Attending Physician: James I. Cipher, MD

S: This new Pt is a 25-year-old female who was involved in a 2-car MVA while driving on the job. She is complaining about some neck pain. She has tingling in her left hand and both feet. She states that her left arm hurts when she tries to pull it overhead. She apparently was told, by a friend, that she should likely need to see a spine doctor, but somehow she came to see me first. PMH is remarkable for kidney trouble. Past bronchoscopy, laparoscopy and kidney stone surgery, otherwise noncontributory as per the medical history form completed by the patient and reviewed at this visit.

O: Ht 5′5″ Wt 179 lb. R 16. Pt presented in a sling. She was told to use it by the same friend. She states if she does not use it, her arm does not feel any different, so I had her remove it. She states that she has not had any prior injury to this area, and has no previous problems with her musculoskeletal system. On exam, HEENT: unremarkable. Neck muscles are taut, particularly on the left side. The left shoulder demonstrates full passive motion, with normal strength testing. No deformity is observable. Pt states there is some tenderness over the left trapezial area. The reflexes are brisk and symmetric. X-rays of her chest 2 views and C spine AP/LAT are relatively benign, as are complete x-rays of the shoulder.

A: Contusion of upper left arm and left shoulder

P: 1. MRI to rule out torn ligament
      2. Rx Naprosyn
      3. Referral to PT
      4. Referral to orthopedist

James I. Cipher, MD

JIC/mg   D: 9/16/08 09:50:16   T: 9/18/08 12:55:01

Find the best, most appropriate E/M code.

_____

_____

_____

CIPHER, VICTORS, & ASSOCIATES
A Complete Health Care Facility
234 MAIN STREET • ANYTOWN, FL 32711 • 407-555-1234

PATIENT: PARKER, PETER
ACCOUNT/EHR #:   PARKPE001
Date: 10/1/08

Attending Physician: Valerie R. Victors, MD

S: This 23-year-old male was brought to the ED by ambulance after he was found unconscious on the living room floor this morning. He regained consciousness within several minutes, however, complained of a severe head-ache and nausea. Pt states that the last thing he remembers he was on a ladder, changing the bulb in the track lighting. He believes he lost his balance trying to reach too far to take out the next light on the track and fell, hitting his head on the coffee table.

O: Ht 5'10" Wt 195 lb. R 16. Head: Scalp laceration on the right posterior parietal bone. Bruise indicates trauma to this area. Eyes: PERL. Neck: Neck muscles are tense; there is minor pain upon rotation of the head. Musculoskel-etal: All other aspects of the shoulders, arms, and legs are unremarkable. X-rays of skull 2 views, and soft tissue of the neck are all benign.

A: Concussion

P: 1. MRI to rule/out subdural hematoma
     2. Repair laceration and bandage

_____

Valerie R. Victors, MD

VRV/mg   D: 10/1/08 09:50:16   T: 10/5/08 12:55:01

Find the best, most appropriate E/M code.

_____

_____

_____

CIPHER, VICTORS, & ASSOCIATES
A Complete Health Care Facility
234 MAIN STREET • ANYTOWN, FL 32711 • 407-555-1234

PATIENT: CRUMPET, KARL
ACCOUNT/EHR #:   CRUMKA001
Date: 10/18/08

Attending Physician: James I. Cipher, MD

S: Karl is an 11-month-old male brought in today by his mother. I last saw this patient at his regular six-month checkup. He has been waking up at night and is irritable. Mother states that he has been tugging at his right ear, and has been running a low-grade fever since yesterday. There has been no cough. Pt has a history of problems with his ears and sinuses. Pt is teething.

O: Ht 2′1″ Wt 25 lb. R 20. T 101.3 HEENT: Purulent nasal discharge, yellow-green in color, is noted. Right TM is erythematous unilaterally, bulging and with purulent effusions. Oropharynx is nonerythematous without lesions. One tooth on the bottom. Tonsils are unremarkable. Neck: Neck is supple with good ROM. Positive cervical adenopathy. Lungs: clear. Heart: Regular rate and rhythm without murmurs.

A: Acute suppurative otitis media, right side.

P: 1. Rx Augmentin 40 mg/kg divided tid 10 days
      2. Bed rest, lots of fluids
      3. Follow-up prn or if no improvement in 10 days

_____

James I. Cipher, MD

JIC/mg   D: 10/18/08 09:50:16   T: 10/23/08 12:55:01

Find the best, most appropriate E/M code.

_____

_____

_____

Part 1   CPT

CIPHER, VICTORS, & ASSOCIATES
A Complete Health Care Facility
234 MAIN STREET • ANYTOWN, FL 32711 • 407-555-1234

PATIENT: TRANSIL, BRENT
ACCOUNT/EHR #:   TRANBR001
Date: 9/29/08

Attending Physician: Benjamin L. Johnston, MD
Referring Physician: James I. Cipher, MD

S: Pt is a 37-year-old male, referred by Dr. Cipher for a consultation regarding a sore on his left temple, at the hairline. Pt states he is very involved in beach and water sports. He knows the importance of sunscreen; however, he does not always remember to put it on. He has not had any dermatological concerns prior to this. Patient states his skin is very dry occasionally and has adult onset acne.

O: Ht 6′1″ Wt 225 lb. R 17. T 98.6 After an examination of the skin along the hairline, as well as the rest of the face and neck, a culture is taken of the lesion. The pathology report confirms a malignant melanoma of the skin of the scalp.

A: Malignant melanoma, scalp

P: 1. Discuss surgical and pharmaceutical options for treatment
     2. Report sent to Dr. Cipher

Benjamin L. Johnston, MD

BLJ/mg   D: 9/29/08 09:50:16   T: 10/1/08 12:55:01

Find the best, most appropriate E/M code.

_____

_____

_____

CIPHER, VICTORS, & ASSOCIATES
A Complete Health Care Facility
234 MAIN STREET • ANYTOWN, FL 32711 • 407-555-1234

PATIENT: ENGLEMAN, LUIS
ACCOUNT/EHR #:   ENGLLU001
Date: 9/29/08

Attending Physician: James I. Cipher, MD

S: Pt is a 77-year-old male requesting a second opinion. His current ophthalmologist, Dr. Quinones, diagnosed him with bilateral senile cataracts three weeks ago. According to the patient, Dr. Quinones is recommending surgical removal of the cataracts and implantation of lens. Pt is concerned about having surgery. He states he has always had excellent vision, but has noticed a decrease in his ability to see clearly over the last year or two. He denies any trauma to the area. Pt has no personal medical history that reveals an unusual risk for this type of surgical procedure. Pt is a social drinker. He denies smoking cigarettes, but states he enjoys a cigar "on occasion." I reviewed the complete medical history form filled out by the patient at the beginning of this visit.

O: Ht 5'9" Wt 225 lb. R 18. T 98.6. A detailed examination of the patient's eyes and visual acuity confirmed the original diagnosis made by Dr. Quinones. Examination of patient's chest reveals no arrhythmia. It appears to be a case of low complexity.

A: Bilateral senile cataracts

P: I told the patient that I confirmed the diagnosis and agreed with Dr. Quinones's recommendation for surgery.

Benjamin L. Johnston, MD

BLJ/mg   D: 9/29/08 09:50:16   T: 10/1/08 12:55:01

Find the best, most appropriate E/M code.

_____

_____

_____

Evaluation and Management Codes, Part 2:

Preventive Medicine, Long-Term Care Services, Critical Care, and Modifiers

5

LEARNING OUTCOMES

- Apply the guidelines for coding different types of evaluation and management services.
- Correctly assign preventive medicine codes, as appropriate.
- Determine the most accurate long-term care service codes.
- Abstract the physician's notes to determine the correct nursing facility service code.
- Calculate the correct code or codes for critical care services.
- Apply evaluation and management modifiers correctly.

KEY TERMS

Anticipatory guidance
Basic personal services
Care plan oversight services
Critical care services
Global surgery package
Hospice
Interval
Nursing home
Preventive
Risk factor intervention

Non-profit organizations
Long-term care facilities
Assisted living facilities
General practice
Hospitals

Physicians' offices
Ambulatory surgery centers
Clinics
Home health agencies
Nursing homes

EMPLOYMENT OPPORTUNITIES

Evaluation and management services go beyond those included in the typical office or hospital visit. Preventive medicine assessments—more commonly called an annual physical, evaluations of patients in short-term and long-term care facilities, coun-seling, and critical care—are just some of the areas of focus that might be required of the attending physician. This chapter reviews these subcategories of evaluation and management codes.

PREVENTIVE MEDICINE

There may be times when the physician's notes do not clearly identify all the individual components (e.g., history, exam, and MDM) of an encounter, such as a patient coming in for an annual physical. In these cases, you should be careful not to force the components or make them up. Instead, you should look at another area of the E/M section. For example, the **Preventive** Medicine section, codes 99381–99429 may be more appropriate.

When provided at the same time as a comprehensive preventive medical examination, preventive medicine service codes 99381–99397 include:

- Counseling
- Anticipatory guidance
- Risk factor reduction interventions

From your own personal experience, you may be familiar with discussions between you and your physician during your annual physical. The talks cover everything from quitting smoking to exercising more and perhaps having a better diet. These are all examples of counseling.

Anticipatory guidance is the physician offering suggestions for behavior modification or other preventive measures related to a patient's high risk for a condition. The concern may be based on specifics in a patient's condition or history (or perhaps a family history or an occupational hazard).

EXAMPLE

Dr. Darby provides anticipatory guidance to Randolph Muldoon with regard to being careful about protecting his respiratory health. Randolph works at an automobile paint shop, and the fumes are very dangerous if a breathing mask is not worn.

Should the physician prescribe a patch to help you quit smoking, or should he or she refer you to a registered dietician to help you with that new diet, that would be categorized as **risk factor intervention.** It means the physician is taking action to intervene with, or help to stop, patient behaviors that put the patient at a higher risk for certain illnesses or conditions.

If such elements such as risk factor reduction intervention or counseling occur at a separate visit (not at the same time as the physical examination), you have to code them separately with a code from the 99401 through 99412 range.

If during the course of the preventive medicine examination, the physician finds something of concern that warrants special and extra attention involving the key components of a problem-oriented E/M service, the extra work should be coded with a separate E/M code, appended with modifier 25. It is only applicable when the same physician does the extra service on the same date.

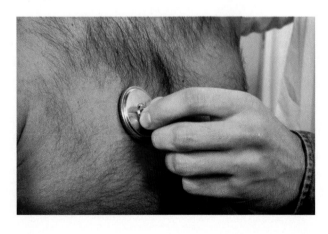

Part 1   CPT

Arlene Barry, a 47-year-old female, comes to see her regular physician, Dr. Fermat, for her annual physical. During the examination, Dr. Fermat finds a mass in her abdomen that concerns him. After the exam, he sits and talks with Arlene about any past or current problems with her abdomen, including pain, discomfort, and other details regarding her abdominal issue. He asks whether any family members have had problems in that area, as well as asking about her alcohol consumption and sexual history as they relate to his concern. Dr. Fermat then goes into his office to analyze the multiple possibilities of diagnoses, evaluates the information in her chart, and reviews the moderate risk of complications that might occur due to her current list of medications. He orders an abdominal CT scan, blood work, and a UA for further input.

Let's Code It!

According to the notes, Dr. Fermat performed an "annual physical exam," also known as a preventive medicine exam, on Arlene, a "47-year-old" female. Let's go to the alphabetic index and look up *Evaluation and Management, Preventive Services,* or go directly to the Evaluation and Management section and look for the Preventive Medicine Services subheading. From the phrase "her regular physician," we know that Arlene is an established patient, bringing us to code:

> 99396 Periodic comprehensive preventive medicine, 40–64 years

Dr. Fermat's notes also tell us that during the exam he found a mass in Arlene's abdomen that he felt needed further investigation. He spent additional time getting details about her personal, family, and social history regarding abdominal problems; he reviewed concerns about multiple possible diagnoses, complications, and treatments. As per the guidelines, this is extra work done on Dr. Fermat's part, and therefore, he is entitled to additional reimbursement, reported with a separate E/M code. As you review the notes, you should be able to determine the best, most appropriate E/M code for the additional service. Dr. Fermat did a comprehensive examination, and his MDM was certainly at a high level of complexity, leading us to:

> 99215 Office or other outpatient visits with comprehensive exam and medical decision-making of high complexity

Plus the modifier:

> -25 Significant, separately identifiable evaluation and management service

The claim form for Dr. Fermat's encounter with Arlene Barry will show 99396, 99215-25. Good job!

99396 will reimburse Dr. Fermat for his time and services for the annual physical, and 99215 will reimburse him for the extra work he did regarding the abdominal mass. The modifier -25 explains that, while unusal, Dr. Fermat did both of these services at the same encounter.

(*Note:* More information on evaluation and management modifiers is given later in this chapter.)

COUNSELING AND/OR RISK FACTOR REDUCTION INTERVENTION

At times the physician will see a patient at a visit, separate from the annual physical or preventive medicine evaluation, for the purposes of helping the patient learn about, understand, and/or adopt better health practices:

- Prevent injury or illness, such as the proper way to lift or the importance of testing one's blood glucose levels regularly.
- Encourage good health, such as nutritional counseling or a new exercise regime.

  Such services are coded from:

  99401–99404 Preventive medicine, individual counseling

  99411–99412 Preventive medicine, group counseling

  99420–99429 Other preventive medicine services

EXAMPLE

Dr. Oppenheimer meets a group of students from the local university to counsel them on preventing sexually transmitted diseases. He spoke with them for 50 minutes. It would be coded using 99412.

HOME SERVICES

If a physician provides evaluation and management services to a patient at the patient's private residence, use codes from 99341–99350. Determine the best, most appropriate code using the same key components as those for E/M services provided in the physician's office.

When a health care professional other than the physician—such as a nurse or respiratory therapist—provides services to a patient at the patient's home, use codes from 99500–99602.

LET'S CODE IT! SCENARIO

Morgan Garrison, a 45-year-old male, suffers from agoraphobia and cannot leave his home. Dr. Lavattney came to the house to examine Morgan because he is complaining of chest congestion. Dr. Lavattney took a problem-focused history, as this was the first time he had seen Morgan. The doctor examined Morgan's HEENT and chest and concluded that Morgan had a chest cold. He told Morgan to get some over-the-counter cold medicine and to call if the symptoms did not go away within a week.

Let's Code It!

We need to find the appropriate code to reimburse Dr. Lavattney for his E/M services to Morgan Garrison. We know that "Dr. Lavattney came to the house," so the location section is titled Home Services. The notes continue to tell us that "this was the first time he had seen Morgan," meaning that Morgan is a new patient, narrowing our choices to codes 99341 through 99345. The book tells us that a new patient home visit requires three key components: history, examination, and MDM. The notes tell us that Dr. Lavattney:

1. Took a problem-*focused history.*
2. Examined his head, ears, eyes, nose, throat (HEENT) and chest: *expanded problem-focused.*
3. Concluded, without tests or additional resources: *straightforward.*

When we assess the levels and use our meet or exceed rule, the most accurate code for the visit is 99341. Good job!

LONG-TERM CARE SERVICES

Specific codes are used to report evaluation and management services provided to patients in residential care facilities.

Use 99304–99318 and 99379–99380 for reporting services to patients in the following places:

Nursing home

Skilled nursing facility (SNF)

Intermediate care facility (ICF)

Long-term care facility (LTCF)

Psychiatric residential treatment center

Use 99324–99340 for reporting services to patients in locations where room, meals, and **basic personal services** are provided but medical services are not included:

Assisted living facilities

Domiciliary

Rest homes

Custodial care settings

Alzheimer's facility

Nursing home

A facility that provides skilled nursing treatment and attention along with limited medical care for its (usually long-term) residents, who do not require acute care services (hospitalization).

Basic personal services

Services that include washing/bathing, dressing and undressing, assistance in taking medications, and getting in and out of bed.

EXAMPLE

Dr. Sanders goes to see William Karlson at the halfway house where William resides. William is autistic, and Dr. Sanders wants to examine him and adjust his medication for asthma. You would report Dr. Sanders's visit to William with code 99334.

Use 99341–99350 for reporting services, by an attending physician, to patients being cared for in a private residence. Some home health agencies employ physicians, others may volunteer, while others only visit established patients who are home-bound.

Care plan oversight services

Evaluation and management of a patient, reported in 30-day periods, including infrequent supervision along with preencounter and postencounter work, such as reading test results and assessment of notes.

Hospice

An organization that provides services to terminally ill patients and their families.

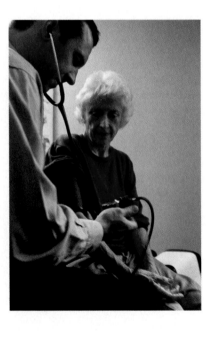

Interval

The time measured between one point and another, such as between physician visits.

Physicians use different methods and tools to assess a patient's status and to create and/or update an appropriate treatment plan for the ongoing care of the individual. Such methods and tools may include:

Resident assessment instrument (RAI)

Minimum data set (MDS)

Resident assessment protocols (RAP)

Care plan oversight services

When a physician provides care plan oversight services, you have to use the appropriate code determined by the length of time involved and the type of facility in which the patient is located.

99339–99340 for patients in assisted living or domiciliary facility.

99374–99375 for home health care patients.

99377–99378 for **hospice** patients.

99379–99380 for residents in a nursing facility—but only if the management of the patient involves repeated direction of therapy by the attending physician.

Admission to the Nursing Facility: 99304-99306

When a patient is admitted into a nursing facility as a continued part of an encounter at the physician's office or the emergency department (on the same day by the same physician), you report only one code (from the nursing facility section of the E/M codes) that will include all the services provided, from all the locations on that day. You may remember from Chap. 4, admission to the hospital from the physician's office or ED is reported all in the one hospital admission E/M code. The same rule also applies to admission to a nursing facility.

However, if the patient has been discharged from inpatient status on the same day as being admitted to a nursing facility, you code the physician's discharge services separately from the admission.

Three key components, similar to other E/M codes, are used to determine the appropriate level of evaluation and management service provided by the attending physician to a patient on the first day at a nursing facility. There is no differentiation made in this section of codes between a new patient and an established patient.

Subsequent Nursing Facility Care

Once the patient is in the facility, it is expected that the physician will continue to review the patient's chart, as well as assess test results and changes in the patient's health status. Notice that the code description for the history key component includes the term **interval.** The physician only needs to evaluate the patient's history back to the last visit to gain a complete, up-to-date picture of the individual's health. The continuing care type of assessment is reported with the most appropriate code from the 99307–99310 range.

If the physician only does an annual assessment of the patient in the nursing facility (typically in cases where the patient is stable, progressing as expected, or recovering), you use code:

99318 Evaluation and management of a patient involving an annual nursing facility assessment

Rita Anne Brigham, a 59-year-old female, was diagnosed with advanced pancreatic cancer and is being cared for at her home, by her family, with the help of a home health agency. Dr. Brosseau is providing care plan oversight services for the first month of care. The plan includes home oxygen, IV medications for pain control management, and diuretics for edema and ascites control. Dr. Brosseau also discusses end-of-life issues, living will directive, and other concerns with the family, nurse, and the social worker. Dr. Brosseau includes documentation of his 45-minute assessment, as well as notes on modifications to the care plan. Certifications of care from the nursing staff, the social worker, the pharmacy, and the company supplying the durable medical equipment for support are also in the record.

Let's Code It!

Dr. Brosseau documented that he provided "care plan oversight services" for Rita Anne Brigham. Turn to the alphabetic index, and look up *Care Plan Oversight Services.* The index instructs you to see *Physician Services.* Turn to *Physician Services,* and you will see *Care Plan Oversight Services.*

As you look at the indented list below that phrase, note that you have to identify the location at which the patient is being cared for. Rita Anne Brigham is being cared for at home, with a home health agency. This will lead you to code 99374.

Physician services

Care plan oversight services

Home health agency care 99374

Next, turn to code 99374:

99374   Physician supervision of a patient under care of home health agency in home, domiciliary or equivalent environment requiring complex and multidisciplinary care modalities involving regular physician development and/or revision of care plans; 15–29 minutes

99375   30 minutes or more

Dr. Brosseau's notes report that he spent 45 minutes. Therefore, the correct code is 99375.

CRITICAL CARE CODES

The management and care of severely ill patients takes a great deal of skill, knowledge, and time. Critically ill or injured patients have a high likelihood of a deteriorating life-threatening condition. Evaluation and management services reported include:

- Highly complex decision-making to assess, manipulate, and support vital system function.

«« CODING TIP

Note that code 99375 was not listed in the alphabetic index. You had to go to the numeric listing to find that 99375 is the most accurate code for the encounter. This instance is a reminder to *never, never, never* code from the alphabetic index, even when there is only one code shown.

- Treating single or multiple vital organ system failure.
- Efforts to avoid additional life-threatening decline of the patient's condition.
- Interpretation of various vital function factors.
- The evaluation of advantages and disadvantages of using advanced technology.

The health care provider must document the amount of time spent so you will know how to code the encounter. The physician may spend his or her time:

- Reviewing test results and films at the nurses' station.
- Discussing the patient's treatment and care with the other members of the medical team.
- Charting (writing in the patient's chart).
- Attending to the patient at bedside.

All such activities are a part of the time spent providing critical care.

Critical care services can be, but do not have to be, provided in a coronary care unit (CCU), an intensive care unit (ICU), a respiratory care unit (RCU), or an emergency care facility.

The codes you choose to report critical care services are determined by the services provided for the critically ill or injured patient, the total length of time of the encounter, and, finally, the age of the patient.

Use the following for coding inpatient services:

99295–99296 for patients who are 28 days of age or less.

99298–99300 for continuing intensive care of neonate patients weighing less than 2500 grams (after the first day of admission).

99293–99294 for patients aged 29 days to 24 months.

99291–99292 for all patients over the age of 24 months.

Use the following for coding outpatient services for the critically ill or injured patient:

99291–99292 regardless of the age of the patient

CODING TIP »»

If the same physician provides critical care services to the same patient on the same date as other E/M services, codes from both subheadings may be reported.

Critical care services

Services for a patient who has a life-threatening condition expected to worsen.

CODING TIP »»

If the same provider provides outpatient and inpatient services for a critically ill or injured patient aged 24 months or younger on the same date, use the inpatient Pediatric or Neonatal Critical Care Services codes.

CODING TIP »»

For neonates who require intense observation but not critical care services, use code 99477.

LET'S CODE IT! SCENARIO

Jason Howard, an 18-year-old male, was brought into the emergency department by ambulance after being involved in a motorcycle accident. He was not wearing a helmet, and his head hit a brick wall. After initial evaluation and testing by the ED physician, Jason was sent to the CCU (critical care unit), and Dr. Oppenheim spent two hours reviewing test results, performing a complete physical exam of Jason, and discussing a care management plan with the rest of the medical team.

Dr. Oppenheim spent "two hours" managing the care of Jason Howard in the "critical care unit." Turn to the Critical Care codes, and let's look at the chart. Two hours *equals* 2 *times* 60 minutes, or 120 minutes. When you look at the chart, you will see that 105–134 minutes (*Note:* 120 minutes is right in the middle of this range) is coded with 99291x1 and 99292x2 (read x2 as reported twice). Look at the following complete description:

> 99291 Critical care, evaluation and management of the critically ill or critically injured patient; first 30–74 minutes

> +99292   each additional 30 minutes

You know that Dr. Oppenheim spent 120 minutes and that 120 minutes *minus* 74 minutes (which is represented by code 99291) leaves 46 minutes unreported. Therefore, you must add 99292 to report an additional 30 minutes. However, 16 minutes still remains. So you must include 99292 again to account for the leftover minutes. The claim form that you complete will show 99291, 99292, 99292 or 99291, 99292x2. Great job!

CASE MANAGEMENT SERVICES

If a patient has several or complex health issues or diagnoses, a team of health care professionals may have to work together to provide proper management and treatment. The team may involve several physicians or the attending physician and a physical therapist, for example, conferencing together. To properly reimburse the health care professional for the time and expertise spent on the patient's behalf with other professionals, you report such services using codes from ranges:

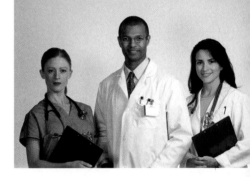

99363–99364	Anticoagulant management
99366–99368	Medical team conferences
99441–99443	for telephone services
99444	for on-line medical evaluation

Arthur Unger, a 73-year-old male, is still having pain and swelling in his hands. Dr. Hertzwell calls Roger Bowen, a physical therapist, to adjust the therapy plan, based on current test results. The call is brief.

Go through the steps of evaluation and management coding, and determine the code that should be reported for the encounter between Dr. Hertzwell and Roger Bowen.

Step 1: Read the case completely.

Step 2: Abstract the notes: Which key words can you identify relating to the E/M service performed?

Chapter 5   Evaluation and Management Codes, Part 2

Step 3: What is the location?

_____

Step 4: What is the relationship?

_____

Step 5: What level of patient history was taken?

_____

Step 6: What level of physical examination was performed?

_____

Step 7: What level of medical decision-making was required?

_____

Answer

Did you find the correct code to be:

> 99367 Medical team conference with interdisciplinary team, 30 minutes or more; participation by physician.

EVALUATION AND MANAGEMENT MODIFIERS

Several modifiers may be used in conjunction with an evaluation and management code to provide additional information about an encounter. Each modifier specifically explains an unusual circumstance that may justify the payment to the provider at a more fitting level.

CPT Level I modifiers are two-digit codes that are listed in Appendix A of the CPT book.

> **21 Prolonged evaluation and management services:** When the face-to-face or floor/unit service(s) provided is prolonged or otherwise greater than that usually required for the highest level of evaluation and management service within a given category, it may be identified by adding modifier 21 to the evaluation and management code number. A report may also be appropriate.

Modifier 21 is used when the time the physician spent with the patient was not only longer than expected but also longer than the highest level of evaluation and management code available. The modifier can *only* be appended to the highest-level code in the subsection. For example, in an office or other outpatient setting, that would be 99205 or 99215.

CODING TIP »»

Note that this is different from using a prolonged services code, reviewed in Chap. 4.

YOU CODE IT! CASE STUDY

Andrea Sorenson, a 23-year-old female, came to see Dr. Tamara about her sore throat. The nurse took a throat culture, and the doctor performed a detailed up-to-date history, as well as a detailed examination.

Andrea has been a patient of Dr. Tamara since she was a teenager. The culture came back positive for syphilis of the throat. While the history and the exam took about 25 minutes, Dr. Tamara spent an additional 30 minutes counseling Andrea about the treatment of her condition, as well as discussing behavior modification that would prevent her contracting the disease again.

You Code It!

Go through the steps of evaluation and management coding, and determine the code that should be reported for the encounter between Dr. Tamara and Andrea Sorenson.

Step 1: Read the case completely.

Step 2: Abstract the notes: Which key words can you identify relating to the E/M service performed?

_____

Step 3: What is the location?

_____

Step 4: What is the relationship?

_____

Step 5: What level of patient history was taken?

_____

Step 6: What level of physical examination was performed?

_____

Step 7: What level of medical decision-making was required?

_____

Answer

Did you find the correct code to be 99215-21?

Andrea went to see Dr. Tamara "at his office," and has been a patient of his "since she was a teenager." Dr. Tamara did a "detailed history" and a "detailed examination." This directs us to code 99214.

Code 99214 indicates a typical time spent of 25 minutes. Our documentation shows that the physician *spent 55 minutes* (25 minutes history and exam and 30 minutes counseling). Using our counseling rule of time (counseling equals more than half of the total time spent), we would then move up to 99215, the highest level of E/M code in this category (location and relationship). Code 99215 indicates a time spent of only 40 minutes. Dr. Tamara spent 55 minutes with this patient, and he deserves to be compensated for that time. Therefore, use the code 99215 (40 minutes), along with the modifier 21 (for the extra 15 minutes), to explain that this E/M encounter was longer than described by the code alone.

24 Unrelated evaluation and management service by the same physician during a postoperative period. The physician may need to indicate that an evaluation and management service was performed during a postoperative period for a reason(s) unrelated to the original procedure. This circumstance may be reported by adding modifier 24 to the appropriate level of E/M service.

As a part of the standard of care, and what is called the **global surgery package,** a physician gets paid for performing surgery and for the time spent checking on the patient, after the surgery, to make certain the body is healing correctly. Modifier 24 would explain that the physician had to see the patient about a totally different concern during this time period.

Global surgery package

A group of services already included in the code for the operation and not reported separately.

YOU CODE IT! CASE STUDY

Dr. Longenstein removed Mark Katzman's gallbladder (a cholecystectomy) on February 27. The global period for this surgical procedure is 90 days. On March 15, Mark came to see Dr. Longenstein because he had been out in his garden and developed a rash on his arms. The physician examines Mark's arms and gives him an ointment for the rash.

You Code It!

Go through the steps of evaluation and management coding, and determine the code that should be reported for the encounter between Dr. Longenstein and Mark Katzman.

Step 1: Read the case completely.

Step 2: Abstract the notes: Which key words can you identify relating to the E/M service performed?

_____

Step 3: What is the location?

_____

Step 4: What is the relationship?

_____

Step 5: What level of patient history was taken?

_____

Step 6: What level of physical examination was performed?

_____

Step 7: What level of medical decision-making was required?

_____

Answer

Did you find the correct code to be 99212-24?

Mark "came to see Dr. Longenstein," meaning the encounter happened at the doctor's office. Considering that Dr. Longenstein "just performed surgery on Mark" two weeks ago, it is very reasonable to consider Mark an established patient. Dr. Longenstein did a "problem-focused examination" (limited exam of the problem area) and his "decision-making was straightforward." This directs us to code 99212.

90 days from February 27 goes all the way to May 27. It means that the visit for the rash, which is a *totally unrelated concern from the gall-bladder surgery,* occurred within the 90-day period. We must explain that Dr. Longenstein should be compensated separately for the encounter because it has nothing to do with the surgery. So our code will be 99212-24.

25 Significant, separately identifiable evaluation and management service by the same physician on the same day of the procedure of other service. It may be necessary to indicate that on the day a procedure or service identified by a CPT code was performed, the patient's condition required a significant, separately identifiable E/M service above and beyond the other service provided or beyond the usual preoperative and postoperative care associated with the procedure that was performed. A significant, separately identifiable E/M service is defined or substantiated by documentation that satisfies the relevant criteria for the respective E/M service to be reported. The E/M service may be prompted by the symptom or condition for which the procedure and/or service was provided. As such, different diagnoses are not required for reporting of the E/M services on the same date. This circumstance may be reported by adding modifier 25 to the appropriate level of E/M service. NOTE: This modifier is not used to report an E/M service that resulted in a decision to perform surgery. See modifier 57.

Certainly this happens quite frequently: A patient goes to see the doctor for a minor procedure in the office. Then the patient says, "Oh, Doc, while I'm here, I want to talk to you about so-and-so." Should that happen, you have to append the E/M code with modifier 25 to explain that there were two visits in one at this encounter.

LET'S CODE IT! SCENARIO

Harriet Robertson goes to see her dermatologist for a scheduled appointment to have a 1.5-cm mole removed from her cheek. Once Dr. Guilley completes the procedure, Harriet asks the doctor to look at a cyst that has developed under her arm. Dr. Guilley does a limited examination of the underarm area and determines that the best course of action is to wait and see what happens with the cyst. He advises Harriet to keep the area clean and to come back in three weeks if the cyst has not gone away.

CODING TIP »»»

In order for modifier 25 to be used correctly, it is best if the E/M code links or relates to a different diagnosis from the procedure performed that day. So there would be at least two diagnosis codes on this same claim form before you consider using this modifier. While different diagnoses are not required, there is concern in the industry about overuse of modifier 25, so this may trigger an audit without a separately identifiable diagnosis.

Harriet met with "her dermatologist," Dr. Guilley, *at her office*. The notes state that Dr. Guilley did a *problem-focused history* and a *problem-focused examination* and her *decision-making was straightforward*. This directs us to code 99212.

But wait! The claim for this encounter is going to include the code for the surgical removal of the mole—*a totally different concern* from the reason prompting the evaluation and management of the patient. In essence, there were two encounters in one here: the first for the removal of the mole and the second for the concern about the cyst. Therefore, the correct code would be 99212-25 (plus the procedure code for the excision of the mole 11312).

32 Mandated services. Services related to mandated consultation and/or related services (e.g., third-party payer, governmental, legislative, or regulatory requirement) may be identified by adding modifier 32 to the basic procedure.

Modifier 32 indicates that a third-party payer, a governmental agency, or other regulatory or legislative action required the encounter, consultation, and/or procedure(s).

LET'S CODE IT! SCENARIO

Elaine Geller, a 53-year-old female, went to see Dr. Overton for a comprehensive physical assessment, as a requirement for her application for life insurance. The insurance carrier would not consider the policy without the examination. She had never seen Dr. Overton before today's visit.

Elaine met with the physician *at his office,* and "had never seen Dr. Overton before," meaning she is a *new patient.* According to the notes, Dr. Overton did an *initial comprehensive preventive medicine* evaluation and management of a "53-year-old" female. That directs us to code 99386.

Notice that the insurance carrier, *a third-party payer, mandated* the evaluation. Therefore, we must add the modifier to the E/M code to get 99386-32.

CODING TIP »»»

Modifier 32 can be used with both E/M codes and procedure or treatment codes.

57 Decision for surgery. An evaluation and management service that resulted in the initial decision to perform the surgery may be identified by adding modifier 57 to the appropriate level of E/M service.

If a physician meets a patient in order to determine whether the patient should have a surgical procedure and the decision is to go ahead and perform the surgery, then the evaluation and management code should be appended with the modifier 57.

Dr. Matson referred Gary Matlin, a 35-year-old male, to Dr. Angelli for a consultation to determine whether or not he needs a prostatectomy. After taking a comprehensive history, performing a comprehensive examination, and reviewing all the previous test results, Dr. Angelli informs Gary that he recommends the procedure. Gary agrees, and they select a date three weeks later for the surgery to be performed.

Let's Code It!

Gary met with the physician *at his office.* He came to see Dr. Matson for a "consultation." Then Dr. Matson did a "comprehensive history" and a "comprehensive examination." His *medical decision-making* was of *moderate complexity.* This directs us to code 99244.

Remember that this encounter *ended in the decision* for Gary *to have the surgery.* Therefore, you must add the modifier 57 to the E/M code, giving us 99244-57.

NEWBORN EVALUATION AND MANAGEMENT CARE

A pediatrician should evaluate a newborn as part of routine health care procedures. These special evaluations are coded in the 99431–99440 range, depending upon where the baby was born and the specifics of the evaluation.

EXAMPLE

Dr. Bryce is a neonatologist. Dr. Opell, an obstetrician, asked Dr. Bryce to be in attendance during the delivery of Cybil Thymes's baby because of a concern over her excessive alcohol consumption during pregnancy. Dr. Bryce was there and stabilized the baby after birth. You would report Dr. Bryce's service with code 99436.

SPECIAL EVALUATION SERVICES

In cases when a patient is about to have a life insurance or disability certificate issued, the insurer often requires the attending physician to provide an evaluation to establish a baseline of data. The visit would not involve any actual treatment or management of the patient's condition—it just creates the appropriate documentation. The codes in range 99450–99456 apply to both new and established patients.

««« **CODING TIP**

When a physician sees a newborn at an office visit after seeing the baby initially at the hospital or other birth location, the visit is coded as an established patient visit (as long as it is within three years, of course).

««« **CODING TIP**

Be aware of codes 99000–99091 in the Special Services, Procedures and Reports subsection—most specifically 99080. Read the notes carefully, as well as the descriptions of the codes, to choose the most accurate.

CHAPTER SUMMARY

In this chapter you learned that the key components of coding for services rendered in a nursing home, long-term care facility, or the patient's home use a different set of codes from those reporting physician services in an office or hospital.

Understand that the elements of the distinct types of encounters, such as annual physicals (preventive medical assessments) and case management services, also use varying sets of parameters.

Your job, as a coding specialist, is to understand the variety of essentials involved in coding evaluation and management services properly and to report those services accurately.

1. A preventive medical E/M encounter may include any of these services except

    a. Counseling.

    b. Admission into the hospital.

    c. Anticipatory guidance.

    d. Risk factor reduction intervention.

2. If the physician finds a health concern during a preventive medicine examination, requiring additional E/M services, you should code this

    a. The preventive medicine code only.

    b. The additional E/M code only.

    c. Whichever is reimbursable at a higher rate.

    d. Separately and additionally.

3. E/M services provided to a patient in an assisted living facility would use a code from the subsection

    a. Nursing Facility.

    b. Home Services.

    c. Domiciliary, Rest Homes, and Custodial Care Settings.

    d. Care Plan Oversight Services.

4. If a patient is discharged from the hospital and admitted into an SNF on the same day by the same physician, code the E/M services with

    a. Admission to the nursing facility E/M code only.

    b. A hospital discharge code and admission to the nursing facility code.

    c. One outpatient E/M services code.

    d. Subsequent nursing facility E/M code.

5. Care plan oversight services provided for a patient in a hospice setting are coded from the

    a. 99339–99340 range.

    b. 99374–99375 range.

    c. 99377–99378 range.

    d. 99379–99380 range.

6. Mary Suppano goes to Dr. Wisabbi's office for an appointment. After a full history, exam, and comprehensive MDM, Dr. Wisabbi recommends that she be admitted into a psychiatric residential treatment center. He takes her over and admits her into the facility that afternoon. You will code the E/M services with

    a. One office visit code.

    b. Admission to nursing facility code.

    c. Both office visit code and admission to nursing facility code.

    d. Domiciliary, rest home, custodial care center code only.

7. Jacob Brassman, a 3-day-old male, was admitted into the NICU for complications of his low birth weight status. Dr. Dakota saw him yesterday, and is in again today. You will code today's E/M services from the

    a. 99295–99296 range.

    b. 99298–99300 range.

    c. 99307–99310 range.

    d. 99210–99215 range.

8. Critical care codes are determined by

    a. Length of time.

    b. Inpatient or outpatient status.

    c. Level of history, exam, and MDM.

    d. New or established patient.

9. Conferencing with other health care professionals regarding management and/or treatment of a patient is

    a. Included in all E/M codes.

    b. Coded as a consultation E/M code.

    c. Coded from 99366–99368.

    d. Coded from 99201–99205.

10. A modifier

    a. Explains an unusual circumstance.

    b. Has five digits.

    c. Begins with the letter M.

    d. Explains how a patient became injured.

1. Dr. Anthony spends approximately one hour on a conference call talking with an oncologist in Texas and a reconstructive specialist in California. The three professionals discussed treatments and options for Zena Johnson, a 37-year-old female, who was recently diagnosed with parosteal osteogenic sarcoma.

   _____

2. Frank Childers, a 72-year-old male in good health, came to see his regular family physician, Dr. Rappoport, for his yearly physical exam.

   _____

3. Premier Life & Health Insurance Company required Tom Cavellini, a 31-year-old male, to get Dr. Louisman, his regular physician, to complete a certificate confirming that Tom's current disability prevents him from working at his regular job and makes him eligible for disability insurance.

   _____

4. Oscar Unger, a 27-year-old male, goes to his family physician, Dr. Carter, for a tetanus shot after stepping on a rusty nail at the beach. While there, he asks Dr. Carter to look at a cut on his left hand. Dr. Carter examines the wound and tells him to keep the wound clean and bandaged.

   _____

5. Catalina King, a 15-month-old female, is admitted today by Dr. Ervin, into the pediatric critical care unit because of severe respiratory distress.

   _____

6. Dr. Lunden spent 2 1/2 hours evaluating Byron Curtis upon his admission into the ICU.

   _____

7. Owen Stabler has been living in the Barton Nursing Center for the last 12 months. Dr. Gilman comes in to do his annual assessment, including a detailed interval history, comprehensive exam, and moderate complexity.

   _____

8. Howard Shires moved into the Barton Assisted Living Center today. Dr. Bowyer, the center's resident physician, introduced himself to Howard and then took a detailed history, performed a comprehensive examination, and found the MDM to be moderate.

   _____

9. Reisa Haven is at home recuperating from surgery on her left hip with the help of Barton Home Health Services. Her attending physician, Dr. Alfaya, comes to her house do a problem-focused interval history and exam.

_____

10. David Magruder was discharged today from the Barton Nursing Center after Dr. Fanelli spent 25 minutes performing a final examination, discussing his stay, and providing instructions to his wife for continuing care.

_____

11. Dr. Servina provided care plan oversight services for Raymond Johnston, one of her patients at the Barton Assisted Living Center. It took her 20 minutes.

_____

12. Ronald Lassier, an 18-year-old male, is the son of two alcoholics. Dr. Foller spends 40 minutes with him providing risk factor reduction behavior modification techniques to help him avoid becoming an alcoholic himself.

_____

13. Makayla Sorensen, a 3-day-old female, currently weighs 2000 grams and requires intensive cardiac and respiratory monitoring. This is her third day in the NICU, and Dr. Pitassin comes in to do his E/M of her condition.

_____

14. Dr. Dodge works in a very small town in Ohio and travels up to 200 miles to see his patients in the surrounding rural areas. His patient, Sarah Matthews, gave birth at her home the day prior to a 6 lb 3 oz baby girl, Amelia Rose. Dr. Dodge sees Amelia Rose for the first time today, does a complete history and exam, and prepares her medical chart. Amelia Rose is a healthy newborn.

_____

15. George Terazzo's legs have finally healed to the point that he can be discharged from the nursing facility, where he has been for the last six weeks. Before he can go home, Dr. Horatio comes in for the final examination and to provide continuing care instructions to his wife, who will be caring for George at home. Dr. Horatio prepares the discharge records and gives a prescription to George for pain medication. This whole process takes Dr. Horatio about 45 minutes to complete.

_____

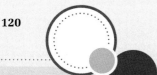

Part 1 CPT

Below and on the following pages, you will see physicians' notes documenting encounters with patients at our textbook's health care facility, Cipher, Victors, & Associates. Carefully read through the notes and find the best E/M code or codes for each of these cases.

CIPHER, VICTORS, & ASSOCIATES
A Complete Health Care Facility
234 MAIN STREET • ANYTOWN, FL 32711 • 407-555-1234

PATIENT: FRANKLIN, FRANCES
ACCOUNT/EHR #: FRANFR001
Date: 10/17/08

Attending Physician: Valerie R. Victors, MD

S: This 57-year-old female came for her routine physical exam. Pt does not smoke, drinks alcohol occasionally, and exercises three times per week. Pt states she has no specific health concerns at this time.

O: Ht 5'3" Wt 145 lb. R 20. HEENT: unremarkable; Respiratory: unremarkable; Musculoskeletal: age appropriate. No sign of osteoporosis. Bone density appropriate. Discussed the importance of keeping up her exercise regimen.

A: Pt is in good health.

P: 1. Follow-up prn
   2. Schedule blood work: comprehensive metabolic panel
   3. Schedule screening mammogram

Valerie R. Victors, MD

VRV/mg   D: 10/17/08 09:50:16   T: 10/23/08 12:55:01

Find the best, most appropriate E/M code.

_____

_____

_____

PATIENT: CASSELTON, BRANDON
ACCOUNT/EHR #: CASSBR001
Date: 10/25/08

Attending Physician: Valerie R. Victors, MD

S: This 85-year-old male is seen this day at Barton Assisted Living Center, where he has been living for the last six months. The last time I saw this patient was right before he moved into the center. Nurse Thomas states that he has been complaining of mild abdominal pain, and some discomfort upon urination. Other than this issue, he has been well and stable.

O: Ht 5'2.5" Wt 145 lb. R 18. Abdomen is unremarkable. No masses or rigidity noted.

A: Suspected bladder infection

P: Order written for UA to rule out bladder infection.

_____

Valerie R. Victors, MD

VRV/mg   D: 10/25/08 09:50:16   T: 10/28/08 12:55:01

Find the best, most appropriate E/M code.

_____

_____

_____

CIPHER, VICTORS, & ASSOCIATES
A Complete Health Care Facility
234 MAIN STREET • ANYTOWN, FL 32711 • 407-555-1234

PATIENT: GREGORY, ALANA
ACCOUNT/EHR #:   GREGAL001
Date: 11/21/08

Attending Physician: Valerie R. Victors, MD

S: This 35-year-old female is seen at her home, where she is on complete bed rest due to complications of her pregnancy. She has hypertension and gestational diabetes. She is at 27 weeks gestation. She states that she has had no problems since my last visit six days ago. She states that she has had no instances of lightheadedness and has had no sense of weakness.

O: Ht 5′5″ Wt 151 lb. R 22 G1 P0. Abdomen is unremarkable. No masses or rigidity noted. B/P 140/97, nonfasting glucose stick 110.

A: Patient improving nicely

P: 1. Continue bed rest
      2. Revisit one week

_____

Valerie R. Victors, MD

VRV/mg   D: 11/21/08 09:50:16   T: 11/23/08 12:55:01

Find the best, most appropriate E/M code.

_____

_____

_____

CIPHER, VICTORS, & ASSOCIATES
A Complete Health Care Facility
234 MAIN STREET • ANYTOWN, FL 32711 • 407-555-1234

PATIENT: BLIGHTON, ELLA
ACCOUNT/EHR #:   BLIGEL001
Date: 10/01/08

Attending Physician: Valerie R. Victors, MD

This 17-month-old female is being admitted to the pediatric critical care unit today. Mother claims that onset of symptoms was sudden. She states that she rushed the child to the ED immediately.

Respiration is shallow. Child is unresponsive. PERL. B/P low. T 102.

Complete blood workup ordered: CBC with diff, tox screen, bilirubin, and basic metabolic panel.

IV fluids to keep hydrated.

Await test results.

_____

Valerie R. Victors, MD

VRV/mg   D: 10/01/08 09:50:16   T: 10/03/08 12:55:01

Find the best, most appropriate E/M code.

_____

_____

_____

Part 1   CPT

CIPHER, VICTORS, & ASSOCIATES
A Complete Health Care Facility
234 MAIN STREET • ANYTOWN, FL 32711 • 407-555-1234

PATIENT: COLES, MARTIN
ACCOUNT/EHR #:   COLEMA001
Date: 11/15/08

Attending Physician: Valerie R. Victors, MD

Infant was born this morning at 0710 to a healthy 27-year-old female in the delivery room of Barton Hospital.
    Full examination of normal newborn; perinatal history; complete notes in medical record created for baby.
    Baby discharged home today 1630.
    Office visit follow-up 10 days.

_____

Valerie R. Victors, MD

VRV/mg   D: 11/15/08 09:50:16   T: 11/17/08 12:55:01

Find the best, most appropriate E/M code.

_____

_____

_____

6

Anesthesia Coding

LEARNING OUTCOMES

- Correctly apply the guidelines for proper anesthesia coding.
- Interpret the types of anesthesia as they relate to the coding process.
- Select the best, most appropriate code for anesthesia services.
- Abstract the notes to determine the correct physical status modifiers.
- Correctly apply qualifying circumstances add-on codes.
- Properly use HCPCS modifiers.

EMPLOYMENT OPPORTUNITIES

Anesthesiologists' offices
Ambulatory surgery centers
Billing companies

Non-profit organizations
Long-term care facilities
Assisted living facilities

The procedure codes for identifying the administration of anesthetics are in the second section of the CPT book, directly after evaluation and management codes. The anesthesiology codes range from 00100 to 01999 and 99100 to 99140.

As a professional coder, you will typically use codes from this section only if you work for an anesthesiologist, in his or her office, or for a billing company that codes and files claims for anesthesiologists. Generally, **anesthesiologists** have their own practices. While almost all their services occur in a hospital or ambulatory surgical center setting, they are not employees of the hospital, and they must submit their own claim forms to the insurance carrier for their services.

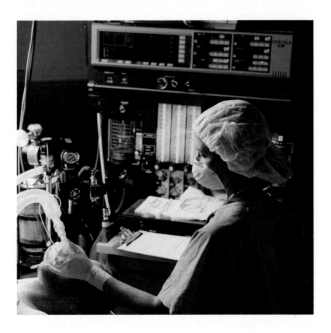

TYPES OF ANESTHESIA

Anesthesia is defined as the suppression of nerve sensations to relieve or prevent the feeling of pain, usually by the use of pharmaceuticals. Essentially, it is more commonly described as the administration of drugs to enable a patient to avoid the feeling of pain. While there are many types of anesthesia, they are all primarily divided into three preliminary categories: topical/local, regional, and general.

1. **Topical** and/or **local anesthesia.** Topical anesthesia refers to the numbing of surface nerves, while local anesthesia refers to the dulling of feeling in a limited area of the body.

EXAMPLE

Dr. Dentmann, a general dentist, rubbed a *topical anesthetic* onto Bernard's gum to prevent him from feeling any pain from the injection of the *local anesthetic*. The local anesthetic will prevent him from feeling pain while the doctor drills the cavity that Bernard has in his left, lower molar.

2. **Regional anesthesia.** Regional anesthesia prevents a section of the body from transmitting pain, and includes epidural, **caudal**, spinal, axillary, stellate ganglion blocks, **regional blocks**, and brachial anesthesia.

EXAMPLE

Dr. Siestaman, an anesthesiologist, was paged to come to the maternity ward to administer *epidural anesthesia* for Robyn Caldwell. After the epidural was given, Robyn was able to proceed with the birth of her baby without the pain of childbirth because the loss of sensation was only from the waist down. She was otherwise awake and alert.

Anesthesiologists

Physicians specializing in the administration of anesthesia.

Anesthesia

The loss of sensation, with or without consciousness, generally induced by the administration of a particular drug.

Topical anesthesia

The application of a drug to the skin to reduce or prevent sensation in a specific area temporarily.

⟪⟪ CODING TIP

Topical: Think *top* for the top layer.

Local anesthesia

The injection of a drug to prevent sensation in a specific portion of the body. Includes local infiltration anesthesia, digital blocks, and pudendal blocks.

⟪⟪ CODING TIP

Local: The effect of the anesthesia stays close to the injection site.

Regional anesthesia

The administration of a drug in order to interrupt the nerve impulses without loss of consciousness.

Caudal

Near the hind part or tail of the body, the sacrum and coccyx areas.

Regional blocks

Areas that include axillary, bier, retobulbar, peribulbar, interscalene, subarachnoid, supraclavicular, and infraclavicular blocks.

General anesthesia

The administration of a drug in order to induce a loss of consciousness in the patient, who is unable to be aroused even by painful stimulation.

3. **General anesthesia.** Also called *surgical anesthesia,* general anesthesia creates a total loss of consciousness and sensation. General anesthesia is given to the patient by inhalation, intravenous (IV) injection, or, on rare occasion, intramuscular (IM) injection.

EXAMPLE

Dr. Jacobs, an anesthesiologist, administered *general anesthesia* to Jamal Johnson after he was brought into the operating room and positioned on the table. Dr. Haverhill was preparing to remove Jamal's gallbladder because of the collection of stones in that organ, and everyone wanted to be certain that Jamal would not feel anything during the surgical procedure.

One additional type of anesthesia that you should know about when coding anesthetic and surgical services is called **conscious sedation.** It is a form of ultralight general anesthesia because it affects the entire body.

Conscious sedation

The use of a drug to reduce stress and/or anxiety.

With conscious sedation, the physician gives the patient medication to reduce anxiety and stress. The patient remains awake and aware of his or her surroundings and what is going on. He or she can answer questions and respond to verbal commands.

Most often, conscious sedation is used for procedures that will not typically cause pain but may be worrisome to patients, causing them to be nervous and frightened. The services of an anesthesiologist are not required for the provision of conscious sedation, so the physician performing the procedure, or a member of the nursing staff, may administer this before the patient goes into the procedure room. This is one of the reasons the codes for this service are not found in the Anesthesia section of CPT, but in the Medicine section.

Codes 99143–99150 report the administration of moderate (conscious) sedation and include:

- Assessing the patient
- Establishing IV access and fluids to maintain patency, when performed
- Administration of the drug
- Maintaining the sedated level
- Monitoring oxygen saturation, heart rate, and blood pressure
- Observation and assessment during recovery

The time spent with the patient under conscious sedation determines the correct code or codes. Intraservice time is measured in an initial 30-minute segment, followed by 15-minute segments. The clock starts when the physician administers the sedative and stops when the patient is discharged and the physician is no longer required to supervise the patient. Total time is calculated only for the minutes the physician continuously spends face to face with the patient.

LET'S CODE IT! SCENARIO

Eunice Harrah, a 37-year-old female, came into Dr. Mancini's office to have a hepatotomy—the open drainage of a cyst. She was very nervous

Part 1 CPT

because she had never had this procedure before. Dr. Mancini gave Eunice an IV of Versed, a sedative to relieve her anxiety. The procedure is not really painful, so there was no need for a full anesthetic or pain-killer. Raymond Elvers, CRNA, sat with Eunice throughout the procedure to ensure her comfort level. Dr. Mancini accomplished the procedure in one stage, taking 30 minutes.

Let's Code It!

Dr. Mancini administered Versed, a mild "sedative," to Eunice before the procedure. When you look at the procedure code for a "hepatotomy" (47010), you will notice that there is no symbol ⊙ next to the code. This absence of this symbol indicates that conscious sedation is not already included and must be coded separately. Let's go to the alphabetic index and find *conscious sedation.*

Note that the CPT book tells you to *see Sedation.*

Under *Sedation,* you find:

Moderate	99143–99150
With independent observation	99143–99145

When you read the complete description of these codes in the numerical section of the CPT book, you should see that code *99144* is the most accurate. This identifies *moderate sedation, administered by the same physician who performed the procedure* (Dr. Mancini), *and includes the presence of an independent trained observer* (Raymond Elvers, CRNA) *to monitor the patient, age 5 years or older, first 30 minutes intra-service.*

So in addition to the code for the *hepatotomy* (47010), you include the code for the *conscious sedation* (99144) on the report and claim form.

In some instances, when conscious sedation is administered, health care professionals prefer that an anesthesiologist is present and monitoring the patient's vital signs throughout the procedure. This is referred to as **monitored anesthesia care (MAC).** Code MAC services from the main anesthesia code section 00100–01999.

CODING ANESTHESIA SERVICES

When coding anesthetic services, you should follow these steps to find the best, most appropriate code.

1. *Confirm* that the physician who performed the procedure for which the anesthesia is necessary is a different professional from the person who administered the anesthesia.

   On those occasions when the same physician who performs the procedure also administers regional or general anesthesia, you must append modifier 47 Anesthesia by Surgeon to the appropriate procedure code. The modifier is not attached to an anesthesia procedure code; it is added to the basic procedure code. No additional code from the Anesthesia section will be used.

Monitored anesthesia care (MAC)

The administration of sedatives, anesthetic agents, or other medications to relax but not render the patient unconscious while under the constant observation of a trained anesthesiologist. Also known as "twilight" sedation.

2. *Identify* the anatomical site of the patient's body upon which the procedure is being performed.

3. *Confirm* the exact procedure performed, as documented in the physician's notes.

4. *Consult* the alphabetic index of the CPT book, look under the heading of Anesthesia, and read down the list to find the anatomical site shown below that heading. Identify the suggested code or codes for this site.

EXAMPLE

Anesthesia

    Skull 00190

5. *Turn* to the numeric portion of the CPT book, Anesthesia section, and find the subsection identifying that anatomical site.

EXAMPLE

00190 Anesthesia for procedures on facial bones or skull; not otherwise specified

00192   radical surgery (including prognathism)

CODING TIP »»

Remember, *never, never, never* code from the alphabetic index. Always confirm the code's full description in the numeric listing.

6. *Read* the descriptions written next to each code option suggested in the alphabetic index carefully. Then compare them to the terms used by the physician in his or her notes documenting the procedure. This will lead you to the best, most appropriate code available.

LET'S CODE IT! SCENARIO

Dr. Jacobs is called in to administer general anesthesia to Miriam Delveccio, a 6-month-old female, diagnosed with congenital tracheal stenosis. Dr. Quartermain is going to perform a surgical repair of her trachea.

Let's Code It!

The notes indicate that Dr. Jacobs *administered the anesthesia* and Dr. Quartermain will be performing a "surgical repair of her trachea." As you will remember, this means that an anesthesia code will be used, not a modifier appended to the procedure code. So let's go ahead and find the best code for the anesthesia service.

Turn to the alphabetic index and look up *anesthesia*. Going down the alphabetic listing of the sites beneath this heading, look for more than a page until you get to the correct anatomical site: *Trachea.*

Trachea   00320, 00326, 00542

    Reconstruction 00539

The physician's notes state that Dr. Quartermain performed a "repair," not a reconstruction, so focus on the codes shown next to *Trachea.* Turn to the numeric listings of the CPT book to find the codes: 00320, 00326, and 00542. Read the descriptions written next to each code, as well as the others found in the sub-section, in order to determine the best, most appropriate code available.

Neck

00320 Anesthesia for all procedures on esophagus, thyroid, larynx, trachea and lymphatic system of neck; not otherwise specified, age 1 year or older

00322 Anesthesia for all procedures on esophagus, thyroid, larynx, trachea and lymphatic system of neck; needle biopsy of thyroid

00326 Anesthesia for all procedures on the larynx and trachea in children less than 1 year of age

00542 Anesthesia for thoracotomy procedures involving lungs, pleura, diaphragm, and mediastinum (including surgical thoracoscopy); decortication

As you review the code descriptions, you can identify which terms or words are most important in matching the code to the physician's documentation of the procedure. Look at the physician's notes one more time and identify the key terms.

Dr. Jacobs is called in to administer general anesthesia *to Miriam Delveccio, a* 6-month-old *female, diagnosed with congenital tracheal stenosis. Dr. Quartermain is going to perform a surgical repair of her* trachea.

The combination of all these terms matches only one of our available code descriptions, doesn't it?

00326 <u>Anesthesia</u> for all procedures on the larynx and <u>trachea</u> in children <u>younger than 1 year</u> of age

You found the best, most appropriate code for the administration of general anesthesia for Miriam Delveccio's surgery.

ANESTHESIA GUIDELINES

The official guidelines specifically intended for coding anesthesia services (general and regional anesthesia) are shown, at length, on the pages at the beginning of the Anesthesia section of the CPT book. Let's go through these guidelines and review how they might help you determine the best, most appropriate anesthesia code.

All the codes within the Anesthesia section of the CPT book include activities that are most often performed by anesthesiologists when they are preparing to administer anesthesia to a patient. The following services are included in the *anesthesia code package* and are not coded separately.

1. *Usual preoperative visits.* Most of the time, the anesthesiologist will stop in to interview the patient, in addition to taking the time to thoroughly read the chart and patient history, prior to administering the anesthesia. It gives the physician the opportunity to discuss any potential reactions or other considerations with the patient.

2. *Anesthesia care during the procedure.* The time and expertise of the anesthesiologist not only to administer the actual anesthetic but also to observe the patient throughout the procedure are a very important part of his or her job responsibilities.

3. *Administration of fluids.* The anesthesiologist gives the patient fluids, as well as analgesics (liquid form), as needed during the procedure.

4. *Usual monitoring services* (e.g., ECG, temperature, BP). As a part of the natural course of the anesthesiologist's duties, he or she must monitor the patient's vital signs throughout the procedure and make certain that there are no unexpected affects from the anesthesia.

5. *Usual postoperative visits.* The anesthesiologist normally visits the patient while in recovery, to ensure that there are no lingering affects of the anesthesia and there are no other concerns as a result of the anesthesia.

When multiple procedures are performed during the same operative session, the anesthesia should be coded for the most complicated procedure only.

Time reporting may be used for billing anesthesia services (for general anesthesia) in certain areas around the country or by certain third-party payers. If this is the custom in your local area, the clock begins when the anesthesiologist starts to prepare the patient for the administration of the anesthetic drug *in the operating room* and is measured in 15-minute increments. The time ends when the anesthesiologist is no longer required to be present, once the patient has been safely transferred to postoperative supervision. When multiple procedures are completed during the same operative session, the time calculated should be the total time for all the procedures performed. A formula is used to calculate the amount of compensation the anesthesiologist will receive. The formula is:

$$\text{Compensation} = (B + T + M) \times \text{CF}$$

where B = base unit

T = time spent by the anesthesiologist with the patient

M = modifying factors

CF = conversion factor

The base unit is assigned by the American Society of Anesthesiologists (ASA), as published in the annual *Relative Value Guide*. The unit includes reimbursement for the usual time and services performed by the anesthesiologist preoperatively and postoperatively. Modifying factors are any adjustments made to allow for the additional challenges presented by the physical status of the patient at the time anesthesia is administered. The conversion factor is the number used to translate units into dollars.

Sometimes special circumstances, also called qualifying circumstances, cause the anesthetic process to be more complicated than usual. In these cases, a second—or add-on—code is used to identify that circumstance.

The available add-on codes for qualifying circumstances are:

- +99100 Patient of extreme age . . . younger than 1 year or older than 70 years. This add-on code is *not* to be used when the code description already includes an age definition, such as codes 00326, 00834, or 00836.

- +99116 Anesthesia complicated by total body hypothermia. Hypothermia is defined as *extremely low body temperature,* below 36.1°C (97°F). Because monitoring vital signs, including body temperature, is an important part of the anesthesia process, a very low body temperature would make the safe administration of anesthesia more complicated.

- +99135 Anesthesia complicated by controlled hypotension. Hypotension is defined as *abnormally low blood pressure.* The critical connection between blood pressure and heart rate makes this situation very intricate for the anesthesiologist.

- +99140 Anesthesia complicated by emergency conditions. An emergency is characterized as a situation in which the patient's life, or an individual body part, would be threatened if there were any delay in providing treatment. In such a case, the anesthesiologist may not have the time to get the patient history or other information necessary to do his or her job most efficiently or effectively.

Coding for the administration of conscious sedation also has a few guidelines to help you determine the best, most appropriate code:

1. If the same physician performing the procedure also administers the conscious sedation, use a code from the 99143–99145 range (located in the Medicine section of the CPT book).

2. If the conscious sedation is administered by a physician other than the one performing a procedure listed in Appendix G, in a facility (hospital, ambulatory surgical center, or skilled nursing facility), use the appropriate code(s) from 99148–99150. However, if this second professional provides the service in a physician's office or freestanding imaging center, the conscious sedation service is not separately reported. If a procedure is performed but not listed in Appendix G and a second physician administers conscious sedation, use the appropriate code from the main anesthesia section, 00100–01999.

3. Note that some CPT codes already include the administration of conscious sedation in the original code. In such cases, you are not permitted to use a separate sedation code. The CPT codes that include conscious sedation are identified in the numerical listing of the CPT book with the symbol ⊙ (a circle with a dot in the center) in front of the code and are listed in Appendix G.

EXAMPLES

⊙ 33010 Pericardiocentesis; initial

⊙ 92953 Temporary transcutaneous pacing

Unusual circumstances might require the administration of general anesthesia for a procedure that typically requires either local anesthesia or no anesthesia. In these cases, the modifier 23 Unusual Anesthesia must be appended to the procedure code for that basic service (not to the anesthesia code). In these cases, you will not assign a code from the Anesthesia section of CPT.

LET'S CODE IT! SCENARIO

Margaret Cabaña, a 68-year-old female, arrives for the insertion of a permanent pacemaker, atrial with transvenous electrodes. Dr. Fowler notices that Margaret has been diagnosed with Parkinson's disease, causing her to have uncontrollable tremors. Dr. Fowler decides that conscious sedation (which is included with the procedure code) is insufficient to ensure the patient's safety. Therefore, he believes that general anesthesia would be more appropriate and administers the anesthesia himself.

Let's Code It!

Dr. Fowler decides that Margaret needs *general anesthesia* for this procedure, *even though it is not the standard,* because her Parkinson's disease makes the procedure unsafe without it. He is *inserting a permanent pacemaker, atrial with transvenous electrodes.*

The alphabetic index shows:

Insertion

    Pacemaker

        Fluoroscopy/Radiography 71090

        Heart   33206–33208, 33212–33213

Look through the descriptions for the codes in the first range, 33200–33208. Do any of the descriptions match the notes?

33206 Insertion or replacement of permanent pacemaker with transvenous electrode(s); atrial

Before you move on to the next section, remember that Dr. Fowler administered general anesthesia. You can tell from the symbol ⊙ next to procedure code 33206 that conscious sedation is included with the code. It indicates that general anesthesia would be unusual. How will you ensure Dr. Fowler's reimbursement for the administration of the anesthesia? This is what modifiers do—identify unusual circumstances. Modifier 23 is specifically for a case when unusual anesthesia is used.

In this case, the correct code is 33206-23.

If the same physician performing the procedure also administers either regional or general anesthesia, the modifier 47 Anesthesia by Surgeon must be appended to the procedure code for that basic service (not to the anesthesia code). In such cases, an anesthesia code would not be reported. However, it is permissible to report a code for the injection of the anesthetic drug.

Part 1   CPT

So, to completely and accurately report Dr. Fowler's care of Margaret, the correct code is 33206-23-47. This tells the third-party payer that Dr. Fowler inserted a permanent atrial pacemaker with transvenous electrodes with unusual anesthesia that he administered himself. This one code with two modifiers tells the whole story of this encounter. [Of course, you should include a letter explaining why the unusual anesthesia had to be administered in the first place.]

YOU CODE IT! CASE STUDY

Marshall Levine, a 27-year-old male, came to see Dr. Houghton for a repair of his extensor tendon in his right wrist. Dr. Houghton administered a regional nerve block and then performed the repair.

You Code It!

Go through the steps of coding, and determine the codes that should be reported for this encounter between Dr. Houghton and Marshall Levine.

Step 1: Read the case completely.

Step 2: Abstract the notes: Which key words can you identify relating to the procedures performed?

_____

Step 3: Query the provider, if necessary.

Step 4: Diagnosis: Torn tendon, wrist.

Step 5: Code the procedure(s).

_____

Step 6: Link the procedure codes to at least one diagnosis code.

Step 7: Back code to double-check your choices.

Answer

Did you find the correct codes to be:

25270-47 Repair, tendon or muscle, extensor, forearm and/or wrist; primary, single, each tendon or muscle, regional anesthesia administered by surgeon

64450 Injection, anesthetic agent; other peripheral nerve or branch

Excellent!

PHYSICAL STATUS MODIFIERS

The American Society of Anesthesiologists (ASA) established six levels of measuring the physical condition of a patient with regard to the administration of anesthesia. Each level, identified by the letter "P" and a number from 1 to 6, denotes issues that may increase the complexity of delivering anesthetic services and are measured at the time the anesthetic is about to be administered. The anesthesiologist is the professional who determines the correct physical status modifier. However, you, as the coding specialist, must be certain to look for the information and include it on the claim form.

Physical status modifiers are mandatory with every code from the Anesthesia section of the CPT book and are placed directly after the five-digit CPT code (with a hyphen between the two). (*Note:* Physical status modifiers are different from, and have nothing to do with, the regular CPT and HCPCS modifiers shown in Appendix A of the CPT book.)

Following are the physical status modifiers that are only to be used with anesthesia codes:

P1 (*a normal healthy patient*). Modifier P1 indicates that the patient to whom the anesthetic was given had no medical concerns that would interfere with the anesthesiologist's responsibilities for keeping the patient sedated and safe.

EXAMPLE

Dr. Tomberg administered general anesthesia to Sarah Robbins, a 17-year-old otherwise healthy female gymnast, before Dr. Navarro performed an arthroscopic extensive debridement of her shoulder joint. The correct code is 01630-P1.

P2 (*a patient with mild systemic disease*). When a patient has a disease that may affect the general workings of the patient's body, it must be taken into consideration with regard to administering anesthesia. However, if the disease is under control, then its involvement is less of a concern.

EXAMPLE

Dr. Geller administered general anesthesia to Roberta Ferrara, a 37-year-old female with controlled type I diabetes mellitus, for her radical mastectomy with internal mammary node dissection, to be performed by Dr. Jackson. The correct code is 00406-P2.

P3 (*a patient with severe systemic disease*). In this case, the patient's disease is serious throughout his or her body and is an important factor for the anesthesiologist to contend with, in addition to the reason for the procedure.

EXAMPLE

Dr. Holloran administered general anesthesia to Vern Amberdeen, a 59-year-old male with benign hypertension due to Cushing's disease. Vern came today for Dr. Colombo to perform a laparoscopic cholecystectomy with cholangiography for acute cholecystitis. The correct code is 00790-P3.

P4 (*a patient with severe systemic disease that is a constant threat to life*). Modifier P4 describes any patient having medical problems that have invaded or affected multiple systems of the body. The large number of issues regarding the effects of the disease, along with existing medications and treatments that have been ongoing in the patient's system, and the potential interactions with the anesthetic make it a very complex case.

EXAMPLE

Dr. Ellerbee administered general anesthesia to Carl Umber, a 61-year-old male. Carl has advanced esophageal cancer that has metastasized throughout his body. Dr. Torres will be performing a partial esophagectomy. The correct code is 00500-P4.

P5 (*a moribund patient who is not expected to survive without the operation*). This is a life or death situation, but not necessarily an emergency. In such cases, the patient is in critical condition, and there are serious medical complications that make administering anesthesia more challenging.

EXAMPLE

Dr. Spinosa administered general anesthesia to Debra Ann Brodsky, a 41-year-old female with acute arteriosclerosis. Dr. Chesterfield was called back in from vacation to perform a heart/lung transplant this morning. The correct code is 00580-P5.

P6 (*a declared brain-dead patient whose organs are being removed for donor purposes*). This modifier is provided by the ASA for use with brain-dead patients. Individuals in this condition need to have anesthesia administered to slow bodily functions and give the transplant team time to harvest the viable organs.

YOU CODE IT! CASE STUDY

Elba Carter, an 83-year-old female, came to see Dr. Jacobs for a total knee arthroplasty due to acute arthritis. Dr. Sinonna is called in to administer the general anesthesia for the procedure. Elba is in otherwise good health.

You Code It!

Go through the steps of coding, and determine the codes that should be reported for this encounter between Dr. Sinonna and Elba Carter.

Step 1: Read the case completely.

Step 2: Abstract the notes: Which key words can you identify relating to the procedures performed?

_____

Step 3: Query the provider, if necessary.

Step 4: Diagnosis: acute arthritis.

Step 5: Code the procedure(s): The administration of the anesthesia.

_____

Step 6: Link the procedure codes to at least one diagnosis code.

Step 7: Back code to double-check your choices.

Answer

Did you find the correct codes to be:

01402-P1 Anesthesia for open or surgical arthroscopic procedures on knee joint; total knee arthroplasty; a normal healthy patient

99100 Anesthesia for patient of extreme age, younger than 1 year and older than 70

HCPCS LEVEL II MODIFIERS

Certified registered nurse anesthetist (CRNA)

A registered nurse (RN) who has taken additional, specialized training in the administration of anesthesia.

Specific HCPCS Level II modifiers are designated for use with anesthesia service codes. The codes are only used if the insurance carrier, such as Medicare, accepts HCPCS codes and modifiers. It is your responsibility, as a professional coder, to know the rules for the different third-party payers with which you will work.

AA Anesthesia services performed personally by the anesthesiologist.

AD Medical supervision by an anesthesiologist for *more than four concurrent anesthesia procedures* being administered by qualified professionals, such as a **certified registered nurse anesthetist (CRNA)** (five or more cases at the same time).

G8 Monitored anesthesia care (MAC) during a deep complex, complicated, or markedly invasive surgical procedure. This modifier might indicate that the procedure was exceptionally lengthy.

G9 Monitored anesthesia care (MAC) for a patient who has a history of a severe cardiopulmonary condition. Certainly, acute problems with the heart and lungs would require more intricate supervision on behalf of the anesthesiologist.

QK Medical direction by an anesthesiologist of *two, three, or four concurrent anesthesia procedures* being administered by other qualified individuals, such as a CRNA.

QS Monitored anesthesia care (MAC).

QY Medical direction of one certified registered nurse anesthetist (CRNA) by an anesthesiologist. This modifier would be used to indicate that an anesthesiologist was available and oversaw the administration of anesthesia services provided by someone else, such as a CRNA. The QY modifier is for the supervision of *one case at a time.* QK is used for two to four cases at one time, and AD is for more than four cases at one time.

If your office uses a CRNA to provide anesthesia services, there are two additional modifiers that might be used with the codes for the services they provide.

QX CRNA service with medical direction by a physician.

QZ CRNA service without medical direction by a physician.

CPT © 2007 American Medical Association. All Rights Reserved.

CHAPTER SUMMARY

For the most part, anesthesia coding is for the purposes of submitting health insurance claim forms on behalf of the anesthesiologist or a member of his or her staff, such as a CRNA.

To find the best, most appropriate code that accurately represents the anesthesia services administered, you must first know which type of anesthesia was used. Then you must determine the anatomical site upon which the procedure was performed and exactly which procedure was provided to the patient. In addition, you must know who administered the anesthesia to the patient: Was it the physician who also performed that procedure, or was it a different health care professional? When using HCPCS modifiers, you also need to know whether the physician who administered the anesthetic was an anesthesiologist.

Once you determine the best, most appropriate code for the dispensation of the anesthesia, you also have to append the correct modifiers, when applicable.

1. Health care professionals permitted to administer anesthetics include

    a. Anesthesiologists.
    b. Certified registered nurse anesthetists.
    c. Surgeons.
    d. All of the above.

2. The categories of anesthesia include all except

    a. Topical/local.
    b. Conscious sedation.
    c. Regional.
    d. General.

3. Topical anesthesia is administered

    a. To the skin.
    b. Intravenously.
    c. Intramuscularly.
    d. Via inhalation.

4. MAC is an acronym that stands for

    a. Medically administered care.
    b. Mutually accessible care.
    c. Monitored anesthesia care.
    d. Medical anesthetic characters.

5. Conscious sedation is provided in order to

    a. Eliminate pain.
    b. Reduce anxiety.
    c. Render the patient unconscious.
    d. Block the nerve sensations to an extremity.

6. When the same physician performing the procedure administers regional or general anesthesia, modifier 47 should be appended to

    a. The correct anesthesia code.
    b. The correct procedure code.
    c. Either (a) or (b).
    d. Modifier 47 should not be used in this circumstance.

7. The anesthesia code package includes all except

    a. Preoperative visits.
    b. Postoperative visits.
    c. Usual monitoring services.
    d. Home health follow-up.

8. When reporting anesthesia services using time reporting, the formula used is

    a. $(B + T + M) \times CF$
    b. $(B + Q + CF) \times T$
    c. $(Q + T + CF) \times B$
    d. $(CF + B + T) \times M$

9. Qualifying circumstances are conditions that might require more work on the part of the anesthesiologist, including all except

    a. Extreme age.
    b. Emergency conditions.
    c. Severe systemic disease.
    d. Total body hypothermia.

10. A physical status modifier describes issues that may increase the complexity of delivering anesthetic services, including

    a. Emergency situation.
    b. Mild systemic disease.
    c. Extreme age.
    d. Controlled hypotension.

Find the best anesthesia code for each of these scenarios.

1. Tammy Mirandosa, a healthy 31-year-old female, received anesthesia before delivering her daughter at the hospital. It was a vaginal delivery.

   _____

2. Dr. Adams administered general anesthesia to Manny Perez, an otherwise healthy 29-year-old firefighter. Dr. Zelmono performed a third-degree burn excision, followed by a skin grafting on Manny's chest where 9% of his body surface was burned while he was rescuing a little boy from a house fire.

   _____

3. Karen Walkins, a 41-year-old female, was previously diagnosed with benign hypertension due to morbid obesity. Dr. Masters administers general anesthesia so that Dr. Morgenstern can perform a direct venous thrombectomy on her lower left leg.

   _____

4. Dr. Beaumont administered anesthesia to Annalee McDonald, a 37-year-old female, diagnosed with a malignant neoplasm of the uterus. Her gynecologist, Dr. Billingsley, performed a vaginal hysterectomy.

   _____

5. Dr. Alexander administered anesthesia to Thomas Valentine, a 9-month-old male, requiring a hernia repair in the lower abdomen. Dr. Georges, the neonatologist, noted that, without the surgery, Thomas was not expected to survive.

   _____

6. Miriam Worshille, a 71-year-old female, with a history of hypertension and diabetes mellitus, is brought into the operating room for Dr. Auerbach to perform a corneal transplant. Dr. Yankovich administers the anesthesia.

   _____

7. Dr. Quanarian is preparing to perform a ventriculography with burr holes on Benjamin Elliston, a 10-year-old male, who fell off the monkey bars onto a cement floor yesterday. Dr. Yorkshire administers the anesthesia.

   _____

8. Dr. Frankfurt administers anesthesia so that Dr. Clausson can perform a diagnostic lumbar puncture on Franklin Keiths, a 45-year-old male. Over the course of the last year, Franklin, a construction worker, has developed essential hypertension, which is currently controlled by diet. This lumbar puncture is to confirm the suspected diagnosis of bacterial meningitis.

   _____

9. John Kinekopsi, a 23-year-old male, plays professional basketball and is given anesthesia by Dr. O'Neill before having a diagnostic arthroscopy of his right knee by Dr. Malone.

   _____

10. Peter Siskowsky, a 15-year-old male, was in a go-kart accident and fractured his upper arm three months ago. Today, Dr. Longine operated on him to repair the malunion of his humerus. Dr. Carole administered the anesthesia.

    _____

11. Juana Ramirez brought her 4-year-old daughter, Sasha, into the emergency room with a deep laceration of her scalp, above her right ear, measuring 2.25 cm. Sasha was distraught, crying, and combative, kicking at the physician and the nurse as they attempted to clean the wound. At the recommendation of Dr. Ferrara, Juana held Sasha in her lap, while the physician administered 10 mg of Versed intranasally. Once the sedation took effect, Dr. Ferrara was able to perform a layered repair of the laceration, while the nurse monitored Sasha's vital signs. The entire procedure took 25 minutes.

    _____

12. Suzanna St. James, a healthy 31-year-old female, was given an epidural during labor, with the expectations of a vaginal delivery. After a time, Dr. Wolfe, her obstetrician, determined that the labor was obstructed and notified the hospital staff, including Dr. Amandon, the anesthesiologist, that they would have to do a cesarean (c-section).

    _____

13. Dr. Reddington administered anesthesia to Carla Corderez, a 47-year-old female, in preparation of the breast reconstruction with TRAM flap to be performed by Dr. Shapiro. Carla has a history of breast cancer and is postmastectomy.

    _____

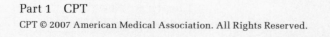

14. Dr. Harrison brought Jared Johannson, a 9-month-old male, into the OR for repair of his complete transposition of the great arteries under cardiopulmonary bypass. Pump oxygenation was used, and Jared was not expected to survive without the surgery. Dr. Leistner administered the anesthesia.

_____

15. Sharita Solington, a 76-year-old female, was given anesthesia by Dr. Welbill in preparation for the repair of her ventral hernia in her lower abdomen, to be performed by Dr. Chen. Sharita has uncontrolled diabetes mellitus and essential hypertension.

_____

YOU CODE IT! Simulation
Chapter 6. Anesthesia Coding

On the following pages, you will see physicians' notes documenting encounters with patients at our textbook's health care facility, Cipher, Victors, & Associates. Find the best anesthesia code for each of these reports. You are coding for the anesthesiologist.

CIPHER, VICTORS, & ASSOCIATES
A Complete Health Care Facility
234 MAIN STREET • ANYTOWN, FL 32711 • 407-555-1234

PATIENT:	CHEN, YVONNE
ACCOUNT/EHR #:	CHENYV001
Date:	10/15/08
Preoperative DX:	Locked right knee, rule out medial meniscus tear
Postoperative DX:	1. Grade 2 Tear, anterior, cruciate ligament
	2. Medial meniscus tear, anterior, horn
	3. Grade 2 Chondrosis, medial femoral condyle
Procedure:	1. Arthroscopy
	2. Partial anterior cruciate ligament debridement
	3. Partial medial meniscectomy
Attending Physician:	James I. Cipher, MD
Anesthesia:	General
Anesthesiologist:	Richard Kastor, MD

Indications: The patient is a 31-year-old female who was in her usual state of good health until about 10 days ago when she sustained a twisting injury to the right knee with inability to fully extend the knee, with pain and swelling.

Procedure: Estimated blood loss: None. Complications: None. Tourniquet time: See anesthesia notes. Specimens: None. Drains: None. Disposition: To the recovery room in stable condition.

Pt taken to surgery and was placed on the operating room table in the supine position. After adequate general anesthesia was administered, she received a gram of intravenous Kefzol preoperatively. A proximal thigh tourniquet was applied. Examination revealed no significant Lachman or drawer and a moderate effusion. No varus or valgus instability. Distal pulses intact. The right lower extremity was placed in the arthroscopic leg holder; shaved, prepped, and draped in the usual meticulously sterile fashion for lower extremity surgery. Esmarch exsanguinations of the limb were performed, and the tourniquet was inflated. Proximal medial, antero-medial, and anterolateral portals were fashioned. A systematic evaluation of the knee was performed. The undersurface of the patella demonstrated normal tracking with no chondrosis.

The suprapatellar pouch, medial, and lateral gutters were well within normal limits and in the notch a grade 2 tear of the anterior cruciate ligament was identified. There were some bloody fragments of the ACL that seemed to be impinging in the medial compartment. This was meticulously debrided. Approximately 50% of the ACL appeared to be intact. Attention was turned to the lateral compartment. The articular surface of the meniscus was normal. On the medial side, a grade 2 lesion in medial femoral condyle, lateral side, was noted. This was not debrided. As well as an anterior tear of the medial meniscus which was frayed and torn, and was another potential source of impingement. This was meticulously debrided to a smooth, stable mechanical limb, and the wound was irrigated and closed with 4-0 nylon simple interrupted sutures. Xeroform, 4x 4s, Webril and Ace bandage from the tips of the toes to the groin completed the sterile dressing. There were no intraoperative or immediate postoperative complications. The prognosis is good, although may be limited by potential for arthritis and instability in the future.

Richard Kastor, MD

RK/mg   D: 10/15/08 09:50:16   T: 10/23/08 12:55:01

Find the best, most appropriate anesthesia code.

CIPHER, VICTORS, & ASSOCIATES
A Complete Health Care Facility
234 MAIN STREET • ANYTOWN, FL 32711 • 407-555-1234

PATIENT: MASTERSON, ROBERT
ACCOUNT/EHR #:   MASTRO001
Date: 10/21/08
Preoperative DX: C5–C6 and C6–C7 herniated nucleus pulposus
Postoperative DX: Same

Procedure: C5–C6 and C6–C7 anterior cervical diskectomy and fusion with cadaver bone and plate

Attending Physician: James I. Cipher, MD
Anesthesia: General endotracheal
Anesthesiologist: Richard Kastor, MD

Indications: The patient is a 38-year-old male with a history of neck and arm pain. MRI scan showed disk herniation at C5–C6 and C6–C7. The patient failed conservative measures and was subsequently set up for surgery.

Procedure: The patient was taken to the operating room. The pt was induced and an endotracheal tube was placed. A Foley catheter was placed. The pt was given preoperative antibiotics. The pt was placed in slight extension. The left neck was prepped and draped in the usual manner. A linear incision was made above the C6 vertebral body. The platysma was divided. Dissection was continued medial to the sternocleidomastoid to the prevertebral fascia. The longus colli were cauterized and elevated. The C5–C6 disk space was addressed first. A retractor was placed. A large anterior osteophyte was removed with a large Leksell and drill. Distraction pins were then placed. The disk space was drilled out. Large bone spurs were drilled posteriorly. The posterior longitudinal ligament was removed. A free fragment was removed from beneath the ligament. The dura was visualized. A piece of bank bone was measured and slightly countersunk. The C6–C7 disk space was then addressed. Distraction pins were placed. A large anterior osteophyte was removed with a large Leksell and drill. The disk space was drilled out. Large bone spurs were drilled posteriorly. The Kerrison punch was used to remove the posterior longitudinal ligament. The dura was visualized. A piece of bank bone was in the C5, 1 in the C6, and 2 in the C7 vertebral bodies. The locking screws were tightened. The wound was irrigated. A drain was placed. The platysma was approximated with simple interrupted Vicryl. The dressing was applied. The patient was placed in a soft collar. The patient tolerated the procedure without difficulty. All counts were correct at the end of the case. The patient was extubated and transferred to recovery.

Richard Kastor, MD

RK/mg   D: 10/21/08 09:50:16   T: 10/23/08 12:55:01

Find the best, most appropriate anesthesia code.

_____

_____

_____

CIPHER, VICTORS, & ASSOCIATES
A Complete Health Care Facility
234 MAIN STREET • ANYTOWN, FL 32711 • 407-555-1234

PATIENT: SORENSON, GILBERT
ACCOUNT/EHR #:   SOREGI001
Date: 11/7/08
Preoperative DX: Inguinal hernia, right
Postoperative DX: Inguinal hernia, right, direct and indirect

Procedure: Repair of right inguinal hernia with mesh

Attending Physician: James I. Cipher, MD
Anesthesia: General
Anesthesiologist: Richard Kastor, MD

Procedure: The patient is a 45-year-old male and was taken to the operating room, and prepped in the usual sterile fashion. After satisfactory anesthesia, a transverse incision was made above the inguinal ligament and carried down to the fascia of the external oblique, which was then opened and the cord was mobilized. The ilio-inguinal nerve was identified and protected. A relatively large indirect hernia was found. However, there was an extension of the hernia, such that one could definitely tell there had been a long-standing hernia here that probably had enlarged fairly recently. The posterior wall, however, was quite dilated and without a great deal of tone and bulging as well, and probably fit the criteria for a hernia by itself. Nonetheless, the hernia sac was separated from the cord structures, and a high ligation was done with a purse string suture of 2-0 silk and a suture ligature of the same material prior to amputating the sac. The posterior wall was repaired with Marlex mesh, which was sewn in place in the usual manner, anchoring two sutures at the public tubercle tissue, taking one lateral up the rectus sheath and one lateral along the shelving border of Poupart's ligament past the internal ring. The mesh had been incised laterally to accommodate the internal ring. Several sutures were used to tack the mesh down superiorly and laterally to the transversalis fascia. Then the two limbs of the mesh were brought together lateral to the internal ring and secured to the shelving border of Poupart's ligament. The mesh was irrigated with Gentamicin solution. The subcutaneous tissue was closed with fine Vicryl, as was the internal oblique. Marcaine was infiltrated in the subcutaneous tissue and skin. The wound was closed with fine nylon. The patient tolerated the procedure well.

Richard Kastor, MD

RK/mg   D: 11/7/08 09:50:16   T: 11/11/08 12:55:01

Find the best, most appropriate anesthesia code.

_____

_____

_____

PATIENT: HAVERSTROM, OLIVIA
ACCOUNT/EHR #:   HAVEOL001
Date: 11/15/08
Preoperative DX: Chronic cholelithiasis
Postoperative DX: Chronic cholelithiasis; subacute cholecystitis

Procedure: Laparoscopic cholecystectomy; intraoperative cholangiogram

Attending Physician: Valerie R. Victors, MD
Anesthesia: General endotracheal
Anesthesiologist: Richard Kastor, MD

Procedure: The patient, a 53-year-old female, was taken to the operating room. The pt was induced and an endo-tracheal tube was placed, and placed in the supine position. The abdomen was prepped and draped in the usual fashion. The pt had several previous lower midline incisions and right flank incision; therefore, the pneumoperito-neum was created via epigastric incision to the left of the midline with a Verres needle. After adequate pneumo-peritoneum, the 11-mm trocar was placed through the extended incision in the left epigastrium just to the left of the midline. The trocar was placed, and the laparoscope and camera were in place. Inspection of the peritoneal cavity revealed it to be free of adhesions, and an 11-mm trocar was then placed under direct vision through a small infraumbilical incision. The scope and camera were then moved to this position, and the gallbladder was easily visualized. The gallbladder was elevated, and Hartmann's pouch was grasped. Using a combination of sharp and blunt dissection, the cystic artery was identified. The gallbladder was somewhat tense and subacutely inflamed. Therefore, a needle was passed through the abdominal wall into the gallbladder, and the gallbladder was aspirated free until it collapsed. One of the graspers was held over this region to prevent any further leakage of bile. Again, direction was turned to the area of the triangle of Calot. The cystic duct was dissected free with sharp and blunt dissection. A small opening was made in the duct, and the cholangiogram catheter was passed. The cholangiogram revealed no stones or filling defects in the bile duct system. The biliary tree was normal. There was good flow into the duodenum, and the catheter was definitely in the cystic duct. The catheter was removed, and the cystic duct was ligated between clips, as was the systic artery. The gallbladder was then dis-sected free from the hepatic bed using electrocautery dissection, and it was removed from the abdomen through the umbilical port. Inspection of the hepatic bed noted that hemostasis was meticulous. The region of dissection was irrigated and aspirated dry. The trocars were removed, and the pneumoperitoneum was released. The inci-sions were closed with Steri-strips, and the umbilical fascial incision was closed with 2-0 Maxon. The patient tol-erated the procedure well; there were no complications. She was returned to the recovery room awake and alert.

Richard Kastor, MD

RK/mg   D: 11/15/08 09:50:16   T: 11/19/08 12:55:01

Find the best, most appropriate anesthesia code.

_____

_____

_____

CIPHER, VICTORS, & ASSOCIATES
A Complete Health Care Facility
234 MAIN STREET • ANYTOWN, FL 32711 • 407-555-1234

PATIENT: ANDERSON, WAYNE
ACCOUNT/EHR #:   ANDEWA001
Date: 12/1/08
Preoperative DX: Sensory deficit of common digital nerve; tendon laceration
Postoperative DX: Same

Procedure: Repair of digital nerve, right hand
                             Repair of tendon laceration

Attending Physician: Valerie R. Victors, MD
Anesthesia: General
Anesthesiologist: Richard Kastor, MD

Indications: The patient is an 18-year-old male who was stabbed in the right hand during a street fight. Examination showed a sensory deficit of the thumb and index finger due to an injury to the common digital nerve, and a tendon laceration involving the abductor pollicis and first dorsal interosseous. He was taken immediately to the operating room for repair.

Procedure: The patient was taken to the operating room. General anesthesia was administered, a tourniquet was applied, and the wound was explored. The common digital nerve to the thumb was identified and found to be divided at the level just proximal to the first metacarpal. The digital nerve to the radial aspect of the index finger was also divided. The abductor pollicis and the first dorsal interosseous tendons were then repaired with 3-0 Vicryl to the fascia.

    Following this, both digital nerves were repaired using interrupted 9-0 Nylon, suturing epineurium to the epineurium. When completed, the wound was thoroughly irrigated with saline solution and the skin was closed with interrupted Ethilon. A dorsal splint was applied to the thumb and remains in IP flexion at about 30 degrees and slight adduction. Tourniquet time totaled 190 minutes.

Richard Kastor, MD

RK/mg   D: 12/1/08 09:50:16   T: 12/4/08 12:55:01

Find the best, most appropriate anesthesia code.

_____

_____

_____

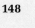

Surgery Coding, Part 1:

The Global Surgical Package, Surgical Modifiers, and Surgery Guidelines–Integumentary System

7

KEY TERMS

Complex closure (repair)

Donor area (site)

Excision

Full-thickness

Global period

Harvesting

Intermediate closure (repair)

Recipient area (site)

Simple closure (repair)

Standard of care

LEARNING OUTCOMES

- Interpret the guidelines for coding surgical procedures.
- Determine which services are included in the global surgical package.
- Identify unusual services and treatments and report them accurately.
- Distinguish between biopsies, excisions, and wound repair.
- Apply the guidelines to determine the best, most appropriate code.
- Decide how and when to use modifiers.

General surgeons' offices

Cardiologists' offices

Neurologists' offices

Plastic/reconstructive surgeons' offices

Colorectal surgeons' offices

Thoracic surgeons' offices

Nephrologists' offices

Hand surgeons' offices

Podiatrists' offices

Ophthalmologists' offices

Vascular surgeons' offices

Maxillofacial surgeons' offices

Surgical oncologists' offices

EMPLOYMENT OPPORTUNITIES

Typically, a surgical procedure can be performed in any one of several locations: the physician's office, an ambulatory care center, or a hospital. Of course, the location will most often be determined by the intensity or complexity of the procedure. You certainly would not expect an entire operating room at the hospital to be used for a physician repairing a simple laceration (cut), and no one could imagine agreeing to have a heart transplant in a physician's office. As a coding specialist, your responsibilities will vary, depending upon where you work, when it comes to coding surgical procedures. In addition, there may be more than one coding specialist involved reporting in one procedure.

Coding operative reports and procedure notes becomes easier with experience because the longer you work for a physician or facility, the more you will learn about the procedures and services. Experience will train you to decipher which services are included in procedures and which are not.

Throughout this chapter and the next, the guidelines and specifications for coding the various types of surgical and non-surgical procedures are reviewed.

THE SURGICAL PACKAGE

One of the trickiest portions of coding surgical events is distinguishing which services and procedures are included in the code and which services and procedures might need to be coded separately for additional reimbursement. While the services included in each surgical protocol may vary with the procedure itself, some elements are already integrated in most CPT codes.

Services Always Included

CODING TIP »»

The Global Surgical Package is the same package of services as described here, and in your Surgery Guidelines under the subheading, "CPT Surgical Package Definition."

CODING TIP »»

Remember that an encounter that ends with an agreement to have surgery is coded with an E/M code appended with modifier 57.

Let's begin by reviewing services that are *always included* in the CPT surgical procedure code.

Once the physician and patient agree to move forward with the operation or procedure, the surgical package includes the following elements.

1. *Evaluation and management encounters provided* after *the decision to have surgery.* These visits may begin the day prior to the surgical procedure (for more complex procedures) or the day of the procedure (for minor procedures), as needed.

2. *Local infiltration, metacarpal/metatarsal/digital block, or topical anesthesia.* You learned about the different types of anesthesia in Chap. 6. The surgical package includes specific types of local and regional anesthesia services and only when they are provided by the surgeon (the same professional who will be performing the procedure).

3. *The operation itself, along with any services normally considered a part of the procedure being performed.* This would include supplies as well as applying sutures, bandages, casts, etc., to enable the patient to leave the operating room safely after the procedure.

4. *Immediate postoperative care.* The care includes assessing the patient in the recovery area; attending to any complications exhibited by the patient (not including any additional trips to the operating room); dictating or writing the operative notes; talking with the patient, the patient's family, and other health care professionals; and writing orders.

5. *Follow-up care.* It includes postoperative visits; pain management; dressing changes; removal of sutures, staples, tubes, casts, etc.; and any other services considered to be the **standard of care,** during the **global period** for the specific surgical procedure. However, be careful. Some procedures may require a longer period of postoperative care by the surgeon. The period is determined by the accepted standard of care guidelines for each specific procedure and the details regarding the particular patient's health.

6. *Supplies provided in a physician's office.* With a few specific exceptions, included supplies are determined by the insurance carrier.

Services Not Included

Some elements that are commonly performed when a patient is going to have, or has had surgery, are *not included* in the surgical package. When such services and/or procedures are performed, you must code them separately.

1. *Diagnostic tests and procedures.* Tests or procedures that the physician needs to confirm the medical necessity for the surgery or investigate other issues related to the surgery are coded separately.

EXAMPLE

Diagnostic tests and procedures include biopsies, blood tests, and x-rays.

2. *Postoperative therapies.* Examples of postoperative therapies include immunosuppressive therapy after an organ transplant or chemotherapy after cancer surgery.

3. *A more comprehensive version of the original procedure.* If the physician attempted to use a less extensive procedure first that was not sufficient to treat the patient, the second, more extensive procedure would be coded separately, with its own surgical package; it is not an extension of the first procedure. Also, the CPT code for the second event would be appended with modifier 58.

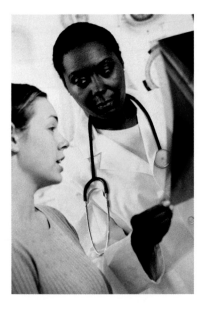

EXAMPLE

Dr. Jeppapai performed a lumpectomy on Sandra Wattell's left breast. The biopsy of the tissue removed during the lumpectomy showed that the malignancy had spread farther through the breast. Dr. Jeppapai had to take Sandra back into the OR for a simple, complete mastectomy. The code for the mastectomy is appended with modifier 58.

19301 Mastectomy, partial (e.g., lumpectomy, tylectomy, quadrantectomy, segmentectomy);

19303 Mastectomy, simple, complete; staged or related procedure or service by the same physician during the postoperative period

CPT © 2007 American Medical Association. All Rights Reserved.

4. *Staged or multipart procedures.* Each stage or operation has its own surgical package and global period for aftercare. You must add modifier 58 to the second, and all following, procedure code.

58 **Staged or related procedure or service by the same physician during the postoperative period.** It may be necessary to indicate that the performance of a procedure or service during the postoperative period of the first procedure, was planned as a staged, series of procedures (*see Services Not Included #4*) or a more extensive version of the original procedure (*see Services Not Included #3*). This modifier is not to be used for procedures to treat complications resulting from the first procedure (*see Services Not Included #5*).

EXAMPLE

Jacob Simmons, a 29-year-old male, suffered a fracture to his upper arm that severely damaged the radial head of his right humerus. Dr. Bearmann decides to do a bone graft to support the healing process of the fracture first, and follow that with a second surgical procedure—an arthroplasty. This is a staged, or multipart surgical procedure.

24665 Open treatment of radial head or neck fracture, includes internal fixation or radial head excision, when performed;

24365–58 Arthroplasty, radial head; staged or related procedure or service by the same physician during the postoperative period

5. *Management of postoperative complications that require additional surgery.* As you may remember from *Services Always Included #4* of the surgical package, the physician's attention to any postoperative complications is included in the original package *unless* those complications require the patient to return to the operating room. In such cases, you must use a modifier with the CPT code for the procedure performed.

76 **Repeat procedure by the same physician.** It may be necessary to indicate that a procedure or service was repeated subsequent to the original procedure or service. This circumstance may be reported by adding modifier 76 to the repeated procedure or service.

78 **Unplanned Return to the Operating/Procedure Room by the same physician following initial procedure for a related procedure during the postoperative period.** When the physician performs a different procedure to treat a complication of the first procedure, you must add this modifier to the correct CPT code for the new procedure.

EXAMPLE

MaryAnn Mason, a 15-year-old female, was burned on her left forearm when she missed catching a flaming baton during cheerleading practice. Five days ago, Dr. Loginella applied a skin allograft to the burned area. MaryAnn is admitted today because the graft is not healing properly, and Dr. Loginella is going to apply a new allograft of 95 sq cm.

15300-76 Allograft skin for temporary wound closure, trunk, arms, legs; first 100 sq. cm or less; repeat procedure by the same physician during the postoperative period

77 **Repeat procedure by another physician.** The physician may need to indicate that a basic procedure or service performed by another physician had to be repeated. This situation may be reported by adding modifier 77 to the repeated procedure/service.

Joseph Johnson, a 17-year-old male, was stabbed in the chest during a fight. Dr. Sanger performed a complex repair of a 6-cm laceration of the chest. The next day, Dr. Sanger left for a medical conference. The guy who stabbed Joseph showed up at the hospital, and Joseph got out of bed, against doctor's orders, and engaged in another fight, ripping open his stitches. Dr. Addison, filling in for Dr. Sanger, had to take Joseph back into the OR and redo the repair. Dr. Addison will send the claim with the following code:

13101-77 Repair, complex, trunk; 2.6 cm to 7.5 cm; repeat procedure by another physician

6. *Unrelated surgical procedure during the postoperative period.* If the same physician must perform an unrelated surgical procedure during the postoperative period, you have to include a modifier to explain that this procedure has nothing to do with the first.

79 **Unrelated procedure or service by the same physician during the postoperative period.** This may be used for any treatment or service provided by the same physician to the same patient, as long as it has nothing to do with the surgery.

Elyse Codwell, a 37-year-old female, had a gastric bypass performed by Dr. Rosenberg 10 days ago. She comes to see him today because she has a fever and pain radiating across her abdomen. Dr. Rosenberg examines her, calls an ambulance, and takes her to the hospital and up to the OR where he performs an appendectomy to remove her ruptured appendix. The global postoperative period for a gastric bypass is 90 days. Dr. Rosenberg performed Elyse's appendectomy during the postoperative period for the bypass, and it had nothing to do with the first procedure. Therefore, our correct code would be

44960-79 Appendectomy; for ruptured appendix with abscess or generalized peritonitis; unrelated procedure or service by the same physician during the postoperative period

7. *Supplies.* In certain cases, for certain procedures performed in a physician's office, a separate code is permitted for supplies, such as a surgical tray, casting supplies, splints, and drugs. You have to check the reimbursement rules for the specific third-party payer.

99070 Supplies and materials (except spectacles), provided by the physician over and above those usually included with the office visit or other services rendered (list drugs, trays, supplies, or materials provided)

SERVICES PROVIDED BY MORE THAN ONE PHYSICIAN

It is expected that the same physician will provide all of the surgical package's elements. This is an umbrella that only covers one health care professional.

Occasionally, however, more than one physician will be involved in providing all the necessary services for one patient having one operation. In such cases, modifiers explain to the third-party payer who did what and when.

54 **Surgical care only.** You must add this modifier to the correct CPT surgical procedure code when your physician is only going to perform the procedure itself, and not provide or be involved in any preoperative or postoperative care of the patient.

55 **Postoperative management only.** This modifier is added to the CPT code for the surgical procedure included on a claim from the physician who only cares for the patient after the operation.

56 **Preoperative management only.** When a physician, other than the surgeon who performed the procedure, cares for the patient from the decision to have surgery, up to but not including the operation itself, modifier 56 is appended to the CPT code for the procedure.

LET'S CODE IT! SCENARIO

Rahima Gonzalez, a 43-year-old female, was on vacation, hiking through the mountains, when she fell over a log and wrenched her knee very badly. She was flown to the nearest hospital and placed under the care of Dr. Peterman. After the diagnostic tests were completed, Dr. Peterman recommended arthroscopic surgery to treat the knee. Dr. Peterman called in Dr. Mathews, an orthopedic surgeon, to perform the procedure. Dr. Mathews performed a surgical arthroscopy and repaired the medial meniscus. Immediately after the surgery, Rahima flew home, and she went to her family physician, Dr. Donaldson, for the follow-up appointments.

Let's Code It!

The notes indicate that Dr. Peterman, Dr. Matthews, and Dr. Donaldson were all involved, to some extent, in caring for Rahima during the procedure—*surgical arthroscopy* and *repair of the medial meniscus*. Let's go to the alphabetic index and look up the procedure.

Find *arthroscopy.* As you go down the list, you will see the subcategories Diagnostic and Surgical. We know from the notes that this was

Part 1   CPT
CPT © 2007 American Medical Association. All Rights Reserved.

surgical. Continue down and find the anatomical site for this procedure: Knee . . . 29871–29889. Indented under knee, you will find additional listings that don't really match, so let's go to the codes shown next to knee and begin at 29871.

29871 Arthroscopy, knee, surgical; for infection, lavage and drainage

The description is correct, up to the semicolon. So continue down the page to find any additional information that might be applicable to the case, according to our documentation. (*Remember:* We read up to the semicolon on the code, because it is at the margin, and then finish the description with each indented description.)

Continue reading until you see:

29882   with meniscus repair (medial OR lateral)

The complete description of this code is:

29882 Arthroscopy, knee, surgical; with meniscus repair (medial OR lateral)

This matches our notes exactly, doesn't it? It does! Good job!

As you have learned, the surgical package for this procedure includes all the services and treatments that Rahima received. However, instead of just one physician, Rahima actually had three doctors caring for her throughout. Each physician will send his or her own claim form in an effort to get paid for the services he or she provided. You need to supply some explanation to the third-party payer, so it can understand receiving three claim forms for one procedure provided to the one patient.

- Dr. Peterman will have the 29882-56 modifier to indicate he only provided the preoperative care.
- Dr. Mathews will have the 29882-54 modifier to indicate he only performed the surgery.
- Dr. Donaldson will have the 29882-55 modifier to indicate she only provided the postoperative care

UNUSUAL SERVICES AND TREATMENTS

Every service and treatment or procedure has an industry standard of care. Included in the assessment of each service is a calculation of how much work and how long it will take to complete the procedure. It is all part of the formula used by third-party payers to determine how much to pay the health care professional. As you might expect, though, particularly in health care, things do not always go exactly as planned. There may be an issue with a patient that requires more work on the physician's part. When this happens, the physician should receive additional compensation. Therefore, you have to attach the modifier 22 to the procedure code to identify an unusual circumstance. You also have to attach documentation that fully explains the circumstances.

- 22 **Increased procedural service.** The modifier 22 can be used with any procedure code in the CPT book to indicate that the service provided was substantially greater than normally required.

Douglas Bamberger, a 15-year-old male, is 5 ft. 6 in., 365 lb. Dr. Oswald performs a partial colectomy with anastomosis. The procedure, however, takes several hours longer than usual due to the fact that Douglas is morbidly obese.

You Code It!

Go through the steps of coding, and determine the codes that should be reported for this encounter between Dr. Oswald and Douglas Bamberger.

Step 1: Read the case completely.

Step 2: Abstract the notes: Which key words can you identify relating to the procedures performed?

_____

Step 3: Query the provider, if necessary.

Step 4: Diagnosis: Ulcerative colitis; morbid obesity.

Step 5: Code the procedure(s).

_____

Step 6: Link the procedure codes to at least one diagnosis code.

Step 7: Back code to double-check your choices.

Answer

Did you find the correct code to be:

44140-22 Colectomy, partial; with anastomosis; increased procedural service

Then you should attach a letter of explanation with the claim to explain the condition that complicated the procedure.

SURGERY GUIDELINES

Separate Procedure

Throughout the CPT book, you will see code descriptions that include the notation "separate procedure." Such services and treatments are generally performed along with a group of other procedures. When this happens, you will be able to find a combination, or bundled, code that includes all the treatments together. However, this particular procedure can also be performed alone. If so, you would use the code for the "separate procedure."

LET'S CODE IT! SCENARIO

Dr. Torres performed a repair of the secondary tendon flexor in Bobby Morton's right foot. He first performed an open tenotomy and then did the repair with a free graft.

The *repair* that Dr. Torres performed on Bobby Morton actually includes the *tenotomy*. Therefore, we will use the one combination code for the entire procedure.

Go to the alphabetic index, and look up the procedure *repair*. Under repair, let's find the anatomical site *foot*. Under foot, let's find the part of the foot that was treated: *tendon*. The index gives us the code range 28200–28226, 28238.

Let's go to the first one.

28200 Repair, tendon, flexor, foot; primary or secondary, without free graft, each tendon

28202   secondary with free graft, each tendon (includes obtaining graft)

It seems we have found the code description that matches the physician's notes.

28202 Repair, tendon, flexor, foot; secondary with free graft, each tendon (includes obtaining graft)

Great job!

Had Dr. Torres performed the tenotomy only, the correct code would be:

28230 Tenotomy, open, tendon flexor; foot, single or multiple tendon(s) (separate procedure)

On occasion, you may find that the "separate procedure" is performed along with other procedures, not those in the bundle. Should this be the situation, you have to add the modifier 59 to the "separate procedure" code.

59 **Distinct procedural service.** When the physician performs a procedure or service that is not normally performed with the other procedures or services, modifier 59 should be added to the second procedure.

LET'S CODE IT! SCENARIO

Barbara Bracken brought her daughter, Darlene, a 5-year-old female, to her pediatrician's office after they had attended a friend's birthday party in the park. After a cursory examination, Dr. Jackson removed a jellybean from Darlene's nose. Then Dr. Jackson removed a splinter from Darlene's hand.

Dr. Jackson *removed a jellybean* and a *splinter* from Darlene.

Go to the alphabetic index, and look up the first procedure *removal*. Under removal, let's find the key term. In this case, Dr. Jackson removed a jellybean, which is a foreign body, from Darlene's nose, so we look up *foreign body*. Under foreign body, let's find the anatomical site *nose*. The index suggests code 30300.

Let's go look at the code's description.

30300 Removal foreign body, intranasal; office type procedure

Good. Now let's do the second procedure.

Go to the alphabetic index, and look up the second procedure *removal*. Under removal, let's find the key term. In this case, Dr. Jackson removed a *foreign body* (the splinter) from Darlene's hand. Under foreign body, let's find the anatomical site *hand*.

So, let's go back to the list under removal, and find the literal anatomical site *subcutaneous tissue*. The index gives us the code range 10120–10121. Go to these codes in the numeric listing and read the descriptions.

10120 Incision and removal of foreign body, subcutaneous tissues; simple

Great! We have one more point to address. And that is the removal of the splinter actually had nothing to do with the removal of the jellybean. Without an explanation, the third-party payer may think that these two procedures, that have nothing to do with each other, must be reported in error. To confirm that this is not an error, and these two procedures were actually performed on the same patient at the same encounter, you have to add the modifier 59. The second code will be reported as:

10120-59 Incision and removal of foreign body, subcutaneous tissues; simple; distinct procedural service

The claim form you prepare for Dr. Jackson's services to Darlene Bracken for this encounter will include two codes: 30300 and 10120-59.

CODING TIP »»

Technically, Dr. Jackson did not remove the splinter from Darlene's hand; he removed it from her subcutaneous tissue (underneath her skin).

INTEGUMENTARY SYSTEM

Biopsies

Although a specimen of tissue may be excised, shave removed, or destroyed and then sent to pathology for testing, it does not automatically indicate the need for a separate or special biopsy code. The guidelines state that you would only use a biopsy procedure code when the procedure is conducted individually, or distinctly separate from any other procedure or service performed at the same time.

LET'S CODE IT! SCENARIO

Ethan Monahan, a 73-year-old male, came to see Dr. Greenberg for the removal of some skin tags on his left cheek. Dr. Greenberg administered a local anesthetic and then electrosurgically destroyed the nine tags. The tags were sent to pathology for testing.

Let's Code It!

Go to the alphabetic index, and let's find our key term for the procedure: *removal*. Now, what did the physician remove? *Skin tags*. Let's find that indented under Removal . . . skin tags . . . 11200–11201. Turn to the numeric listing of the book, in the Surgery section, and look for those codes. You will see:

11200 Removal of skin tags, multiple fibrocutaneous tags, any area; up to and including 15 lesions

+11201   each additional ten lesions (list separately in addition to code for primary procedure)

(Use 11201 in conjunction with 11200.)

The next question is, How many skin tags (lesions) did the physician remove from Ethan's face? When you reread the notes, you will see that he removed *nine tags.* This confirms the correct code is 11200.

The notes also indicate that the lesions were sent to pathology, meaning a biopsy. Should we add another code for the biopsy? Remember that the guidelines state that a separate code for the biopsy is only used when the biopsy has its own procedure, not a part of another service. In this case, the biopsy was a part of the removal of the skin tags and does not require a second code.

Excisions

When the physician removes a lesion from a patient, you must code the **excision** of each lesion separately. Codes for the excision, or **full-thickness** removal, of lesions are determined first by the anatomical site from where the lesion was removed and then by the size of the lesion removed. The code for the excision includes the administration of a local anesthetic and a **simple closure** of the excision site, as mentioned in the definition.

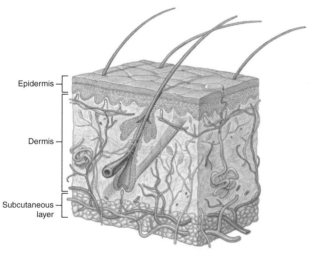

Epidermis

Dermis

Subcutaneous layer

To correctly measure what was excised, you must look at the dimensions of the lesion itself *plus* a proper margin around the lesion. That will give you the total amount actually excised by the physician and lead you to the correct code. In order to find the correct size of the lesion excised, we must do the following: Add the size of the lesion (2.0 cm—the largest measurement of the lesion) *plus* the size of the margin (0.2 cm) added twice (margins *all around* mean that the diameter will have a margin on each side).

The formula is

Coded size of lesion = size of lesion + (size of margins × 2)

Excision

The full-thickness removal of a lesion, including margins; includes (for coding purposes) a simple closure.

Full-thickness

A measure that extends from the epidermis to the connective tissue layer of the skin.

Simple closure (repair)

A method of sealing an opening in the skin (epidermis or dermis), involving only one layer. It includes the administration of a local anesthesia and/or chemical or electrocauterization of a wound not closed.

««« CODING TIP

1 centimeter (cm) = 10 millimeters (mm) = 0.4 inch

1 millimeter (mm) = 0.1 centimeter (cm) = 0.04 inch

1 inch (in.) = 2.54 cm

Dr. Vitali excised a lesion measuring 2.0 cm by 1.0 cm, with 0.2-cm margins all around, from Benita Corraldo's neck. The pathology report confirmed that the lesion was benign.

Let's Code It!

Go to the alphabetic index, and find the suggested code or codes.

Look up *excision* for the procedure and then *neck* for the anatomical site, right? Well, you will see that there is no listing for *neck* under *excision.* What should you do now? Analyze what you see in the physician's notes. Where exactly is the lesion? It isn't really on her *neck;* it is on her *skin.* So look at *excision, skin.* Aha! Under *skin,* you will see *lesion.* Good. And now, check *benign,* as per the notes. This leads us to the code range of 11400–11471.

When you go to the numeric listing, you will see the description for the first code in our range.

> 11400 Excision, benign lesion including margins, except skin tag (unless listed elsewhere), trunk, arms or legs; excised diameter 0.5 cm or less

The description for code 11400 matches our physician's notes except for the mention of the anatomical sites: trunk, arms, or legs. Our patient had the lesion on her neck. Continue looking down the listings, and take a look at the description for code 11420.

> 11420 Excision, benign lesion including margins, except skin tag (unless listed elsewhere), scalp, neck, hands, feet, genitalia; excised diameter 0.5 cm or less

This matches our physician's notes. Next, you must determine the size of the lesion. Remember our formula

Coded size of lesion = size of lesion + (size of margins × 2)

To the size of the lesion (2.0 cm, which is its largest measurement), we add the size of the margin (0.2 cm) times 2 (margins *all around* mean that the diameter will have a margin on each side). With the figures in place, our formula becomes

$$\text{Coded size of lesion} = 2.0 \text{ cm} + (0.2 \text{ cm} \times 2)$$
$$= 2.4 \text{ cm}$$

Therefore, the total size of the lesion excised is 2.4 cm. Now find the descriptions indented underneath 11420.

> 11423 Excision, benign lesion including margins, except skin tag (unless listed elsewhere), scalp, neck, hands, feet, genitalia; excised diameter 2.1 to 3.0 cm

This matches exactly. We have found our code: 11423.

You may find that the physician's notes indicate that the excision of the lesion was complicated or unusual in some way. Should this be the situation, remember to add modifier 22 to the procedure code. The difficulty is related to the process of excising the lesion, not the closure.

If the closure of the excision site becomes more involved than a simple closure, and is described as an **intermediate** or **complex closure,** the

---

CODING TIP »»

Some surgeons include the measurement of the margins in their operative notes. In other cases, you may need to review the pathologist's report to determine an accurate measurement.

Intermediate closure (repair)

A multilevel method of sealing an opening in the skin involving one or more of the deeper layers of the skin. (*Note:* Single-layer closure of heavily contaminated wounds that required extensive cleaning or removal of particulate matter also constitutes intermediate repair.)

Complex closure (repair)

A method of sealing an opening in the skin involving a multilayered closure and a reconstructive procedure such as scar revision, debridement, or retention sutures.

---

repair is no longer included in the code for the excision procedure. You have to code a more intricate closure separately.

LET'S CODE IT! SCENARIO

Dr. Simmons excised a lesion measuring 3.1 by 3.0 cm, with 0.3-cm margins on each side, from Raymond Fulbright's left forearm. Due to the lesion's proximity to the wrist bone, performing the excision took more exactness than the typical procedure. Finally, the lesion was successfully removed. The pathology report confirmed that the lesion was benign.

Let's Code It!

The notes tell you that Dr. Simmons performed an *excision; skin; lesion; benign.* The alphabetic index suggests the code range of 11400–11471.

When you go to the numeric listing, you will need to look for the code that identifies the correct anatomical site of the lesion that was excised: *forearm.* You find the following:

> 11400 Excision, benign lesion including margins, except skin tag (unless listed elsewhere), trunk, arms or legs; excised diameter 0.5 cm or less

The first code matches perfectly. Now, you must determine the exact size of the lesion plus margins that was excised. The largest measurement of the lesion is 3.1 cm, and the margins are 0.3 cm. Fit the numbers into our formula:

$$\text{Coded size of lesion} = 3.1 \text{ cm} + (0.3 \text{ cm} \times 2) = 3.7 \text{ cm}$$

The coded size will direct you to the correct code for our procedure:

> 11404 Excision, benign lesion including margins, except skin tag (unless listed elsewhere), trunk, arms or legs; excised diameter 3.1 to 4.0 cm

Excellent! However, there is one other thing mentioned in the notes. The physician wrote that the "excision took more exactness than the typical procedure." The writing indicates that this was an *unusual procedure,* meaning that we must add the appropriate modifier. Our final correct code is 11404-22.

LET'S CODE IT! CASE SCENARIO

Dr. Burgoud excised a lesion measuring 2.1 by 3.0 cm, with 0.5-cm margins on each side, from Wanda Wainright's abdomen. Wanda is clinically obese, and the excess fatty tissue around the lesion required a complex closure of the excision site. The pathology report confirmed that the lesion was malignant.

Let's Code It!

The alphabetic index will direct you to a slightly different group of codes—*excision, skin, lesion, malignant*—giving us the code range of

11600–11646. Just as before, you will need to find the code in this range that identifies the correct anatomical location of the lesion.

11600 Excision, malignant lesion including margins, trunk, arms or legs; excised diameter 0.5 cm or less

The abdomen is a part of the trunk, so this code is OK. Next, you will need to add up the size of the lesion.

$$\text{Coded size of lesion} = 3.0 \text{ cm} + (0.5 \text{ cm} \times 2) = 4.0 \text{ cm}$$

The answer 4.0 cm brings us to the code:

11604 Excision, malignant lesion including margins, trunk, arms or legs; excised diameter 3.1 to 4.0 cm

Excellent! Wanda's case was not as complicated as Raymond's, so modifier 22 will not be required. However, Dr. Burgoud did note that Wanda's procedure "required a complex closure of the excision site." The guidelines tell us that only a simple closure is included in the excision code. A complex closure, just like an intermediate closure, is coded in addition to the code for the excision. So let's code it!

Go back to the alphabetic index and look up the key term *closure.* None of the indented descriptors seems to match, so you should investigate the code range shown next to the word *closure:* 12001–13160.

You will notice the heading immediately above the first code in the range: 12001. It reads "Repair–Simple." But we are looking for a complex closure, so let's continue down the page. The next section, above code 12031, is "Repair–Intermediate." This is closer to what we need, but not exact. Above code 13100, you find the heading you have been looking for: "Repair–Complex."

Remember that Wanda's lesion was located on her abdomen (trunk). Look at the codes in this section, and find the best code for the *complex closure* of her excision site.

13100 Repair, complex, trunk; 1.1 cm to 2.5 cm

Excellent! You have found the correct level of closure (repair) for the correct anatomical site (trunk). Now, you must find the correct size of the excision site. Our calculation totaled 4.0 cm, which brings us to the correct code:

13101 Repair, complex, trunk; 2.6 cm to 7.5 cm

Excellent! You now know that, for this one procedure on Wanda, the claim form will include the codes:

11604 Excision, malignant lesion including margins, trunk, arms or legs; excised diameter 3.1 to 4.0 cm

13101 Repair, complex, trunk; 2.6 cm to 7.5 cm

Good job!

Reexcision

In the case of malignant lesions, the pathology report may indicate that the physician did not cut around the lesion (the margins) widely enough to get all the malignancy. This may require an additional excision procedure to ensure that the entire tumor was removed.

If the reexcision is performed during the same operative session, then you must adjust the total size of the lesion being coded to include the new total measurement. You use just the one code, with the largest measurement shown in the operative or procedure notes.

If the reexcision is performed during a subsequent, or later, encounter, during the postoperative period, you have to attach modifier 58 to the correct procedure code. The reexcision to remove additional tissue around the original site during the postoperative period would directly apply to modifier 58's description: *more extensive than the original procedure.*

Wound Repair

When multiple wounds are repaired with the same complexity on the same anatomical site(s) as indicated by the code descriptor, add all the lengths together to use one code for the total repair.

»» CODING TIP

The multiple wound repair guideline differentiates wounds from lesions. Remember that with lesions, each lesion is coded separately. With wounds, you have one code for the total length of all wounds being repaired on the same anatomical site.

LET'S CODE IT! SCENARIO

Quentin Alexander, a 19-year-old male, got into a bar fight and sustained multiple wounds to his hand and arm. Dr. Havilland performed intermediate repair of a 5- by 2-cm wound and a 3.1- by 1-cm wound on Quentin's right hand and a simple repair to a 3.2- by 1-cm wound to his right forearm.

Let's Code It!

You can see by Dr. Havilland's notes that Quentin had two wounds, treated with intermediate closures, on his right hand, and one wound, with a simple repair, on his right forearm. These facts will lead you to the alphabetic index to look up *repair, wound, intermediate* (leading you to 12031–12057) and *repair, wound, simple* (12001–12021).

The intermediate repairs were done to the right *hand,* so turn to the numeric listing for the code range 12031–12057. Find the best code for the correct anatomical site.

> 12041 Layer closure of wounds of neck, hands, feet and/or external genitalia;
>   2.5 cm or less

Now, you must find the correct size of the wound or wounds being repaired (the first is 5 by 2 cm and the second 3.1 by 1 cm). You must match the anatomical sites: Quentin's hand has two wounds, one 5 cm × 2 cm and another 3.1 cm × 1 cm. Both of these wounds are on the hand and both of these wounds received intermediate repair. The guidelines state that because the wounds are on the same anatomic site as per the code description (*hands*), you must add them together. Therefore, add the two longest measurements together (5 cm + 3.1 cm), and we have 8.1 cm. This brings us to the correct code:

> 12044 Layer closure of wounds of neck, hands, feet and/or external genitalia;
>   7.6 cm to 12.5 cm

CPT © 2007 American Medical Association. All Rights Reserved.

Good job! Now, the last wound on Quentin's forearm is different. It is a simple repair, rather than an intermediate repair, and the wound is on his arm, not his hand. Therefore, the wound repair will have its own code. Follow the code descriptions, and see if you can come up with the correct answer. Did you get the following:

> 12002 Simple repair of superficial wounds of scalp, neck, axillae, external genitalia, trunk and/or extremities (including hands and feet); 2.6 cm to 7.5 cm

That's great! You did excellent work!

When multiple wound repairs are performed, the codes should be listed in order from the most complex to the simplest. All additional repairs, after the first, should have the modifier 51 appended to the procedure code.

EXAMPLE

Now that you know the guideline regarding multiple wound repairs, do you think any adjustments should be made to the claim form you are preparing for Dr. Havilland to be reimbursed for his work on Quentin? Yes, the codes will look like this:

> 12044 (The intermediate repair tells us this was the more severe or complicated procedure. Therefore, this code is first.)

> 12002-51 (This was the simple repair of a smaller wound, making it less complicated in this case. Therefore, the code is listed second and appended with the modifier 51.)

Debridement or decontamination of a wound is included in the code for the repair of that wound. However, if the contamination is so extensive that it requires extra time and effort, it should be coded separately. Also, if the debridement is performed and the wound is not closed or repaired during the same session, code the debridement separately.

YOU CODE IT! CASE STUDY

A woman was screaming in a parking lot and calling for help. She had accidentally locked her keys in the car, along with her infant son. It was a hot day, and she was very concerned about her child. Martin Hendry came along and used a rock to break a window on the other side of the car, reached in through the broken glass, and unlocked the door. Without question, Martin is a hero, but he also cut his wrist on the broken glass. At his physician's office, Dr. Albertson discovered that the cut (the skin and the subcutaneous tissue) was littered with tiny shards of glass. Dr. Albertson administered a local anesthetic. It took Dr. Albertson quite a long time to debride the wound of all the glass, before he sutured the 5.3-by 1.6-cm wound.

Go through the steps of coding, and determine the codes that should be reported for this encounter between Dr. Albertson and Martin Hendry.

Step 1: Read the case completely.

Step 2: Abstract the notes: Which key words can you identify relating to the procedures performed?

_____

Step 3: Query the provider, if necessary.

Step 4: Diagnosis: Laceration.

Step 5: Code the procedure(s).

_____

Step 6: Link the procedure codes to at least one diagnosis code.

Step 7: Back code to double-check your choices.

Answer

Did you find the correct code to be:

11042   Debridement; skin, and subcutaneous tissue

12002-51 Simple repair of superficial wounds of scalp, neck, axillae, external genitalia, trunk and/or extremities (including hands and feet); 2.6 cm to 7.5 cm; multiple procedures

Excellent! You are really learning how to code!

Skin Replacement Surgery and Flaps

The codes for skin grafts are determined by three aspects:

1. The size of the **recipient area** (the size of the wound to be grafted)
2. The location of the recipient area (the anatomical site)
3. The type of graft (e.g., pinch graft, split graft, full-thickness graft, etc.)

The codes include a simple debridement, or avulsion, of the recipient site.

Grafts can be taken, or **harvested,** from another part of the patient's body, from another body (a live donor), a cadaver (a deceased person), skin substitutes (e.g., neodermis, synthetic skin), or another species (e.g., a porcine graft). You have to know where the graft came from in order to determine the best, most appropriate code.

It is not uncommon for skin grafts to be planned, from the beginning, to be done in stages. When this is the case, the second and subsequent portions of the staged procedure should be appended with modifier 58. This is directly described in CPT's modifier 58 description: *planned prospectively at the time of the original procedure (staged).*

If the **donor site** requires a skin graft or a local flap to repair it, it should be coded as an additional procedure.

When evaluating the size of the wound that has been grafted, the measurement of *100 sq cm* (square centimeters) is used with patients

Recipient area (site)

The area or site of the body receiving a graft of skin or tissue.

Harvesting

The process of taking skin or tissue (on the same body or another).

Donor area (site)

The area or part of the body from which skin or tissue is removed with the intention of placing that skin or tissue in another area or body.

aged 10 and older. The code descriptor referring to a *percentage of the body area* only applies to patients under the age of 10.

EXAMPLE

15002 Surgical preparation or creation of recipient site by excision of open wounds, burn eschar, or scar (including subcutaneous tissues, or incisional release of scar contracture, trunk, arms, legs); first *100 sq cm* or *1% of body area of infants and children*

In the subheading relating to flaps and grafts, when the physician attaches a flap, either in transfer or to the final site, the anatomical sites identified in the code's description is the *recipient* site, not the donor site.

EXAMPLE

15732 Muscle, myocutaneous, or fasciocutaneous flap; *head and neck* (e.g., temporalis, masseter muscle, sternocleidomastoid, levator scapulae)

When a tube is formed to be used later, or when "delay" of flap is done before the transfer, the anatomical sites indicated in the code description refer to the *donor* site, not the recipient site.

EXAMPLE

15620 Delay of flap or sectioning of flap (division and inset); at forehead, cheeks, chin, mouth, neck, axillae, genitalia, hands or feet

When extensive immobilization is performed, such as large plaster casts or traction, the application of the immobilization device should be coded as a separate procedure. However, make note that the procedure codes in the range 15570–15738 already include small or standard immobilization, such as a sling or splint.

YOU CODE IT! CASE STUDY

Rudy Fetland, an 11-year-old male, had burn eschar on his face from an accident. Dr. Imatione performed a surgical preparation of the area. Two days later, Dr. Imatione applied a dermal autograft to the 30 sq cm area.

You Code It!

Read Dr. Imatione's notes on the procedures performed on Rudy. Find the best, most appropriate code or codes to report all of Dr. Imatione's work.

Step 1: Read the case completely.

Step 2: Abstract the notes: Which key words can you identify relating to the procedures performed?

Step 3: Query the provider, if necessary.

Step 4: Diagnosis: Burn eschar.

Step 5: Code the procedure(s).

Step 6: Link the procedure codes to at least one diagnosis code.

Step 7: Back code to double-check your choices.

Answer

Did you find codes?

15004 Surgical preparation or creation of recipient site by excision of open wounds, burn eschar, or scar (including subcutaneous tissues), or incisional release of scar contracture, face, scalp, eyelids, mouth, neck, ears, orbits, genitalia, hands, feet, and/or multiple digits; first 100 sq cm or 1% of body area of infants and children

15135-58 Dermal autograft, face, scalp, eyelids, mouth, neck, ears, orbits, genitalia, hands, feet, and/or multiple digits; first 100 sq cm or less, or 1% of body area of infants and children; staged procedure

Great work!

Destruction

Destruction is the term used for the removal of diseased or unwanted tissue from the body by surgical or other means, such as surgical curettement (scraping for the purposes of removing abnormal tissue), laser treatment, electrosurgery, chemical treatment, or cryosurgery. The codes in the destruction subheading of the surgical section include the administration of local anesthesia.

LET'S CODE IT! SCENARIO

Frank Mulrooney, a 43-year-old male, came to see Dr. Johnston, his podiatrist, for the removal of a benign plantar wart from the sole of his left foot. Dr. Johnston administered a local anesthetic and then destroyed the wart using a chemosurgical technique. A protective bandage was applied to the foot, and Frank was sent home with an appointment to return in one week for a follow-up check.

Let's Code It!

The notes indicate that Frank had a *benign plantar wart* which Dr. Johnston *destroyed* using *chemosurgery*.

Let's go to the alphabetic index and look up *destruction*.

Under destruction, you will see an alphabetical list that includes both anatomical sites as well as skin conditions, such as cysts and lesions. You know from the notes that Dr. Johnston destroyed a wart on Frank's foot. There are no listings for foot or sole of foot. However, there is a listing for Warts, flat . . . 17110–17111. Do you know if a plantar wart is a flat wart? Because this is our only choice here, let's go to the codes suggested and see if the numeric listing can provide us with more information.

The code descriptions read:

17110 Destruction (e.g., laser surgery, electrosurgery, cryosurgery, chemosurgery, surgical curettement), of benign lesions other than skin tags or cutaneous vascular proliferative lesions; up to 14 lesions

17111 15 or more lesions

The descriptions do not really answer our question about whether a plantar wart is a flat wart or a benign lesion. But before you query the doctor, go to the beginning of this subsection and read down. Directly below the description for code 17003 is a notation:

(For destruction of common or plantar warts, see 17110, 17111.)

This is an excellent example of how you must investigate all possibilities and really give the CPT book a chance to point you toward the correct code.

Dr. Johnston destroyed with chemosurgery Frank's benign lesion that was not a skin tag or a cutaneous vascular proliferative lesion, and he only had one. 17110 is perfect!

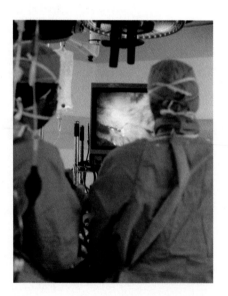

MOHS MICROGRAPHIC SURGERY

The group of codes for Mohs micrographic surgery will only be used should you be coding for a physician specially trained in this type of procedure because it requires one doctor to act as *both* surgeon and pathologist. If two different professionals perform these functions, the codes cannot be used.

If a repair is performed, during the same session, the repair procedures should be coded separately.

If a biopsy is performed on the same day as the Mohs surgery, because the physician suspects that the patient has skin cancer, it should be reported separately, as well, appended with modifier 59.

CHAPTER SUMMARY

When coding surgical procedures, you have the challenge of determining which services are included in the procedure code, which services are part of the global package, and which services must be coded separately.

In addition, it is important to remember that the Surgery section of the CPT book not only includes codes for reporting services provided in an operating room under general anesthesia but also includes codes for reporting simple and small procedures such as removing a splinter.

1. The global surgical package includes all except

    a. Preprocedure evaluation and management.
    b. General anesthesia.
    c. The procedure.
    d. Follow-up care.

2. The global period is determined by

    a. The type of anesthesia provided.
    b. The size of the excision.
    c. The location of the donor site.
    d. The standard of care.

3. The following is an example of a diagnostic test not included in the global package:

    a. Closure.
    b. Local infiltration.
    c. Biopsy.
    d. Metacarpal block.

4. When a procedure is planned as a series of procedures, each service after the first should be appended with the modifier

    a. 76.
    b. 79.
    c. 58.
    d. 59.

5. When a surgeon does not provide preoperative or postoperative care to the patient upon whom he or she operates, the procedure code should be appended with modifier

    a. 54.
    b. 55.
    c. 56.
    d. 77.

6. Excision of lesions are reported with

    a. Total measurement of all lesions removed in one code.
    b. Only the largest lesion measured is coded.
    c. Each lesion coded separately.
    d. As a part of the total surgical procedure.

7. The code for the excision includes this type of repair:

    a. Intermediate.
    b. Complex.
    c. None.
    d. Simple.

8. If the surgeon performs a reexcision of a lesion during a later encounter with the patient, append the procedure code with modifier

    a. 58.
    b. 59.
    c. 51.
    d. 77.

9. If multiple wounds located on the same anatomical site are repaired with the same complexity, report this procedure by

    a. Coding each wound separately.
    b. Coding only the largest wound.
    c. Adding all the lengths together and code the total.
    d. Coding the average of all the wounds repaired.

10. The elements of determining the most accurate code for a skin graft includes all except

    a. The size of the recipient area.
    b. The type of donor.
    c. The location of the recipient area.
    d. The type of graft.

1. Dr. Quartermain performed a rhinoplasty to correct the nasal deformity on Frank Chestnut, a three-year-old male born with a cleft palate. The tip, septum, and osteotomies were all treated.

   _____

2. Roger Appleton, a 27-year-old male, cut his thumb at work on a construction site three weeks ago. He did not get any treatment for the wound, which became infected. Today, Dr. Kenny will amputate the thumb. The procedure is made more complicated by the spread of the infection to the surrounding tissues, as Dr. Kenny fights to save as much of the hand as possible.

   _____

3. Two weeks ago, Dr. Sweetzer performed an ureteroneocystostomy with cystoscopy and ureteral stent placement laparoscopically on Patricia Worster. However, today he must perform an open procedure on her to drain a renal abscess that was discovered. Code the drainage of Patricia's renal abscess.

   _____

4. On May 1, Dr. Monmouth performed a percutaneous core needle biopsy on Stephan English. Two days later, after reviewing the results of the biopsy, Dr. Monmouth performs a complete thyroidectomy on Stephan. Code both procedures.

   _____

5. Dr. Macintosh performed a lumbar laminectomy on Rick Greenlaw on September 15. One month later, as originally planned, Dr. Macintosh brought Rick back into the operating room to implant an epidural drug infusor with a subcutaneous reservoir. Code both procedures.

   _____

6. Warren Samuels, a 47-year-old male, owns a landscaping business. While he was reviewing some property to write a proposal, the family's toy poodle bit him on the leg. While the 12-cm wound was not severe, Warren wanted Dr. Dawson to check it out. Dr. Dawson performed a simple repair and applied a bandage.

   _____

7. Jackie Thurman, a 35-year-old female, was seen by her regular physician, Dr. Callman, after she spilled a pot of boiling water on her stomach and legs. Thankfully, her apron and corduroy dress absorbed most of the heat, and she only had first-degree burns. Dr. Callman performed initial local treatment and sent her home.

_____

8. Colleen Sizmauski, a 59-year-old female, came to Dr. Lafferty's office to have an epidermal facial chemical peel performed.

_____

9. Mark Matthews, a 32-year-old male, was seen by Dr. Rothstein, his regular physician, because Mark smashed his finger with a hammer while installing wallboard. Dr. Rothstein performed an evacuation of a subungual hematoma.

_____

10. Cletus Jones, a 23-year-old male, was in a fight at a hockey game and was hit in the head with a bottle, which caused some deep lacerations in his scalp. Dr. Fairchild performed a layered closure of the wounds: one 2.0 cm; one 4.5 cm; and two lacerations that were 1.0 cm each in length.

_____

11. Cassandra Twillinger, a 29-year-old female, is postmastectomy and comes in today so Dr. Edwin can perform a breast reconstruction with free flap.

_____

12. Jason McCall, a 51-year-old male, has a pilonidal cyst. Dr. Bonneti performs an I&D (incision and drainage).

_____

13. Denita Tauber found a sore on her neck. The lab test identified it as a malignant lesion, and Dr. Capp excised the lesion, measuring 2.9 cm with margins.

_____

14. Hannah Lopez, a 63-year-old female, is bedridden with two broken legs in traction. Dr. Quinn excised an ischial pressure ulcer with a primary suture.

_____

15. Ruth Ann Marcelle, a 9-year-old female, had a partial thickness burn on her hand. Dr. Assiss performed a debridement and dressing of the injury.

_____

YOU CODE IT! Simulation
Chapter 7. Surgery Coding, Part 1

Below and on the following pages, you will see physicians' notes documenting encounters with patients at our textbook's health care facility, Cipher, Victors, & Associates. Find the best, most appropriate codes from the Surgery section of the CPT book for each of these reports.

CIPHER, VICTORS, & ASSOCIATES
A Complete Health Care Facility
234 MAIN STREET • ANYTOWN, FL 32711 • 407-555-1234

PATIENT:	JABELONE, JAMAL
MRN:	JABELA01
Admission Date:	9 October 2008
Discharge Date:	9 October 2008
Date:	9 October 2008
Preoperative DX:	Lacerations of arm, hand, and leg
Postoperative DX:	same
Procedure:	Layered repair of leg laceration; simple repair of arm and hand lacerations
Surgeon:	Geoff Conner, MD
Assistant:	None
Anesthesia:	General

Indications: The patient is a 4-year-old male brought to the emergency room by his father. He was helping his father install a new window when the window fell and shattered. The boy suffered lacerations on his left hand, left arm, and left leg.

Procedure: The patient was placed on the table in supine position. Satisfactory anesthesia was obtained. The area was prepped and attention to the deeper laceration of the left thigh, right above the patella, was first. A layered repair was performed, and the 5.1-cm laceration was closed successfully with sutures. The lacerations on the upper extremity, 2-cm laceration on the left hand at the base of the fifth metacarpal, and the 3-cm laceration on the left arm, just below the joint capsule in the posterior position, were successfully closed with 4-0 Vicryl, as well. The patient tolerated the procedures well, and was transported to the recovery room.

10/9/08 11:47:39

Find the best, most appropriate code(s).

_____

_____

_____

CIPHER, VICTORS, & ASSOCIATES
A Complete Health Care Facility
234 MAIN STREET • ANYTOWN, FL 32711 • 407-555-1234

PATIENT: RUDERMAN, LILLIE ANN
MRN: RUDELI01
Admission Date: 15 October 2008
Discharge Date: 15 October 2008

Date: 15 October 2008
Preoperative DX: Augmentation of lips
Postoperative DX: same
Procedure: Collagen injections

Surgeon: Wayne Fleeter, MD
Assistant: None
Anesthesia: Local

Indications: The patient is a 41-year-old female with a low self-image. She presents today for enhancement of her lips.

Procedure: The patient was placed on the table in supine position. Local anesthesia was administered. As soon as patient stated a complete loss of feeling in the area, the injections were given subcutaneously—a total of 2.3 cc.

10/15/08 11:47:39

Find the best, most appropriate code(s).

_____

_____

_____

PATIENT: HODGES, MARJORIE
MRN: HODGMA01
Admission Date: 1 November 2008
Discharge Date: 1 November 2008

Date: 1 November 2008
Preoperative DX: Toxic epidermal necrolysis
Postoperative DX: same
Procedure: Xenogaft

Surgeon: Wayne Fleeter, MD
Assistant: None
Anesthesia: Local

Indications: The patient is a 26-year-old female with a diagnosis of toxic epidermal necrolysis as a result of a reaction to procainamide, previously prescribed by a physician no longer in attendance.

Procedure: The patient was placed on the table in supine position. Local anesthesia was administered. As soon as patient stated a complete loss of feeling in the left forearm, the dermal xenograft proceeded. Procedure repeated for right forearm.

A total of 150 sq cm of grafting was successfully completed.

Bandages were applied. A prescription for Darvocet N100 po q4-6h prn was given to the patient before discharge.

Follow-up appointment in office scheduled for 10 days.

11/1/08 17:47:39

Find the best, most appropriate code(s).

_____

_____

_____

Part 1   CPT

PATIENT: MORALES, MARVIN
MRN: MORAMA01
Admission Date: 09 September 2008
Discharge Date: 09 September 2008

Date: 09 September 2008
Preoperative DX: Plantar warts, sole, left foot
Postoperative DX: same
Procedure: Electrodesiccation

Surgeon: Wayne Fleeter, MD
Assistant: None
Anesthesia: Local

Indications: The patient is a 37-year-old male with pain from a plantar wart located at the ball of the left foot.

Procedure: The patient was placed on the table in supine position. 1% Lidocaine injected under and around the lesion. Three warts are successfully electrodesiccated and removed with a curette. After wart tissue is completely removed on each, light desiccation is used to control bleeding and prevent the wart from reoccurring.
     Sterile bandage is applied with instructions to patient for care and replacement.
     Tylenol suggested for pain management, should patient feel discomfort.

     Follow-up appointment recommended for one week.

09/09/08 11:47:39

Find the best, most appropriate code(s).

_____

_____

_____

CIPHER, VICTORS, & ASSOCIATES
A Complete Health Care Facility
234 MAIN STREET • ANYTOWN, FL 32711 • 407-555-1234

PATIENT: RUMBLESS, WILLIAM
MRN: RUMBWI01
Admission Date: 23 September 2008
Discharge Date: 23 September 2008

Date: 23 September 2008
Preoperative DX: Third-degree burns, palm of right hand
Postoperative DX: same
Procedure: Allograft

Surgeon: Wayne Fleeter, MD
Assistant: None
Anesthesia: General

Indications: The patient is a 19-year-old male with electrical burns on the palm of his right hand.

Procedure: The patient was placed on the table in supine position. Anesthesia is administered. Skin grafted from a healthy cadaveric donor was prepared and applied to resurface the palm of the hand. Total of 75 sq cm used.
   Sterile bandage is applied with instructions to patient for care and replacement.
   A prescription for Darvocet N100 po q4h prn was given to the patient before discharge.

   Follow-up appointment recommended for one week.

09/23/08 11:47:39

Find the best, most appropriate code(s).

_____

_____

_____

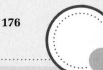

Surgery Coding, Part 2:

Surgery Guidelines—Musculoskeletal, Respiratory, Cardiovascular, Digestive, Urinary, Genital, Nervous, Visual, and Auditory Systems

8

LEARNING OUTCOMES

- Correctly apply the guidelines for coding surgical procedures.
- Recognize when an add-on code is required.
- Identify services included in a procedure code.
- Distinguish separately reportable services.
- Ascertain the elements of coding an organ transplant.
- Determine how and when to use modifiers.

EMPLOYMENT OPPORTUNITIES

General surgeons' offices

Cardiologists' offices

Dermatologists' offices

Neurologists' offices

Plastic/reconstructive surgeons' offices

Colorectal surgeons' offices

Thoracic surgeons' offices

Nephrologists' offices

Hand surgeons' offices

Podiatrists' offices

Ophthalmologists' offices

Vascular surgeons' offices

Maxillofacial surgeons' offices

Surgical oncologists' offices

In CPT, the term *surgery* does not limit itself to only those services and treatments performed in an operating room or even in a hospital. Within this section of the CPT book, codes are listed that report:

- Incision and drainage of a cyst

- Debridement

- Simple repair of a superficial wound

All these services can easily be performed in a physician's office. In addition, many procedures are now performed at an ambulatory surgical center or outpatient department.

In Chap. 7, you began learning about coding surgical procedures involving the integumentary system. Chapter 8 continues from that point through the balance of the Surgery section of the CPT.

Cervical vertebrae

Thoracic vertebrae

Lumbar vertebrae

Sacrum

Coccyx

CODING TIP »»

If a thoracotomy or laparotomy is performed, then those procedures should be coded instead of an exploration code (20100-20103).

Fascia lata graft

The transplanting of a connective tissue that encases the thigh muscles.

Arthrodesis

The immobilization of a joint using a surgical technique.

Laminectomy

The surgical removal of a vertebral posterior arch.

MUSCULOSKELETAL SYSTEM

The Musculoskeletal System subsection of codes reports procedures and treatments performed on the bones, ligaments, cartilage, muscles, and tendons in the human body.

The Code Package

Codes in this subsection already include the application and removal of a cast or traction device, as a part of the procedure performed.

If a second cast or traction device is required during the total course of treatment for the injury or condition, then the application and removal of any additional cast or traction device would be coded separately, from the Applications of Casts and Strapping subsection, codes 29000–29799.

Penetrating Trauma Wounds

The CPT book distinguishes between wounds and penetrating trauma wounds. A penetrating trauma wound requires:

1. Surgery to explore the wound
2. Determination of the depth and complexity of the wound
3. Identification of any damage created by the penetrating object (e.g., the stabbing from a knife or the wound from a bullet)
4. Debridement of the wound to remove any particles, dirt, and foreign fragments
5. Ligation or coagulation of minor subcutaneous tissue, muscle fascia, and/or muscle (not severe enough to require a thoracotomy or laparotomy)

You will use codes 20100–20103 to report the exploration of such wounds. Then code whichever repair the physician actually performs, as documented in the notes.

Bone Grafts and Implants

Medical science and technology have progressed amazingly. Be certain to differentiate between skin grafts (as reviewed in Chap. 7) and bone, cartilage, tendon, and **fascia lata grafts** that are coded from the musculoskeletal subsection.

Spine

As you may remember from anatomy class, the human spine is referred to in sections: cervical (at or near the neck); thoracic (the chest area); lumbar (at the waist and lower back); and sacral. References to the individual vertebrae are most often identified by their alphanumeric identifiers, such as C1 (cervical vertebra number 1), L5 (lumbar vertebra number 5), or S3 (sacral vertebra number 3).

Arthrodesis can be performed alone or in combination with such other procedures as bone grafting, osteotomy, fracture care, vertebral corpectomy, or **laminectomy**.

When arthrodesis is done at the same time as another procedure, modifier 51 Multiple Procedures should be appended to the code for the arthrodesis. This applies to almost all procedures, with the exception of bone grafting and instrumentation. Modifier 51 is not used in those cases because bone grafts and instrumentation are never performed without arthrodesis.

LET'S CODE IT! SCENARIO

Jamica Jones, a 51-year-old female, was diagnosed with degenerative disc disease three months ago. She is admitted today for Dr. Veronic to perform a posterior arthrodesis of L5–S1 (transverse process), utilizing a morselized autogenous iliac bone graft harvested through a separate fascial incision. Jamica tolerates the procedure well and is returned to her hospital room after two hours in recovery.

Let's Code It!

Pull out the description of the procedures that Dr. Veronic performed. First, we have the "posterior arthrodesis of L5–S1" and then the "morselized autogenous iliac bone graft harvested through a separate fascial incision."

Let's begin with the alphabetic index for arthrodesis. The designation of L5–S1 tells us this was done to Jamica's spine. However, *spine* isn't listed under arthrodesis. Keep reading and you will see *vertebra* listed, *lumbar* underneath that, and *posterior* beneath that. However, the physician noted "transverse process," which is listed here as well. Let's investigate code 22612, as suggested by the index.

22612 Arthrodesis, posterior or posterolateral technique, single level; lumbar (with or without lateral transverse technique)

This matches the physician's notes.

Now, let's move to the next procedure performed.

Look in the alphabetic index under *bone graft.* Read through the list until you reach the item that reflects what was done for Jamica: *spine surgery.* Indented below that we see *autograft* (the same as *autogenous*) and then *morselized.* The index suggests code 20937. Let's look at the code's description:

+20937 Autograft for spine surgery only (includes harvesting the graft); morselized (through separate skin or fascial incision)

Notice the symbol to the left of code 20937: +. The plus sign means this is an add-on code and it cannot be used alone. However, the notation below 20937 indicates that you are permitted to use this code along with 22612.

In addition, the guidelines state that when arthrodesis is performed with another procedure, you need to add modifier 51 to the arthrodesis code *except* when the other procedure is a bone graft. This is the case in Jamica's record, so our claim form for Jamica Jones's surgery will show procedure codes 22612 and 20937—with no modifiers. Great job!

Fractures and Dislocations

Many different types of treatments may be provided for a fracture and/or dislocation. Be careful not to confuse the diagnosed state of the fracture (e.g., **closed, open,** or compound) with the description of the treatment (e.g., **percutaneous skeletal fixation** or **manipulation**) provided by the physician.

Closed treatment

A fracture treated without surgically opening the affected area.

Open treatment

Surgically opening the fracture site, or another site in the body nearby, in order to treat the fractured bone.

Benjamin Zabine, a 17-year-old male, plays basketball on his high school team. While practicing in his driveway, he falls and fractures his knee. Dr. Casson, the orthopedist on duty at the emergency room, is able to use a closed treatment because it was just a hairline fracture of the patella. No manipulation was required.

Let's Code It!

Percutaneous skeletal fixation

The insertion of fixation instruments (e.g., pins) placed across the facture site. It may be done under x-ray imaging for guidance purposes.

Turn to the alphabetic index. This time, we won't look up the procedure by the type of treatment (*closed*), but we will look at the condition that was treated: *fracture.* Under *fracture,* find the anatomical site of the fracture—*patella*—and then the *closed treatment without manipulation.* The index suggests code 27520. Let's check the description in the numeric listing:

27520 Closed treatment of patellar fracture, without manipulation

That's exactly what Dr. Casson did. Great job!

YOU CODE IT! CASE STUDY

Manipulation

The attempted return of the fracture or dislocation to its normal alignment manually by the physician.

Hannah Rosensweig, a 71-year-old female, fell and sustained a fracture to the proximal end, neck, of her femur. Due to the position of the actual fracture, Dr. Plant was able to use a percutaneous skeletal fixation of the femur (without having to expose the fracture) and put her through a surgical procedure.

You Code It!

Go through the steps of coding and determine what codes should be reported for this encounter between Dr. Plant and Hannah Rosensweig.

Step 1: Read the case completely.

Step 2: Abstract the notes: What key words can you identify relating to the procedures performed?

Step 3: Query the provider, if necessary:

Step 4: Diagnosis: Fracture, femur, proximal end, neck.

Step 5: Code the procedure(s).

Step 6: Link the procedure codes to at least one diagnosis code.

Step 7: Back code to double-check your choices.

Answer

Did you find the correct code to be:

27235 Percutaneous skeletal fixation of femoral fraction, proximal end, neck

Great job!

RESPIRATORY SYSTEM

The organs and tissues involved with bringing oxygen into the body and discharging gases make up the respiratory system. Procedures and treatments affecting this sector are coded from the Respiratory System subsection.

Lung Transplantation

Special guidelines help you report any lung transplant. However, as soon as you begin to read the notation shown before codes 32850–32856, you will see that the editors of the CPT book use the term lung **allo-transplantation** in addition to **transplantation.** These words have a very similar meaning.

A lung transplant requires three steps that can be performed by a single physician or a team of physicians, with each physician submitting his or her own claim. Each step has its own code.

Cadaver Donor Pneumonectomy

Because a human cannot live without lungs, the donor would have to be deceased (a cadaver) prior to the harvesting of the organ. This portion of the transplant, or allotransplantation, procedure would be identified with the code:

32850 Donor pneumonectomy (including cold preservation), from cadaver donor

Backbench Work

The actual preparation of the cadaver donor lung allograft prior to the transplant procedure is coded using either of the following:

32855 Backbench stand preparation of cadaver donor lung allograft prior to transplantation . . . ; unilateral

or 32856 Backbench stand preparation of cadaver donor lung allograft prior to transplantation . . . ; bilateral

Allotransplantation

The relocation of tissue from one individual to another (both of the same species) without an identical genetic match.

Transplantation

The transfer of tissue from one site to another.

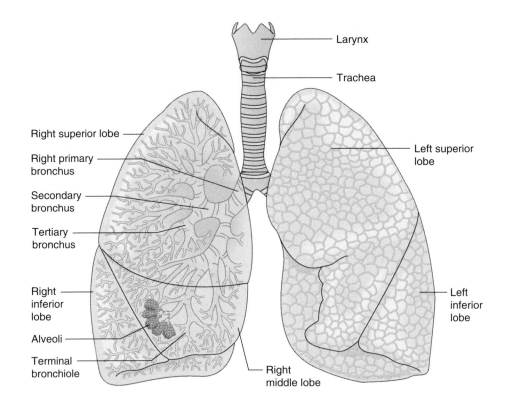

Larynx

Trachea

Right superior lobe

Right primary bronchus

Secondary bronchus

Tertiary bronchus

Right inferior lobe

Alveoli

Terminal bronchiole

Left superior lobe

Left inferior lobe

Right middle lobe

Recipient Lung Allotransplantation

The final code for the entire operation identifies the placement of the allograft into the patient (the recipient). The selection of a code from the range 32851–32854 is determined by whether the procedure is performed unilaterally or bilaterally and with or without a cardiopulmonary bypass.

LET'S CODE IT! SCENARIO

Ilonia Gonzalez, a 15-year-old female, was diagnosed three years ago with idiopathic pulmonary fibrosis, a chronic interstitial pulmonary disease. Corticosteroid therapy has not improved her condition, so Dr. Lancer has admitted her today for a double-lung transplantation. The harvesting of the allograft and the preparation of the cadaver donor double lung allograft was done by Dr. Cannon. Dr. Lancer will only be performing the actual lung transplant, en bloc, along with a cardiopulmonary bypass. Ilonia tolerated the procedure well and has an excellent prognosis.

Let's Code It!

The notes indicate that Dr. Lancer only performed one of the three steps. Therefore, we will only have one code on his claim form for Ilonia's surgery.

Let's go to the alphabetic index and look for *transplant*. Read down until you find *lung*. We know that Ilonia received a *double-lung* transplant, *en bloc, with a bypass.* It leads us to the suggested code 32854. Let's go to the numeric listing to check the complete code description.

32854 Lung transplant, double (bilateral sequential or en bloc); with cardio-pulmonary bypass

Terrific! It matches the notes.

CARDIOVASCULAR SYSTEM

Treatments and procedures on the heart as well as the entire network of veins, arteries, and capillaries are coded from the Cardiovascular System subsection.

Pacemakers

When a physician inserts a single-chamber pacemaker system into a patient, it includes the pulse generator and one electrode inserted into *either* the atrium or ventricle.

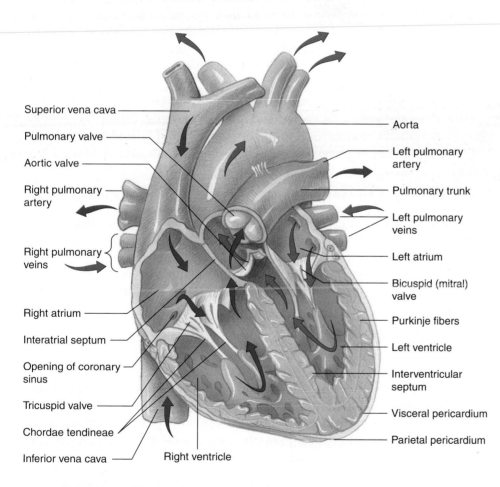

Superior vena cava

Pulmonary valve

Aortic valve

Right pulmonary artery

Right pulmonary veins

Right atrium

Interatrial septum

Opening of coronary sinus

Tricuspid valve

Chordae tendineae

Inferior vena cava

Right ventricle

Aorta

Left pulmonary artery

Pulmonary trunk

Left pulmonary veins

Left atrium

Bicuspid (mitral) valve

Purkinje fibers

Left ventricle

Interventricular septum

Visceral pericardium

Parietal pericardium

Oxygenated blood

Deoxygenated blood

When a dual-chamber pacemaker system is placed, the system includes the pulse generator and one electrode into *both* the right atrium and the right ventricle.

Occasionally, the physician will insert *an additional electrode* into the left ventricle, as well as the dual-chamber insertion. This is called *biventricular pacing*. The insertion of the pacing electrode is coded separately, using code 33224 and possibly 33225.

> 33224 Insertion of pacing electrode, cardiac venous system, for left ventricular pacing, with attachment to previously placed pacemaker or pacing cardioverter-defibrillator pulse generator (including revision of pocket, removal, insertion and/or replacement of generator)

> +33225 Insertion of pacing electrode, cardiac venous system, for left ventricular pacing, at time of insertion of pacing cardioverter-defibril-lator or pacemaker pulse generator (including upgrade to dual chamber system) (List separately in addition to code for primary procedure.)

Pacing Cardioverter-Defibrillators

Pacing cardioverter-defibrillator systems are similar to pacemaker systems. While they also consist of a pulse generator and electrodes, the units may use several leads inserted into a single chamber (ventricle) or into dual chambers (atrium and ventricle). The system is actually a combination of antitachycardia pacing, low-energy cardioversion, or defibrillating shocks to address a patient's ventricular tachycardia or ventricular fibrillation.

In some cases, an additional electrode may be needed to regulate the pacing of the left ventricle, called *biventricular pacing*. When this occurs, the placement of the electrode transvenously should be coded separately, using either 33224 or possibly 33225, just as with the pacemaker.

Battery Replacement

Commonly, battery replacement is referred to as replacing the battery in the pacemaker or cardioverter-defibrillator, but it is actually the removal of the old pulse generator and the insertion of a new pulse generator. These two actions should be coded individually—one code for the removal of the old and another code for the insertion of the new.

Bypass Grafting

Venous Grafts

When a venous graft is performed, you use codes from the range 33510–33516. All these codes include a **saphenous vein** graft.

However, if the graft is harvested from an upper extremity (arm) vein, you need to code this separately, using code 35500, in addition to the code for the bypass procedure itself.

> +35500 Harvest of upper extremity vein, one segment for lower extremity or coronary artery bypass procedure (List separately in addition to code for primary procedure.)

Saphenous vein

Either of the two major veins in the leg that run from the foot to the thigh near the surface of the skin.

Part 1   CPT

If the graft comes from a femoropopliteal vein, use code 35572 in addition to the bypass procedure code.

> +35572 Harvest of femoropopliteal vein, one segment, for vascular reconstruction procedure (e.g., aortic, vena caval, coronary, peripheral artery) (List separately in addition to code for primary procedure.)

Combined Arterial-Venous Grafts

When both venous grafts and arterial grafts are used during the same procedure, you will use two codes. First, code the combined arterial-venous graft from the range 33517–33523. Just like the codes for the venous grafts, these include getting the graft from the saphenous vein. Second, code the appropriate arterial graft from the range 33533–33536. Harvesting the arterial vein section is included in those codes.

Arterial Grafts

When an arterial graft is performed, you use codes from the range 33533–33545. All those codes include the use of grafts from the internal mammary artery, gastroepiploic artery, epigastric artery, radial artery, and arterial conduits harvested from other sites. For example, examine the following code description:

> 33533 Coronary artery bypass, using arterial graft(s); single arterial graft

Use one of the following codes (in addition to the code for the bypass procedure) if the graft is harvested from another site:

- From an upper extremity artery, add code 35600.
- From an upper extremity vein, add code 35500.
- From the femoropopliteal vein, use code 35572.

Composite Grafts

When two or more vein segments are harvested from a limb other than that part of the body undergoing the bypass, you must use the best, most appropriate code from the range 35682–35683 to report the harvesting and anastomosis of the multiple vein segments.

> +35682 Bypass graft; autogenous composite, two segments of veins from two locations (List separately in addition to code for primary procedure.)

> +35683 Bypass graft; autogenous composite, three or more segments of vein from two or more locations (List separately in addition to code for primary procedure.)

A little confusing? Hopefully, Table 8-1 will help you organize all the rules for coding bypass grafts.

Heart/Lung Transplantation

Similar to the components of the lung transplantation that we reviewed earlier in this chapter, a heart transplant, with or without a lung allotransplantation, requires three steps to be performed by a single physician or a team of physicians. Each step has its own codes.

««« **CODING TIP**

The same exceptions apply as before: If the graft is harvested from an upper extremity artery, code it separately from the bypass procedure, using code 35600. And if the graft is obtained from the femoropopliteal vein, code it with 35572 in addition to the code for the bypass procedure.

TABLE 8-1 Bypass Grafts

Graft	Harvested From	Use Code(s)
Venous graft	Saphenous vein	Choose from 33510–33516
Venous graft	Upper extremity vein	Choose from 33510–33516; + 35500
Venous graft	Femoropopliteal vein	Choose from 33510–33516; + 35572
Arterial-venous	Saphenous vein	Choose from 33517–33523; + Choose from 33533–33536
Arterial-venous	Upper extremity vein	Choose from 33510–33516; + Choose from 33533–33536 + 35500
Arterial-venous	Upper extremity artery	Choose from 33510–33516; + Choose from 33533–33536 + 35600
Arterial-venous	Femoropopliteal vein	Choose from 33510–33516; + Choose from 33533–33536 + 35572
Arterial graft	Internal mammary artery Gastroepiploic artery Epigastric artery Radial artery Arterial conduits from other sites	Choose from 33533–33545
Arterial graft	Upper extremity vein	Choose from 33533–33545; + 35500
Arterial graft	Upper extremity artery	Choose from 33533–33545; + 35600
Arterial graft	Femoropopliteal vein	Choose from 33533–33545; + 35572
Composite graft	Two or more segments from another part of body	+ 35682 or 35683

Cadaver Donor Cardiectomy with or without a Pneumonectomy

A human cannot live without a heart or lungs, so the donor has to be deceased (a cadaver) prior to any organ harvesting. This portion of the transplant or allotransplantation procedure is identified with the code 33930 (heart and lungs) or 33940 (heart alone):

33930 Donor cardiectomy-pneumonectomy (including cold preservation)

or 33940 Donor cardiectomy (including cold preservation)

Backbench Work

The actual preparation of the cadaver donor heart, or heart and lung, allograft prior to the transplant procedure is known as *backbench work.* The second portion of the transplant is coded using either of the following:

> 33933 Backbench standard preparation of cadaver donor heart/lung allograft

> or 33944 Backbench standard preparation of cadaver donor heart allograft

Recipient Heart with or without Lung Allotransplantation

The third code for the entire operation identifies the placement of the allograft into the patient (the recipient). Select the code from either of the following:

> 33935 Heart-lung transplant with recipient cardiectomy-pneumonectomy

> or 33945 Heart transplant with or without recipient cardiectomy

The codes for the insertion of the transplanted organs include the removal of the damaged or diseased organs.

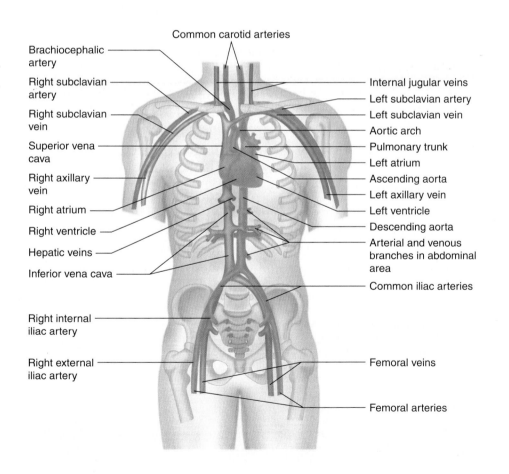

Arteries and Veins

The primary vascular procedure codes 34001–37799 include:

1. Ensuring both the inflow and the outflow of the arteries and/or veins involved
2. The operative arteriogram that is performed by the surgeon during the procedure
3. Sympathectomy for aortic procedures

The repair of an abdominal aortic aneurysm, codes 34800–34826, includes several procedures, such as:

1. Placement of an endovascular graft for an abdominal aortic aneurysm repair
2. Open femoral or iliac artery exposure
3. Manipulation and deployment of the device used
4. Closure of the arteriotomy site(s)
5. Balloon angioplasty and/or stent deployment, as long as it is within the target treatment area for the endoprosthesis

When the notes indicate that any or all of these procedures were done at the same time as the abdominal aortic repair, they *are not* coded separately.

However, several other procedures may be performed at the same time which *are* coded separately (in addition to the code for the repair itself):

1. The introduction of guidewires and/or catheters (36140, 36200, 36245–36248)
2. Extensive repair or replacement of an artery (35226 or 35286)
3. Renal transluminal angioplasty (i.e., the enlargement of the renal artery, when it has become narrowed using a balloon-tip catheter)
4. Arterial embolization (i.e., blocking an artery with a material such as gelatin or sponge, to stop uncontrollable internal bleeding)
5. Intravascular ultrasound
6. Balloon angioplasty (i.e., reconstruction of a blood vessel)
7. Stenting of the native artery outside of the endoprosthesis area (when done before or after deployment of a graft)
8. Fluoroscopic guidance in conjunction with the repair (75952 or 75953)

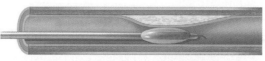

Narrowed artery with balloon catheter positioned.

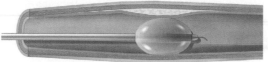

Inflated balloon presses against arterial wall.

Blood vessel   Stent

Endovascular repair of an iliac aneurysm has similar guidelines to the coding process for the abdominal aortic aneurysm repair. First, let's look at the list of procedures that are included in the code 34900 and that *are not* coded separately.

1. Introduction, positioning, and operation of an endovascular graft of the iliac artery (common, hypogastric, or external)
2. All balloon angioplasty and/or stent deployments within the treatment area

There are also procedures frequently performed along with an iliac aneurysm repair that *are* coded separately. These procedures include:

1. Open femoral or iliac artery exposure (code 34812 or 34820)
2. Introduction of guidewires and/or catheters (code 36200, 36215, 36216, 36217, or 36218)
3. Extensive repair or replacement of the artery (a code from the range 35206–35286, as appropriate)
4. Transluminal angioplasty outside the aneurysm area
5. Arterial embolization
6. Intravascular ultrasound
7. Fluoroscopic guidance in conjunction with the iliac aneurysm repair (Use code 75954.)

LET'S CODE IT! SCENARIO

Zena Quinones, a 15-week-old female, was diagnosed with ventricular septal defect (VSD) after her pediatrician, Dr. Osterman, ordered an echocardiography. A large VSD was identified in the septum. Due to the size of the defect, Dr. Osterman admits Zena, today, into the hospital to close the defect with a patch graft.

Let's Code It!

Review the notes, and abstract the key terms. Then go to the alphabetic index and look up *closure,* which is the actual procedure being performed. Under the word *closure,* you will find *septal defect,* which suggests the code 33615.

While we are in the alphabetic index, let's try one other way to look up the code. Go to *heart,* which of course is the anatomical site where the procedure is being performed. When you read the column below *heart,* you will see *closure, septal defect,* which again suggests code 33615. However, just out of curiosity, continue reading down the columns until you get to *repair* (another word for the procedure being done). As you read everything listed under *repair,* keep going past *septal defect,* all the way to *ventricular septum*—33545, 33647, 33681–33688, 33692–33697, 93581. *Ventricular septum* is a much better match to the physician's notes than *septal defect,* isn't it? Not certain? That's great, because we need to let the actual code descriptions in the numeric listing give us more details before we make a decision.

This is where time and patience are important to the coding process. Read carefully through the description of each code suggested by the alphabetic index. Do you agree that the best, most appropriate code is:

33681 Closure of ventricular septal defect, with or without patch

Great job!

DIGESTIVE SYSTEM

Beginning at the mouth and traveling through the body all the way to the anus is the digestive tract. The organs along the pathway process food and nourishment, so cells can absorb nutrients and eliminate waste. The digestive tract is also referred to as the alimentary canal or the gastrointestinal (GI) tract.

Endoscopic Procedures

There are times when a physician needs to examine the interior of an organ, such as the throat, stomach, or bladder in order to make a more accurate diagnosis. In these cases, an endoscope may be used.

Endoscopy can be used for therapeutic procedures, as well, like when Dr. Sanger had to remove a penny (foreign body) from little Billy's esophagus after he tried to swallow the coin, code 43247.

Intestinal Transplantation

Much like the components that we have reviewed for lung and heart transplants, an intestinal allotransplantation involves three separate service components.

Donor Enterectomy

A human can live without a portion of the intestine, so the donor can be either deceased (a cadaver) or living.

44132 Donor enterectomy (including cold preservation), open; from cadaver donor

or 44133 Donor enterectomy (including cold preservation), open; partial, from living donor

Backbench Work

The backbench work code reports the actual preparation of the intestine allograft prior to the transplant procedure. This portion of the transplant would be coded using:

44715 Backbench standard preparation of cadaver or living donor intestine allograft

In certain cases, some reconstruction of the intestine will be required prior to the transplantation. If the notes indicate that a venous and/or arterial anastomosis was also performed, then you have to use:

44720 Backbench reconstruction of cadaver or living donor intestine allograft prior to transplantation; venous anastomosis, each

ACCESSORY ORGANS

ALIMENTARY CANAL

Mouth
Mechanical breakdown
of food; begins chemical
digestion of carbohydrates

Salivary glands
Secrete saliva, which contains
enzymes that initiate breakdown
of carbohydrates

Pharynx
Connects mouth with
esophagus

Esophagus
Peristalsis pushes
food to stomach

Liver
Produces bile, which
emulsifies fat

Stomach
Secretes acid and
enzymes. Mixes food
with secretions to
begin enzymatic
digestion of proteins

Small intestine
Mixes food with bile
and pancreatic juice.
Final enzymatic breakdown
of food molecules;
main site of
nutrient absorption

Gallbladder
Stores bile and
introduces it into
small intestine

Pancreas
Produces and secretes
pancreatic juice, containing
digestive enzymes and
bicarbonate ions,
into small intestine

Large intestine
Absorbs water and
electrolytes to form feces

Rectum
Regulates elimination
of feces

Anus

Recipient Intestinal Allotransplantation with or without Recipient Enterectomy

The third code for the entire operation identifies the placement of the allograft into the patient (the recipient). Select either of the following codes:

44135 Intestinal allotransplantation; from cadaver donor

or 44136 Intestinal allotransplantation; from living donor

Liver Transplantation

Again, the components that we have reviewed for the other organ transplants are involved with a liver allotransplantation.

Donor Hepatectomy

A human can live without a portion of the liver, so the donor can be either deceased (a cadaver) or living. The best code for this portion of the transplant process is determined by whether or not the donor is living; and if living, what percentage or portion of the liver is donated.

> 47133 Donor hepatectomy (including cold preservation), from cadaver donor
>
> or 47140 Donor hepatectomy (including cold preservation), from living donor; left lateral segment only
>
> or 47141 Donor hepatectomy (including cold preservation), from living donor; total left lobectomy
>
> or 47142 Donor hepatectomy (including cold preservation), from living donor; total right lobectomy

Backbench Work

The actual preparation of the whole liver graft prior to the transplant procedure is coded using:

> 47143 Backbench standard preparation of cadaver donor whole liver graft

In certain cases, and almost always if the donor is living, some reconstruction of the liver will be required prior to the transplantation. If the notes indicate that a venous and/or arterial anastomosis was also performed, then you will need to use:

> 47146 Backbench reconstruction of cadaver or living donor liver graft prior to allotransplantation; venous anastomosis, each

Recipient Liver Allotransplantation

The third code for the entire operation identifies the placement of the allograft into the patient (the recipient). This code is determined by the placement of the allograft: orthotopic (normal position) or heterotopic (other than normal position).

> 47135 Liver allotransplantation; orthotopic, partial or whole, from cadaver or living donor, any age
>
> or 47136 Liver allotransplantation; heterotopic, partial or whole, from cadaver or living donor, any age

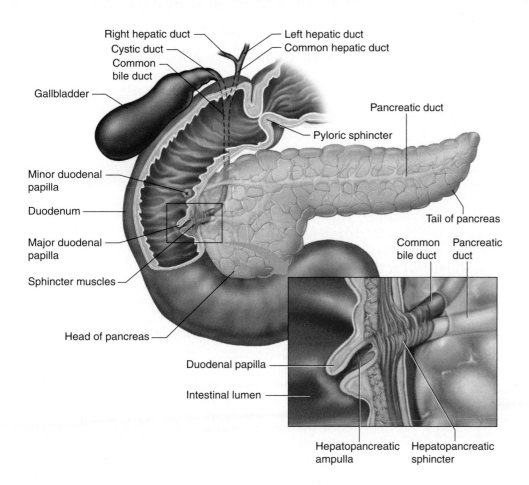

Right hepatic duct
Cystic duct
Common bile duct
Gallbladder
Minor duodenal papilla
Duodenum
Major duodenal papilla
Sphincter muscles
Head of pancreas

Left hepatic duct
Common hepatic duct
Pancreatic duct
Pyloric sphincter
Tail of pancreas

Common bile duct
Pancreatic duct

Duodenal papilla
Intestinal lumen
Hepatopancreatic ampulla
Hepatopancreatic sphincter

Pancreas Transplantation

Again, the components that we have reviewed for the other organ transplants are involved with a pancreatic allotransplantation.

Cadaver Donor Pancreatectomy

A pancreas graft has to come from a deceased (a cadaver) donor.

> 48550 Donor pancreatectomy (including cold preservation), with or without duodenal segment for transplantation

Backbench Work

When the preparation of the pancreas graft prior to the transplant procedure is routine, you use the following code:

> 48551 Backbench standard preparation of cadaver donor pancreas allograft

However, in certain cases, some reconstruction of the pancreas will be required prior to the transplantation. If the notes indicate that a venous and/or arterial anastomosis was performed, then you have to use:

> 48552 Backbench reconstruction of cadaver donor pancreas allograft prior to allotransplantation; venous anastomosis, each

Recipient Pancreatic Allotransplantation

The final code for the entire operation identifies the placement of the allograft into the patient (the recipient). For this, use the following code:

48554 Transplantation of pancreatic allograft

LET'S CODE IT! SCENARIO

Paul Williamson, a 57-year-old male, was suffering from fecal incontinence, diarrhea, and constipation. He came to the Ambulatory Care Center so that his gastroenterologist, Dr. Apterman, could perform a colonoscopy. Demerol and Versed were given IV, and the patient was brought into the examination room. The pediatric variable flexion Olympus colonoscope was introduced into the rectum and advanced to the cecum. In the midsigmoid colon, a 3-mm sessile polyp was destroyed. Paul tolerated the procedure well and was told to return to Dr. Apterman's office in one week for the results of the biopsies.

Let's Code It!

We know that the main procedure was a *colonoscopy,* so let's look that up in the alphabetic index. When you refer to the notes, what else was done for Paul, in conjunction with the colonoscopy? *A polyp was destroyed.*

Find *destruction* beneath *colonoscopy.* Do you know whether a polyp is a lesion or a tumor? It happens to be a lesion; however, you don't have to know this because the index suggests the same code for both: 45383. Let's look at the complete description in the numeric listing.

45383 Colonoscopy, flexible, proximal to splenic flexure; with ablation of tumor(s), polyp(s), or other lesion(s) not amenable to removal by hot biopsy forceps, bipolar cautery, or snare technique

You might think about also coding the moderate sedation that was given to Paul (the Demerol and Versed). However, look at the bull's eye symbol next to 45383 . . . the sedation is included in this code. So, you are not to code the moderate sedation separately. Great job!

URINARY SYSTEM

The urinary system is responsible for maintaining the proper level and composition of fluids in the body.

Renal (Kidney) Transplantation

The same three components exist for renal transplantation as they do for the other organ transplants.

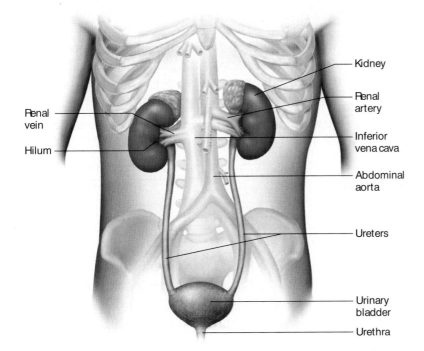

Kidney

Renal artery

Inferior vena cava

Abdominal aorta

Ureters

Urinary bladder

Urethra

Renal vein

Hilum

Donor Nephrectomy

A human can live without one kidney, so the donor can be either deceased (a cadaver) or living.

> 50300 Donor nephrectomy (including cold preservation); from cadaver donor, unilateral or bilateral
>
> or 50320 Donor nephrectomy (including cold preservation); open, from living donor
>
> or 50547 Laparoscopy, surgical; donor nephrectomy (including cold preservation), from living donor

Backbench Work

Performing the routine preparation of the allograft is coded differently, depending upon whether the donor is living or a cadaver.

> 50323 Backbench standard preparation of cadaver donor renal allograft
>
> or 50325 Backbench standard preparation of living donor renal allograft

In certain cases, some reconstruction of the kidney will be required prior to the transplantation. If the notes indicate that a venous, arterial, and/or ureteral anastomosis was performed, then you have to use:

> 50327 Backbench reconstruction of cadaver or living donor renal allograft prior to allotransplantation; venous anastomosis, each
>
> or 50328 Backbench reconstruction of cadaver or living donor renal allograft prior to allotransplantation; arterial anastomosis, each
>
> or 50329 Backbench reconstruction of cadaver or living donor renal allograft prior to allotransplantation; ureteral anastomosis, each.

Recipient Renal Allotransplantation

The final code for the entire operation identifies the placement of the allograft into the patient (the recipient). Choose the code by whether or not a recipient nephrectomy (the removal of the organ being replaced) is performed at the same time by the same physician:

> 50360 Renal allotransplantation; implantation of graft; without recipient nephrectomy
>
> or 50365 Renal allotransplantation; implantation of graft; with recipient nephrectomy

Urodynamics

The codes listed for the procedures in the Urodynamics section, 51725–51798, include the services of the physician to perform the procedure (or directly supervise the performance of the procedure), as well as the use of all instruments, equipment, fluids, gases, probes, catheters, technician's fees, medications, gloves, trays, tubing, and other sterile supplies.

If the physician for whom you are coding did not actually perform the procedure but only interpreted the results, then the appropriate procedure code from this section should be appended with modifier 26 Professional Component.

EXAMPLE

Dr. Klotzkin interprets the voiding pressure study of his patient, Barney Trumm, taken at the lab. Use code 51795-51.

Transurethral Surgery

When a diagnostic or therapeutic cystourethroscopic intervention is performed, the appropriate codes, 52320–52355, include the insertion and removal of a temporary stent. Therefore, those services are not reported separately—when done at the same time as the cystourethroscopy.

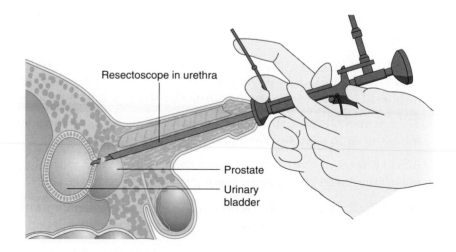

Resectoscope in urethra

Prostate

Urinary bladder

If the physician, however, inserts a self-retaining, indwelling stent during the diagnostic or therapeutic cystourethroscopic intervention, use either of the following:

1. Code 52332 with the modifier 51, along with the code for the cystourethroscopy for a unilateral procedure

2. Code 52332 with modifiers 50 and 51, along with the code for the cystourethroscopy for a bilateral procedure

Note that when the physician removes the self-retaining, indwelling ureteral stent, use either 52310 or 52315 with modifier 58.

LET'S CODE IT! SCENARIO

Anita Jullianni, a 37-year-old female, is admitted today for the surgical removal of a kidney stone. The stone was too big for her to pass, so Dr. Hernandez decided to remove it surgically. The nephrolithotomy, with complete removal of the calculus, went as planned and Anita tolerated the entire procedure well.

Let's Code It!

Dr. Hernandez performed a *nephrolithotomy*, involving the *removal of a kidney stone,* also known as *calculus.* Let's try something direct, and look up *nephrolithotomy* in the alphabetic index.

The index suggests the code range 50060–50075. Let's go to the numeric listing and read the different code descriptions.

Do you agree, that according to the physician's notes, the best, most appropriate code available is:

50060 Nephrolithotomy; removal of calculus

You are getting very good at this.

<<< **CODING TIP**

Read carefully, because there are several different procedures that look very similar in spelling.

MALE GENITAL SYSTEM

There are *no* specific guidelines for the Male Genital System subsection of surgery.

YOU CODE IT! CASE STUDY

Doug Daniels, a 17-year-old male, came to see his regular physician, Dr. Bomgarden, for help. Doug and his friends were fooling around at his father's construction company, and a staple gun went off, projecting a staple into his scrotum. Dr. Bomgarden carefully removed the staple and applied some antibiotic ointment to prevent infection until the two small wounds healed.

Go through the steps of coding, and determine the codes that should be reported for this encounter between Dr. Bomgarden and Doug Daniels.

Step 1: Read the case completely.

Step 2: Abstract the notes: Which key words can you identify relating to the procedures performed?

_____

Step 3: Query the provider, if necessary.

Step 4: Diagnosis: Foreign body in scrotum.

Step 5: Code the procedure(s).

_____

Step 6: Link the procedure codes to at least one diagnosis code.

Step 7: Back code to double-check your choices.

Answer

Did you find the correct code to be:

55120 Removal of foreign body in scrotum

This matches the physician's description perfectly!

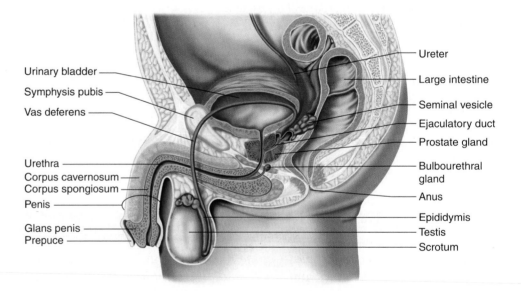

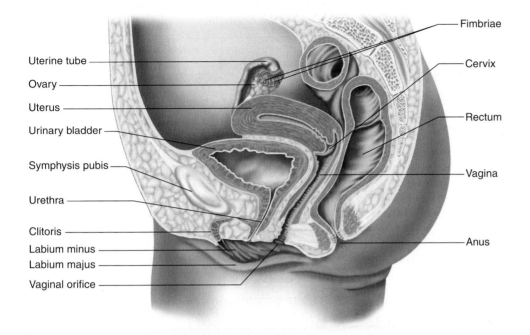

Uterine tube
Ovary
Uterus
Urinary bladder
Symphysis pubis
Urethra
Clitoris
Labium minus
Labium majus
Vaginal orifice

Fimbriae
Cervix
Rectum
Vagina
Anus

FEMALE GENITAL SYSTEM

Vulvectomy

Sometimes physicians use direct terms in their notes, such as "simple," "partial," "radical," or "complete." Such terms actually make finding the best code easier. However, other physicians may be more descriptive in their notes, regarding the procedure. Therefore, you have to know what those terms mean. The CPT book defines them as follows:

Simple: The removal of skin and *superficial* subcutaneous tissues.

Radical: The removal of skin and *deep* subcutaneous tissues.

Partial: The removal of *less than* 80% of the vulvar area.

Complete: The removal of *more than* 80% of the vulvar area.

EXAMPLES

56620 Vulvectomy, simple; partial

The description of this code represents a physician's statement that he or she removed less than 80% of the skin and superficial subcutaneous tissues of the vulvar area.

56633 Vulvectomy, radical; complete

The description of this code represents a physician's statement that he or she removed more than 80% of the skin and deep subcutaneous tissues of the vulvar area.

Procedures performed on the nervous system organs (the brain, spinal cord, nerves, and ganglia) and connective tissues are coded from the Nervous System subsection. These components of the human body are responsible for sensory, integrative, and motor activities.

Skull Surgery

The complexity of surgical treatment of skull base lesions often demands the skills of more than one surgeon during the same session. When one surgeon provides one portion of the procedure and another surgeon a different portion, each surgeon only uses the code for the surgical procedure he or she performed. Typically, the segments include the following:

1. The *approach* describes the tactic of the procedure, such as craniofacial, orbitocranial, or trancochlear:
   a. Anterior cranial fossa, 61580–61586
   b. Middle cranial fossa, 61590–61592
   c. Posterior cranial fossa, 61595–61598

2. The *definitive* describes the procedure itself, such as resection, excision, repair, biopsy, or transection:
   a. Base of anterior cranial fossa, 61600–61601
   b. Base of middle cranial fossa, 61605–61613
   c. Base of posterior cranial fossa, 61615–61616

3. The *repair/reconstruction* identifies a secondary repair, such as:
   a. Extensive dural grafting
   b. Cranioplasty

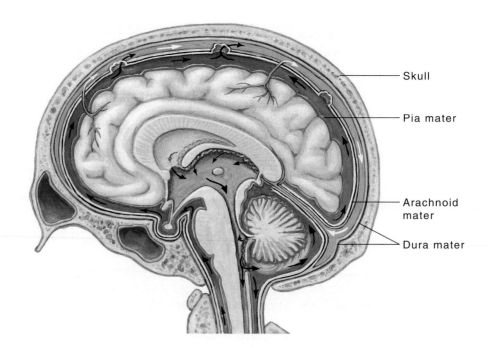

Skull

Pia mater

Arachnoid mater

Dura mater

c. Local or regional myocutaneous pedicle flaps

d. Extensive skin grafts

If one surgeon performs more than one of the above procedures, each segment should be reported separately, with the second (and third, if applicable) appended with modifier 51 to indicate that multiple procedures were performed at the same session by the same physician.

When a surgeon embeds a neurostimulator electrode array and also performs microelectrode recording, the recording is included in the implantation code and shouldn't be coded separately.

Code 62263 includes the following:

- Percutaneous insertion of an epidural catheter
- Removal of the catheter several days later
- Procedure injections
- Fluoroscopic guidance and localization
- Multiple adhesiolysis sessions, over the course of two or more days

The code should be used only once to represent the entire series.

62263 Percutaneous lysis of epidural adhesions using solution injection (e.g., hypertonic saline, enzyme) or mechanical means (e.g., catheter) including radiologic localization (includes contrast when administered), multiple adhesiolysis sessions; 2 or more days

62264   1 day

<< **CODING TIP**

If multiple treatments are provided all in one day, then use code 62264.

LET'S CODE IT! SCENARIO

Barry Gauchier, a 63-year-old male, is admitted for the implantation of a cerebral cortical neurostimulator. Dr. Jackson performed a craniotomy and then successfully implanted the electrodes.

Let's Code It!

Dr. Jackson first performed a *craniotomy*. Let's go to the alphabetic index and look.

Below *craniotomy,* you will see the listing *for implant of neurostimulators.* That matches our notes, so let's go to the numeric listing and check the descriptions for 61850–61875, as suggested. Read through the codes and their descriptions in this section. Do you agree that the following matches our notes the best?

61860 Craniectomy or craniotomy for implantation of neurostimulator electrodes, cerebral, cortical

It does!

EYE AND OCULAR ADNEXA

There are *no* specific guidelines for the Eye and Ocular Adnexa subsection of surgery.

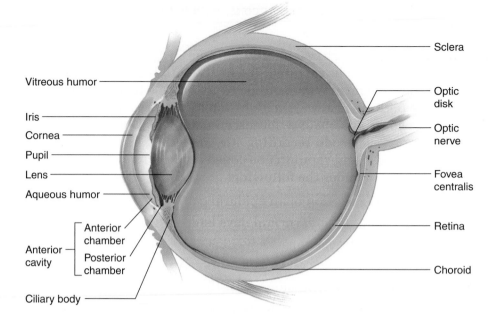

Vitreous humor

Iris

Cornea

Pupil

Lens

Aqueous humor

Anterior cavity
- Anterior chamber
- Posterior chamber

Ciliary body

Sclera

Optic disk

Optic nerve

Fovea centralis

Retina

Choroid

YOU CODE IT! CASE STUDY

Edward Yankovic, a 53-year-old male, was working in a metal shop. As he was trimming a steel bar, some metal splinters got into his eye. Fortunately, Dr. Madison found that the metal pieces presented superficial damage, and had not embedded themselves in Edward's conjunctiva. Dr. Madison removed all the metal pieces and placed a patch over Edward's eye.

You Code It!

Go through the steps of coding, and determine the codes that should be reported for this encounter between Dr. Madison and Edward Yankovic.

Step 1: Read the case completely.

Step 2: Abstract the notes: Which key words can you identify relating to the procedures performed?

_____

Step 3: Query the provider, if necessary.

Step 4: Diagnosis: Foreign body, conjunctiva, superficial.

Step 5: Code the procedure(s).

_____

Step 6: Link the procedure codes to at least one diagnosis code.

Step 7: Back code to double-check your choices.

Answer

Did you find the correct code to be:

65205 Removal of foreign body, external eye; conjunctival superficial

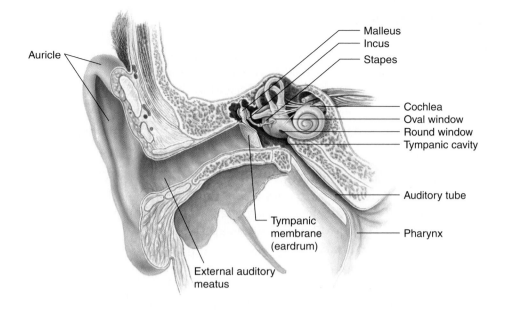

Auricle

Malleus
Incus
Stapes

Cochlea
Oval window
Round window
Tympanic cavity

Auditory tube

Tympanic
membrane
(eardrum)

Pharynx

External auditory
meatus

AUDITORY SYSTEM

There are *no* specific guidelines for the Auditory subsection of surgery.

YOU CODE IT! CASE STUDY

Rochelle McMillian, a 31-year-old female, has been deaf since she was 12. She is admitted today for Dr. Donaldson to put a cochlear implant in her left ear. It is expected that Rochelle will gain back much of her hearing.

You Code It!

Go through the steps of coding, and determine the codes that should be reported for this encounter between Dr. Donaldson and Rochelle McMillian.

Step 1: Read the case completely.

Step 2: Abstract the notes: Which key words can you identify relating to the procedures performed?

Step 3: Query the provider, if necessary.

Step 4: Diagnosis: Deafness, acquired.

Step 5: Code the procedure(s).

Step 6: Link the procedure codes to at least one diagnosis code.

Step 7: Back code to double-check your choices.

Answer

Did you find the correct code to be:

69930 Cochlear device implantation, with or without mastoidectomy

OPERATING MICROSCOPE

When a surgeon performs microsurgery, he or she has to use an operating microscope. In such cases, you must code the microscope, code 69990, in addition to the procedure in which the microscope is used.

> +69990 Microsurgical techniques, requiring use of operating microscope (List separately in addition to code for primary procedure.)

There are two guidelines with regard to this add-on code:

1. Do not append modifier 51 Multiple Procedures to the code for the microscope. In reality, it is not a separate or additional procedure. The code 69990 indicates the use of a special technique or tool. Therefore, modifier 51 would not be appropriate.

2. There are some codes that already include the use of the operating microscope. Therefore, adding code 69990 is redundant. The tough part here is that none of the codes that already include use of the operating microscope include this information in their description. Following is the list of codes with which you are *not* permitted to add code 69990 because it is already included:

15756–15758	31526	49906
15842	31531	61548
19364	31536	63075–63078
19368	31541	64727
20955–20962	31561	64820–64823
20969–20973	31571	65091–68850
26551–26554	43116	
26556	43496	

EXAMPLE

19364 Breast reconstruction with free flap

(Do not report code 69990 in addition to code 19364.)

As you can see, the codes involved are throughout the Surgery section of the CPT. You might want to go though and mark or highlight the codes, should you be coding for a physician who works with an operating microscope.

CHAPTER SUMMARY

When reporting surgical procedures, it is important (1) to identify the components of the operation and (2) determine which services are included in the code's description and which services require a separate code. The Surgery section of the CPT book is divided into subsections identified by the body system upon which the technique was performed.

1. Codes within the musculoskeletal subsection include

   a. X-rays.

   b. Cast.

   c. Medications.

   d. Shoes.

2. Arthrodesis is performed

   a. Alone.

   b. In combination with other procedures.

   c. (*a*) and (*b*).

   d. None of the above.

3. An open treatment of a fracture is performed

   a. Only on a compound fracture.

   b. After the cast is applied.

   c. Surgically.

   d. In the radiology department.

4. Backbench work during a transplant process is

   a. The harvesting of an organ from a donor.

   b. The implantation of the new organ.

   c. The documentation of the surgery.

   d. The preparation of the organ.

5. The cardiovascular system includes all except

   a. Heart.

   b. Veins.

   c. Lungs.

   d. Arteries.

6. Venous grafts harvested from the saphenous vein

   a. Are included in the graft code.

   b. Require an add-on code.

   c. Are coded with a modifier.

   d. Are coded separately.

7. The code for an endovascular repair of an iliac aneurysm includes all except

   a. Introduction of graft.

   b. Stent deployment.

   c. Balloon angioplasty.

   d. Pacemaker.

8. An enterectomy is the harvesting of a donor's

   a. Lung.

   b. Liver.

   c. Intestine.

   d. Artery.

9. A pancreatic donor must be

   a. Living.

   b. Deceased.

   c. Either living or deceased.

   d. A relative.

10. A physician who only interprets the results of a urodynamic procedure must be coded with

   a. Modifier 32.

   b. Modifier 26.

   c. Modifier 53.

   d. Modifier 51.

1. Peter Lynch, a 15-year-old male, came to see Dr. Ferguson for the first time. He was in a fight at school and got punched in the jaw, dislocating his temporomandibular joint. Dr. Ferguson performed a closed treatment of the temporomandibular dislocation. He did not require any wiring or fixation.

   _____

2. Bobby Sherman, a 13-year-old male, was brought to the emergency room by his camp counselor. Two weeks prior, Bobby had broken his arm and had a short-arm cast applied. While walking by the pool, his friends pushed him in, getting the cast wet. Bobby was brought here to have his cast reapplied.

   _____

3. Brad Vitalli, a 49-year-old male, was admitted into the hospital so that Dr. Alden could remove a tumor found on his larynx. Brad tolerated the laryngotomy and the removal of the tumor well.

   _____

4. Dr. Unger ordered a catheter aspiration of Marion Gerstein's tracheobronchial tree. Marion was given some Versed (conscious sedation), and the procedure was performed at her bedside in her hospital room.

   _____

5. Dr. Albertson performed the backbench preparation of a cadaver donor heart allograft prior to Dr. Contini performing the transplantation. Code for Dr. Albertson's work.

   _____

6. Dr. Eldersten performed an endovascular graft on Wanda Popu, a 45-year-old female, diagnosed with an arteriovenous malformation of the iliac artery.

   _____

7. George Jaden, a 59-year-old male, is admitted for a partial colectomy. Dr. Issacson resected a segment of George's colon and performed an anastomosis between the remaining ends of the colon. George tolerated the procedure well.

   _____

8. Patricia Morrison, a morbidly obese 37-year-old female, was admitted for a gastric restrictive procedure. In addition to the gastric bypass performed by Dr. Wattel, Patricia's small intestine was reconstructed to limit absorption.

   _____

9. Israel Ortega, a 51-year-old male, is admitted to the hospital today so that Dr. Warren can perform a total urethrectomy and a cystostomy.

   _____

10. Jan Springer, a 51-year-old male with multiple sclerosis, has been diagnosed with Peyronie disease. He is admitted today so that Dr. Rudner can excise the penile plaque that has developed.

    _____

11. Jack Friedman, an 83-year-old male, had a programmable cerebrospinal fluid shunt inserted six weeks ago by Dr. Girald. Today, Jack comes to the office so that Dr. Girald can reprogram the shunt and make the adjustments as shown necessary by the CT scan taken last week.

    _____

12. Bridgette Smith, a 17-year-old female, was taken to the OR, so that Dr. Payas could perform a twist drill hole in order to evacuate and drain a subdural hematoma that formed after she banged her head on an overhead bar while on a roller-coaster at an amusement park.

    _____

13. Donna Travellina, a 33-year-old female, noticed a lesion on her left eyelid. Over the period of a few months, it not only bothered but also worried her. She was admitted today so that Dr. Charne could excise the lesion. He used a simple, direct closure. Donna's prognosis is excellent.

    _____

14. Jay Ericson, a 41-year-old male, hurt his eye in an accident. Dr. Lucas examined him and noticed that his cornea was scratched. It was not a perforating laceration. Dr. Lucas repaired the laceration of the cornea in the office.

    _____

15. Having trouble hearing, Rodney Loman, a 61-year-old male, came to see Dr. Beariman, an audiologist. After examination, Dr. Beariman removed the impacted earwax from both ears. Rodney was amazed at the improvement in his hearing and left the office feeling much better.

    _____

Below and on the following pages you will find several procedure and operative notes from physicians performing services and treatments for patients. Find the best, most appropriate codes from the Surgery Section of the CPT book for the physician's work from each of these reports.

CIPHER, VICTORS, & ASSOCIATES
A Complete Health Care Facility
234 MAIN STREET • ANYTOWN, FL 32711 • 407-555-1234

PATIENT:	FRIEDMAN, DORIS
MRN:	FRIEDO01
Date:	23 September 2008
Procedure performed:	Colonoscopy
Physician:	Matthew Appellet, MD

Indications: History of inflammatory bowel disease

Procedure: The patient was given no premedication at her request, and the Olympus PCF-130 colonoscope was used. The mucosa of the rectum was essentially normal apart from some mild nonspecific edema. Photographs and biopsies were obtained. The remainder of the rectum was normal. The sigmoid was normal as was the descending colon, splenic flexure, transverse colon, hepatic flexure, right colon and cecum. No evidence of polyps, tumors, masses, or inflammation. The scope was then withdrawn, these findings confirmed. The procedure was terminated, and the patient tolerated it well.

Impression:	Normal colonic mucosa through the cecum.
Plan:	Await results of rectal biopsies.

9/23/08 19:38:17

Matthew Appellet, MD

MA/mg D: 9/23/08 09:50:16 T: 9/25/08 12:55:01

Find the best, most appropriate code(s).

_____

_____

_____

CIPHER, VICTORS, & ASSOCIATES
A Complete Health Care Facility
234 MAIN STREET • ANYTOWN, FL 32711 • 407-555-1234

PATIENT: FRANKS, ELMER
ACCOUNT/EHR #:   FRAEL002

Date of Operation: 06/17/08
Preoperative Diagnosis: Orbital mass, OD
Postoperative Diagnosis: Herniated orbital fat pad, OD
Operation: Excision of mass and repair, right superior orbit

Surgeon: Mark C. Warren, M.D.
Assistant: n/a
Anesthesia: Local

Description of Operative Procedure:

After proparacaine was instilled in the eye, it was prepped and draped in the usual sterile manner and 2 percent Lidocaine with 1:200,000 epinephrine was injected into the superior aspect of the right orbit. A corneal protective shield was placed in the eye. The eye was placed in down-gaze.

The upper lid was everted and the fornix examined. The herniating mass was viewed and measured at 0.75 cm in diameter. Westcott scissors were used to incise the fornix conjunctiva. The herniating mass was then clamped, excised and cauterized. It appeared to contain mostly fat tissue, which was sent to pathology. The superior fornix was repaired using running suture of 6-0 plain gut. Bacitracin ointment was applied to the eye followed by an eye pad. The patient tolerated the procedure well and left the operating room in good condition.

_____

Mark C. Welby, MD

MCW/mg   D: 06/17/08 09:50:16   T: 06/19/08 12:55:01

Find the best, most appropriate code(s).

_____

_____

_____

CIPHER, VICTORS, & ASSOCIATES
A Complete Health Care Facility
234 MAIN STREET • ANYTOWN, FL 32711 • 407-555-1234

PATIENT: ROBART, BETTY
MRN: ROBABE001
Date: 09/23/08

Attending Physician: James Healer, MD

Preoperative Diagnosis: C5 compression fracture
Postoperative Diagnosis: same
Procedure: C5 corpectomy and fusion fixation with fibular strut graft and Atlantis plate
Anesthesia: General endotracheal

This is a 25-year-old female status post assault. The patient sustained a C5 compression fracture. MRI scan showed compression with evidence of posterior ligamentous injury. The patient was subsequently set up for the surgical procedure. The procedure was described in detail including the risks. The risks included but not limited to bleeding, infection, stroke, paralysis, death, cerebrospinal fluid (CSF) leak, loss of bladder and bowel control, hoarse voice, paralyzed vocal cord, death and damage to adjacent nerves and tissues. The patient understood the risks. The patient also understood that bank bone instrumentation would be used and that the bank bone could collapse and the instrumentation could fail, break, or the screws could pull out. The patient provided consent.

  The patient was taken to the OR. The patient was induced. Endotracheal tube was placed. A Foley was placed. The patient was given preoperative antibiotics. The patient was placed in slight extension. The right neck was prepped and draped in the usual manner. A linear incision was made over the C5 vertebral body. The platysma was divided. Dissection was continued medial to the sternocleidomastoid to the prevertebral fascia. This was cauterized and divided. The longus colli was cauterized and elevated. The fracture was visualized. A spinal needle was used to verify the location using fluoroscopy. The C5 vertebral body was drilled out. The bone was saved. The disks above and below were removed. The posterior longitudinal ligament was removed. The bone was quite collapsed and fragmented. Distraction pins were then packed with bone removed from the C5 vertebral body prior to implantation. A plate was then placed with screws in the C4 and C6 vertebral bodies. The locking screws were tightened. The wound was irrigated. Bleeding was helped with the bipolar. The retractors were removed. The incision was approximated with simple interrupted Vicryl. The subcutaneous tissue was approximated and skin edges approximated subcuticularly. Steri-Strips applied. A dressing was applied. The patient was placed back in an Aspen collar. The patient was extubated and transferred to recovery.

James Healer, MD

JH/mgr D: 09/23/08 12:33:08 PM T: 09/25/08 3:22:54 PM

Find the best, most appropriate code(s).

_____

_____

_____

CIPHER, VICTORS, & ASSOCIATES
A Complete Health Care Facility
234 MAIN STREET • ANYTOWN, FL 32711 • 407-555-1234

PATIENT:	BAKER, DORITTA
MRN:	BAKEDO01
Admission Date:	19 September 2008
Discharge Date:	19 September 2008
Date:	19 September 2008
Preoperative DX:	High-grade squamous intraepithelial lesion of the cervix
Postoperative DX:	same
Operation:	Loop electrosurgical excision procedure (LEEP) and ECC (endocervical curettage)
Surgeon:	Rodney L. Cohen, MD
Assistant:	None
Anesthesia:	General by LMA
Findings:	Large ectropion, large non-staining active cervix essentially encompassing the entire active cervix
Specimens:	To pathology
Disposition:	Stable to recovery room

Procedure: The patient was taken to the OR where she was placed in the supine position and administered general anesthesia. She was then placed in cane stirrups and prepped and draped in the usual fashion. Her vaginal vault was not prepped. The coated speculum was then placed and the cervix exposed. It was then painted with Lugol and the whole entire active cervix was nonstaining with the clearly defined margins where the stain began to be picked up. The cervix was injected with approximately 7 cc of lidocaine with 1% epinephrine. Using a large loop, the anterior cervix was excised and then the posterior loop was excised in separate specimens. Because of the size of the lesion one piece in total was not accomplished. Prior to the excision, the endocervical curettage was performed and specimen collected. All specimens sent to pathology. The remaining cervical bed was cauterized and then painted with Monsel for hemostasis. The case was concluded with this. Instruments were removed. The patient was taken down from candy cane stirrups, awakened from the anesthesia, and taken to the recovery room in stable condition.

9/19/08 19:38:17

Find the best, most appropriate code(s).

_____

_____

_____

PATIENT: UNDERWOOD, PRISCILLA
MRN: UNDEPR01

Date: 25 September 2008
Diagnosis: Medulloblastoma
Procedure: Central Venous Access Device (CVAD) insertion

Physician: Frank Vincent, MD
Anesthesia: Conscious sedation

Procedure: Patient is a 4-year-old female, with a recent diagnosis of malignancy. Due to an upcoming course of chemotherapy, the CVAD is being inserted to ease administration of the drugs. The patient was placed on the table in supine position. The patient is given Versed to achieve conscious sedation. The incision was made to insert a central venous catheter, centrally. During the placement of the catheter, a short tract (nontunneled) is made as the catheter is advanced from the skin entry site to the point of venous cannulation. The catheter tip is set to reside in the subclavian vein. The patient was gently aroused from the sedation and was awake when transported to the recovery room.

Frank Vincent, MD

FV/mg   D: 9/25/08 09:50:16   T: 9/25/08 12:55:01

Find the best, most appropriate code(s).

_____

_____

_____

Radiology Coding

9

LEARNING OUTCOMES

- Apply the guidelines to determine the best, most appropriate codes.
- List the various types of imaging techniques.
- Decide when to code radiologic services as a companion to a surgical procedure.
- Distinguish technical components from professional components.
- Correctly apply guidelines regarding the use of additional codes.
- Determine how and when to use modifiers.

KEY TERMS

Angiography
Arthrography
Computerized tomography (CT)
Fluoroscope
Magnetic resonance arthrography (MRA)
Magnetic resonance imaging (MRI)
Nuclear medicine
Radiation
Sonogram
Venography

Hospitals
Ambulatory surgery centers
Clinics
Long-term care facilities
Multispecialty clinics
Interventional radiologists

Diagnostic imaging centers
Portable x-ray suppliers
Orthopedists
Physical medicine and rehabilitation centers

EMPLOYMENT OPPORTUNITIES

Health care professionals use radiologic imaging to see inside the body. Radiologic services, also known as *interventional radiology,* can be used to investigate a potential condition (diagnostically), measure the progress of a disease or condition, or aid in the actual reduction or prevention of disease or other condition (therapeutically).

Many, many years ago, radiology was simply known as x-ray, because this was the extent of the equipment. Now, technology has made tremendous advancements in the science of imaging, and health care professionals can screen, diagnose, monitor, and treat patients much more effectively and efficiently.

TECHNICAL VS. PROFESSIONAL

Essentially, there are two primary components of any radiologic procedure: the technical and the professional (referred to as supervision and interpretation in the CPT). This is not to say that radiologic technicians are not professionals. Not at all. The designation is merely to divide the services provided so that it can be determined which facility or practitioner should be paid for what.

EXAMPLE

Meredith Atkins, a 33-year-old female, was sent to Diagnostic Imaging Center to get an x-ray, three views, of her skull, after she was hit in the head by a bat at a softball game.

The x-ray equipment is owned by the facility. Sarah Carter, the x-ray technician who will operate the equipment, is a member of the facility's staff, and Dr. Rivers, a board-certified radiologist who will interpret the films and send a report of this evaluation to Meredith's physician, is also a staff member of the Center. Therefore, Diagnostic Imaging's coding specialist will ask the insurance company for reimbursement for both the technical procedure (the use of the equipment, materials, and the staff to work and maintain that equipment) and the professional aspect (the cost and work to surpervise and interpret the films).

For Meredith's case, the code to be reported is 70250.

Purchasing (or leasing) and maintaining imaging equipment is very expensive, and cannot be supported by every health care facility. In addition, physicians who are specially trained radiologists are not necessarily staff members of all health care facilities with the equipment. Therefore, circumstances may arise when the technical procedure and the professional service must be billed separately. In those cases, the coder who is responsible for charging for the professional services must use modifier 26 to identify the separation of the components.

26 **Professional Component:** Certain procedures are a combination of a physician component and a technical component. When the physician component is reported separately, the service may be identified by adding modifier 26 to the usual procedure number.

EXAMPLE

Clifford Sienna, a 27-year-old male, was brought into the emergency department of a small hospital near his farm after he fell off a ladder onto his back while working in the barn. The physician sent Clifford to radiology for an entire spine survey study. The hospital does not have a staff radiologist, so Dr. Chen is brought over to evaluate the x-rays and write the report for the physician.

The hospital, which owns the equipment and pays the salary for the technician, will bill the insurance carrier for the technical portion of the examination, using code 72010.

Dr. Chen's coding specialist will send in a claim for Dr. Chen's interpretation only, the professional services he provided. In order to make this clear on the claim form, the modifier 26 Professional Component will be appended to the code for the radiologic examination who will report 72010-26 on his claim form.

As you have already learned, sometimes the CPT book will save you work. Certain radiologic examination codes distinguish the technical component and professional component of services for you. One of the easiest ways to identify such cases is by the notation within the code's description that specifies the code is for radiologic supervision and interpretation only.

«« **CODING TIP**

If the third-party payer accepts HCPCS Level II, you can add the modifier TC Technical Component to the CPT code.

EXAMPLE

> 71040 Bronchography, unilateral, radiological supervision and interpretation

«« **CODING TIP**

Some third-party payers will determine the TC and PC components for payment without the modifier by the place of service code shown on the claim form.

From the example, you can see that code 71040 excludes the technical component. If you are coding for the physician's services only, that makes it easy. If you are coding for the facility for the technical aspect, you may need to add a modifier.

After a while, you will learn the details about the procedures performed by all of the professionals in your health care facility, and you will be able to identify the components easily. It just takes some practice.

LET'S CODE IT! SCENARIO

Derick Norton, an 8-year-old male, is brought into the emergency department by ambulance. He was skateboarding off a homemade ramp and fell on his neck and shoulder. Dr. Defeaux suspects a broken clavicle and orders a complete radiologic exam of the area. The staff radiologist, Dr. Grace, reads the films and sends a report down to Dr. Defeaux confirming the fracture.

Let's Code It!

The physician's notes state that a *radiologic exam* of Derick's *clavicle* was performed. When you turn to the alphabetic index under *radiology*, you note that the choices are not going to satisfy our needs. Therefore, let's try an alternate term for radiology: x-ray. Turn to *x-ray*, and you find a long list of anatomical sites. Next to the word *clavicle* you see only one suggested code. Let's go to the numeric listing and read the complete description.

> 73000 Radiologic examination; clavicle, complete

This is exactly what Dr. Defeaux ordered for Derick. Good job!

LET'S CODE IT! SCENARIO

Marisol Martinez, a 31-year-old female, is 10 weeks pregnant. This is her first pregnancy, and twins run in her family. In order to determine how many fetuses there are, Dr. Phillips orders a sonogram. Brenda Hughes is the technician at the Imaging Center next door to Dr. Phillips's office.

The Imaging Center performs Marisol's real-time transabdominal exam, and sends the documentation to Dr. Phillips so he can read and interpret the results.

Sonogram

The use of sound waves to record images of internal organs and tissues. Also called an ultrasound.

You are Dr. Phillips's coder, and his notes state that a **sonogram** of Marisol was performed at the imaging center. We know that she is pregnant, and this is why she is having the test done, so the anatomical site of the examination is her *pregnant uterus.* Turn to the alphabetic index under *sonography,* and the CPT book tells you to *see echography,* which is the type of technology that sonograms use. Turn to *echography* (caution—not echo*cardio*graphy; this is not of Marisol's heart), and you find a list of anatomical sites. Looking for *pregnant uterus,* you see a range of suggested codes. Let's go to the numeric listing, and read the complete description of the first one.

> 76801 Ultrasound, pregnant uterus, real time with image documentation, fetal and maternal evaluation, first trimester (<14 weeks 0 days), Transabdominal approach; single or first gestation

Great! The very first code seems to match the notes perfectly. However, to make certain you are using the best, most appropriate code, you will want to read through all the suggested codes.

Remember, you are coding for Dr. Phillips. With regard to Marisol's radiologic exam, he provided the interpretation—the professional component only. Therefore, the claim form you prepare should show this code as 76801-26.

VIEWS

Throughout the Radiology section of the CPT book, radiologic examinations are often described by the number of views taken by the technician.

EXAMPLE

> 73060 Radiologic examination, humerus, two views

The "two views" refers to the number of angles, or perceptions, from which the images were taken, such as anterior and posterior. Such codes represent the norm, or standard, in imaging when it comes to these certain anatomical sites.

The most common angles, or pathways, of imaging include:

- AP   *Anteroposterior:* Front to back
- PA   *Posteroanterior:* Back to front
- O   *Oblique:* At an angle
- RAO   *Right anterior oblique:* At an angle from the right front
- RPO   *Right posterior oblique:* At an angle from the right back
- LAO   *Left anterior oblique:* At an angle from the left front

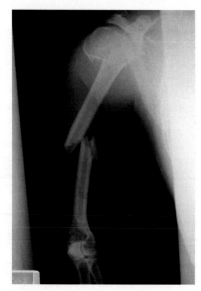

- LPO *Left posterior oblique:* At an angle from the left back
- Lat *Lateral (lat):* From one side to the other side

Should it happen that the radiologist takes fewer than the minimum number of views included in the description, you have to append the radiologic code with modifier 52 Reduced Services.

52 **Reduced Services:** Under certain circumstances a service or procedure is partially reduced or eliminated at the physician's discretion. Under these circumstances, the service provided can be identified by its usual procedure number and the addition of modifier 52, signifying that the service is reduced. This provides a means of reporting reduced services without disturbing the identification of the basic service.

YOU CODE IT! CASE STUDY

Caroline Stephens, an 18-month-old female, is brought into her pediatrician's office, Dr. Katzman, because she fell off the couch onto a hard tile floor. It appears that her hip is painful to her, so Dr. Katzman wants an x-ray of the pelvis and hip to determine if there is a fracture. However, Dr. Katzman orders only the anteroposterior view to be taken. He has a policy of not subjecting his patients to exposure to radiology unnecessarily, and he believes that the one view will tell him what he needs to know. The x-ray does confirm a hairline fracture, and he applies a cast.

You Code It!

Go through the steps of coding, and determine the codes that should be reported for this encounter between Dr. Katzman and Caroline Stephens.

Step 1: Read the case completely.

Step 2: Abstract the notes: Which key words can you identify relating to the procedures performed?

_____

Step 3: Query the provider, if necessary.

Step 4: Diagnosis: Fracture, hip.

Step 5: Code the procedure(s).

_____

Step 6: Link the procedure codes to at least one diagnosis code.

Step 7: Back code to double-check your choices.

Answer

Did you find the correct code to be:

73540-52 Radiologic examination, pelvis and hips, infant or child, minimum of two views; reduced service

Good job!

Arthrography

The recording of a picture of an anatomical joint after the administration of contrast material into the joint capsule.

Fluoroscope

A piece of equipment that emits x-rays through a part of the patient's body onto a fluorescent screen, causing the image to identify various aspects of the anatomy by density.

Computerized tomography (CT)

A specialized computer scanner with very fine detail, to record imaging of internal anatomical sites.

Magnetic resonance arthrography (MRA)

MR imaging of an anatomical joint after the administration of contrast material into the joint capsule.

Magnetic resonance imaging (MRI)

A three-dimensional radiologic technique that uses nuclear technology to record pictures of internal anatomical sites.

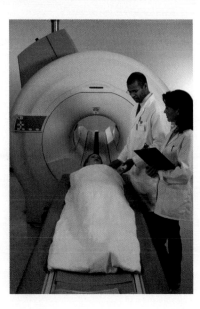

PROCEDURES WITH OR WITHOUT CONTRAST

Some imaging examinations use contrast materials to gain a clearer picture of an organ or anatomical site. The phrase "with contrast" means that the technician or physician gave the patient a substance to enhance the image.

1. When radiographic **arthrography** is performed, use an additional code for the supervision and interpretation of the appropriate joint. This includes the use of a **fluoroscope.**

EXAMPLE

Dr. Goldtree, a radiologist, supervised a radiographic arthrography of Conrad Douglas's ankle and later the interpreted results would be reported using code 73615.

2. Imaging "with contrast" has some guidelines that you have to know in order to code accurately.
   a. If the code description includes the term "with contrast," such as **CT** with contrast, CTA with contrast, **MRA** with contrast, or **MRI** with contrast, the injection of the contrast materials, when administered intravenously, is already included in the code and should *not* be reported separately.
   b. If the contrast material is injected intra-articularly (into a joint) or intrathecally (into a tendon or sheath), an additional code is reported for the appropriate joint injection.
   c. Providing contrast materials orally and/or rectally alone does not constitute an exam "with contrast."

EXAMPLE

Dr. Holmes injected David Rogers's elbow intrathecally with contrast materials to do an radiographic arthrography for his tennis elbow. This is reported with codes 24220, 73085.

3. When a CT or MR arthrography is performed without radiographic arthrography, you will need three different codes:
   a. A code for the imaging guidance (fluoroscopy) of the placement of the needle to inject the contrast material
   b. A code for the injection of the contrast material into the specific joint
   c. A code for the appropriate CT or MR

EXAMPLE

Bernadette Hughes is experiencing pain in her pelvic region. Dr. Mateo orders an MRA of her hip/pelvis with contrast. The material is injected intra-articularly. This is reported using codes 77002, 27093, 72198.

Part 1   CPT

Jason Tennison, a 75-year-old male, has been having problems with his memory and his walking. After an extensive examination, his neurologist, Dr. Grunion, orders an MRI, brain, with and without contrast, to determine if Jason is suffering from hydrocephalus.

Let's Code It!

This is very straightforward. Jason had a *MRI* of his *brain* taken. Let's go to the alphabetic index and look this up. Under *magnetic resonance imaging (MRI)*, we see the list of anatomical sites, including *brain*, which gives us the suggested code range 70551–70553. (Note: *Intraoperative*, indented below *brain*, means that the MRI was performed during surgery. This was not the case for Jason, according to the physician's notes.) Go to the numeric listing and read the descriptions.

> 70551 Magnetic resonance (e.g., proton) imaging, brain (including brain stem); without contrast material
>
> 70552   with contrast material(s)
>
> 70553   without contrast material, followed by contrast material(s) and further sequences

Dr. Grunion's notes state that the MRI is *with* and *without contrast.* That means both types of imaging were done. Code 70551 describes without contrast and code 70552 includes the contrast. When you keep reading, you see that code 70553 is the correct code because, as the notes state, it includes both sequences: without the contrast followed by with contrast materials. Of course, you will also add the appropriate HCPCS level II codes to report the contrast materials used.

««« **CODING TIP**

Appropriate HCPCS Level II codes from the range Q9945-Q9954, based on the number of units, should be assigned to report the contrast materials used.

Other types of radiologic procedures include:

Positron emission tomography (PET): Uses a variety of radiopharmaceuticals that mimic natural sugars, water, proteins, and oxygen and collect in various tissues and organs. It is a time-exposure picture of cellular biological activities.

Bone density scan (DEXA): Used most often for osteoporosis screenings; enables assessment of bone minerals in spine, hip, and other skeletal sites.

Nuclear medicine scan: Used to assess organ system function.

DIAGNOSTIC ANGIOGRAPHY

The coding of the process of imaging the body's blood vessels, diagnostic **angiography**, carries certain guidelines affecting their use.

1. In some cases, interventional coding guidelines don't permit you to report a diagnostic angiography when performed at the same time as a therapeutic interventional procedure. This rule applies, when the patient has already been diagnosed and has scheduled

Angiography

The imaging of blood vessels after the injection of contrast material.

a therapeutic intervention to correct the problem. As you have already learned, you must read the guidelines and the code descriptions carefully.

EXAMPLE

Dr. Aspiras performed a carotid arterial angiography to check for blockage and immediately performed an intervention procedure. You would report this using code 75660, along with the codes for the intervention, the catheterization, and the contrast injection.

2. In other cases, the diagnostic angiography *should be coded separately* even though it is done at the same session as an interventional procedure. This is true if one of the following conditions has been met:

   a. A full diagnostic study is done, no prior catheter-based angiographic study is available, and the decision to intervene is determined by the diagnostic study.

   b. The patient's condition has changed since a previously done study.

   c. The patient's condition changes during the interventional procedure that requires a diagnostic procedure to look at vessels outside of the area.

   d. If the prior diagnostic angiography did not show the applicable anatomy and/or pathology being treated at the session.

EXAMPLE

Denise Casson had a diagnostic angiography of her adrenal gland one year ago. Since then, her condition has deteriorated. Therefore, Dr. Reginald first performs a diagnostic procedure. Because this showed changes at the same session, he performs an interventional procedure.

CODING TIP »»

The CPT book provides diagnostic angiography guidelines in the text directly before code 75600.

3. Diagnostic angiography is included with the code for an interventional procedure and should *not* be coded separately when that diagnostic angiography is performed for any of the following:

   a. Vessel measurement

   b. Postangioplasty or stent angiography

   c. Contrast injections, angiography, road mapping, and/or fluoroscopic guidance for the interventional procedure

LET'S CODE IT! SCENARIO

Norma Washington, a 57-year-old female, has had two mild heart attacks in the past two years. Today, Norma is at the Fairfield Ambulatory Surgical Center for a diagnostic angiography to quantify the degree of blockage suspected in her left renal artery. Dr. Johannson performed the procedure that included placing the catheter directly in the renal artery. Later that day, Dr. Johannson dictated a report indicating that Norma's left renal artery is 50% blocked.

The notes indicate that a *left renal angiography* was performed on Norma. Let's go to the alphabetic index and look up *angiography*. You know that Norma's renal artery was examined, and the index suggests codes 75722–75724. Let's check the complete descriptions in the numeric listings.

75722 Angiography, renal, unilateral, selective (including flush aortogram), radiological supervision and interpretation

75724 Angiography, renal, bilateral, selective (including flush aortogram), radiological supervision and interpretation

The difference between these two code descriptions is that 75722 is for a unilateral procedure and 75724 is for a bilateral procedure. Norma had only her left renal artery examined. One side is unilateral, leading us to the correct code of 75722.

DIAGNOSTIC VENOGRAPHY

The codes for reporting diagnostic **venography** have similar guidelines to those for diagnostic angiography.

Venography

The imaging of a vein after the injection of contrast material.

1. Some interventional procedure codes include the diagnostic venography when done at the same time. You must read the descriptions carefully to determine if this is the case.

2. Diagnostic venography done at the same time, as an interventional procedure *should be coded separately* if one of the following conditions has been met:

   a. A full diagnostic study is done, no prior catheter-based venographic study is available, and the decision to intervene is determined by this diagnostic study.

   b. The patient's condition has changed since a previously done study.

   c. The patient's condition changes during the interventional procedure that requires a diagnostic procedure to look at vessels outside of the area.

   d. If the prior diagnostic venography did not show the applicable anatomy and/or pathology being treated at the session.

3. Diagnostic venography is included with the code for an interventional procedure and should *not* be coded separately when that diagnostic venography is performed for any of the following:

   a. Vessel measurement,

   b. Postangioplasty or stent venography,

   c. Contrast injections, venography, road mapping, and/or fluoroscopic guidance for the interventional procedure.

Natan Fawzi, a 55-year-old male, flew in yesterday from Australia, a 26-hour airplane ride. Since getting off the plane, he has been having pain in his right calf. Dr. Leventhol performed a diagnostic venography to determine if Natan has deep vein thrombosis (DVT). After completing the procedure, he wrote a report with his interpretation, which was sent to Natan's internist.

Let's Code It!

Dr. Leventhol performed a *diagnostic venography* of Natan's *right leg.* Let's go to the alphabetic index and find *venography.* Beneath *venography,* you see the anatomical site *leg* with the suggested code range 75820–75822. Let's look at the code descriptions in the numeric listings.

> 75820 Venography, extremity, unilateral, radiological supervision and interpretation

> 75822 Venography, extremity, bilateral, radiological supervision and interpretation

The difference between these two codes is that 75820 is a unilateral procedure and 75822 is a bilateral procedure. Natan had only his right leg examined, making it a unilateral procedure and making 75820 the correct code.

TRANSCATHETER PROCEDURES

Therapeutic transcatheter radiological supervision and interpretation codes, when associated with intervention, already include:

1. Vessel measurement,
2. Postangioplasty or stent venography,
3. Contrast injections, angiography/venography, road mapping, and/or fluoroscopic guidance for the interventional procedure.

Transcatheter therapeutic radiologic and interpretation services *are* separately reportable from diagnostic angiography/venography done at the same time *unless* they are specifically included in the code descriptor.

Dr. Jerome is in the OR today to perform a transcatheter placement of an intravascular stent, percutaneously, in Gayle Calendar's common iliac.

Let's Code It!

You are Dr. Jerome's coding specialist, so you are only going to code the *radiological supervision and interpretation* of the *transcatheter pro-*

Part 1 CPT

cedure, as well as the placement of the stent itself. Let's go to *trans-catheter* in the alphabetic index. You will notice that if we go to *place-ment* under *transcatheter,* you see *intravascular stents* indented below. Here, the index suggests some category III codes (the T codes, which we review in full detail in Chap. 12) along with code ranges 37205–37208, 37215–37216.

When you turn to the codes, you realize that they are in the Surgery section, not Radiology. However, they are the only codes offered by the index, so let's take a look at the first code:

37205 Transcatheter placement of an intravascular stent(s), (except coronary, carotid, and vertebral vessel), percutaneous; initial vessel

But we are coding for Dr. Jerome's radiological supervision and inter-pretation for the procedure, and the stent placement. Keep reading, and you will see the CPT book's notation in the parentheses directly below code 37205. It says, "(For radiological supervision and interpretation, use 75960)." Check out code 75960, and see that it reads:

75960 Transcatheter introduction of intravascular stent(s), (except coronary, carotid, and vertebral vessel), percutaneous and/or open, radiological supervision and interpretation, each vessel.

Reporting both codes tells the whole story. Perfect!

DIAGNOSTIC ULTRASOUND

The description of an ultrasound exam as being "complete" is determined by the specific number of elements, such as organs or areas, which are to be surveyed during the test. However, sometimes, the full list is not visualized. For example, an organ may have been previously removed surgically, or another organ may be blocking the view of the exam. The report that is submitted for the patient's record, after the exam, should note everything that was studied—as well as those elements that should have been but were not, along with why they were not. As the coding specialist, you must read the report and pay attention to whether the exam was "complete" or "limited" and choose the correct code.

You will find information regarding what is included in a com-plete exam in the instructions shown before each of the ultrasound subheadings.

CODING TIP

If the reason that an organ was not visible is documented in the patient's record, then, you are permitted to code this as "complete."

EXAMPLE

76770 Ultrasound, retroperitoneal (e.g., renal, aorta, nodes), B-scan and/or real time with image documentation; complete

76775   limited

You already know that ultrasound may be called a sonogram. How-ever, there are other definitions that are important for you to know so that you can determine the best, most appropriate code. The following terms identify the actual type of scan:

A-mode indicates a one-dimensional ultrasonic measurement procedure.

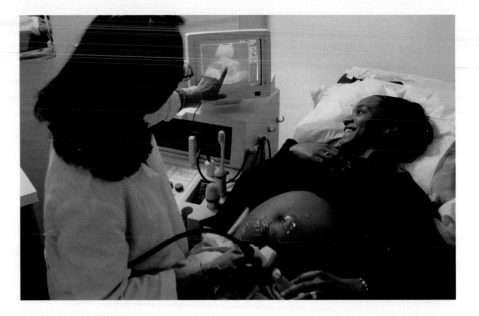

M-mode is also a one-dimensional ultrasonic measurement procedure; however, it includes the movement of the trace so that there can be a recording of both amplitude and velocity of the moving echo-producing structures.

B-scan indicates a two-dimensional ultrasonic scanning procedure with a two-dimensional display.

Real-time scan indicates that a two-dimensional ultrasonic scanning procedure with a display was performed and included both the two-dimensional structure and motion with time.

If the report indicates that a Doppler evaluation of vascular structures was performed, it should be coded separately with the codes from the Noninvasive Vascular Diagnostic Studies subsection, codes 93875–93990.

Should an ultrasound exam be performed *without* a thorough evaluation of an organ or anatomical region, recording of the image, and a final, written report, you are not permitted to code the procedure separately.

YOU CODE IT! CASE STUDY

Roger Kennedy, a 63-year-old male, was sent to the Diagnostic Imaging Center by Dr. Yanksey for a complete ultrasound of his abdominal region due to ongoing pain in the area. After the exam, the report indicated that his gallbladder was not visualized because it had been surgically removed in 1996. This fact is noted in Roger's chart. Dr. Yanksey's report concluded that Roger did appear to have calculus in his kidneys.

You Code It!

Go through the steps of coding, and determine the codes that should be reported for this encounter between Dr. Yanksey and Roger Kennedy.

Step 1: Read the case completely.

Step 2: Abstract the notes: Which key words can you identify relating to the procedures performed?

_____

Step 3: Query the provider, if necessary.

Step 4: Diagnosis: Abdominal pain.

Step 5: Code the procedure(s).

_____

Step 6: Link the procedure codes to at least one diagnosis code.

Step 7: Back code to double-check your choices.

Answer

Did you find the correct code to be:

76700 Ultrasound, abdominal, real time with image documentation; complete

Good job!

RADIATION ONCOLOGY

Radiation oncology, as you probably already know, is performed in the treatment of malignant neoplasm, carcinomas, also known as cancer.

The codes in the subsection already include certain services:

- Initial consultation
- Clinical treatment planning
- Simulation
- Medical radiation physics
- Dosimetry (the determination of the correct dosage)
- Treatment devices
- Special services
- Clinical treatment management procedures
- Normal follow-up care during treatment and for three months following the completion of the treatment

Radiation oncology services may be provided in varying degrees of intensity, and are determined, usually, in the planning process. Therefore, the preparation for the sequence of treatments must be coded accurately. Some professionals may describe the planning as simple, intermediate, or complex. However, others may provide the detail, leaving you to match the components performed with the level of service. Here are the specifics involved in each level:

- *Simple planning* involves one treatment area with one port, or parallel opposed ports, with simple or no blocking.

- *Intermediate planning* will involve two separate treatment areas, three or more converging ports, multiple blocks, or special time dose constraints.

Radiation

The high-speed discharge and projection of energy waves or particles.

Interventional radiologic
services, such as radiation
oncology, are typically provided
in a series over a span of time.
Make certain to code dates of
service accurately.

- *Complex planning* involves three or more separate treatment areas, highly complex blocking, custom shielding blocks, tangential ports, special wedges or compensators, rotational or special beam consideration, or a combination of therapeutic methods.

Just to keep you on your toes, you will find the same terms (simple, intermediate, complex) also used to describe the simulation applied. The good news is that the same terms relate to the same elements involved in the process. With simulation, we have one additional descriptor:

- *Three-dimensional computer-generated* reconstruction of the size and mass of the tumor and the normal tissues that surround the tumor site

If you work in a facility that provides proton beam treatments and/or clinical brachytherapy for patients, you will note that the CPT book has additional definitions for the same three terms: simple, intermediate, and complex.

NUCLEAR MEDICINE

Nuclear medicine

Treatment that includes the injection or digestion of isotopes.

One important point that you have to know as a coding specialist working with **nuclear medicine** procedures is that the codes presented in the CPT book do not include diagnostic or therapeutic radiopharmaceuticals (the drugs or isotopes used in the treatments). Therefore, you have to code them separately. If the insurance carrier accepts HCPCS Level II codes, you will use them. You learn all about HCPCS Level II codes in Part 2 of this textbook.

The administration of nuclear drugs, whether given to the patient orally, intravenously, intracavitarily, interstitially, or intra-arterially, are reported with codes 79005–79999.

Also note that any chemical pathology or chemical analysis done in connection with the provision of nuclear medicine treatments should be coded separately from the Pathology and Laboratory section of the CPT book.

YOU CODE IT! CASE STUDY

Florence Spevack, a 37-year-old female, had gained a great deal of weight recently with no change in her diet or exercise regimen. After a thorough examination, Dr. Sundance ordered nuclear imaging of her thyroid, with uptake. Radiopharmaceuticals were administered intravenously. The report came back to Dr. Sundance with the multiple determinations of Florence's exam.

You Code It!

Go through the steps of coding, and determine the codes that should be reported for this encounter between Dr. Sundance and Florence Spevack.

Step 1: Read the case completely.

Step 2: Abstract the notes: Which key words can you identify relating to the procedures performed?

_____

Step 3: Query the provider, if necessary.

Step 4: Diagnosis: Unexplained weight gain.

Step 5: Code the procedure(s).

_____

Step 6: Link the procedure codes to at least one diagnosis code.

Step 7: Back code to double-check your choices.

Answer

Did you find the correct code to be:

78007 Thyroid imaging, with uptake; multiple determinations

Great job!

CHAPTER SUMMARY

Health care technology has advanced tremendously in the area of radiology and imaging. As a coding specialist, it is important that you understand the differences between the types of radiological methods, as well as the components of each. With contrast and without contrast, CT scans, MRIs, sonograms, and so many more enable professionals to look inside the patient in a noninvasive manner, and it is your job to obtain the correct reimbursement for each and every procedure.

1. The professional component of radiological services includes

    a. Repair of the equipment.

    b. Interpretation of the imaging.

    c. Supplies.

    d. Training.

2. Interventional radiologic services are provided with the intent of all except

    a. Diagnosing a condition.

    b. Preventing the spread of a disease.

    c. Measuring the progress of a disease.

    d. Testing the equipment.

3. Sonograms use _____ to record images.

    a. nuclear isotopes

    b. radiation

    c. 3-D contrast reflection

    d. sound waves

4. The term "with contrast" means that the technician or radiologist

    a. Administered a substance to enhance the image.

    b. Used a black background behind the patient.

    c. Took the image a second time, to compare to the first.

    d. Used a blue background beneath the patient.

5. If the code description includes the term "two views" and the radiology reports only one view was taken, you should code the service

    a. With that code alone.

    b. With that code plus the modifier 52.

    c. With that code plus the modifier 53.

    d. With that code plus the modifier 22.

6. Angiography is the imaging of

    a. Bone.

    b. Internal organs.

    c. Blood vessels.

    d. Anatomical joint.

7. RPO stands for

    a. Right procedure operation.

    b. Regional protocol obstetric.

    c. Right posterior oblique.

    d. Right preventive oblique.

8. Radiation for the treatment of a malignant neoplasm is most often used for

    a. Diagnostic purposes.

    b. Therapeutic purposes.

    c. Research purposes.

    d. Prevention purposes.

9. An x-ray is the same as a

    a. CTA.

    b. CT.

    c. MRI.

    d. None of the above.

10. MRI stands for

    a. Magnetic radiological image.

    b. Medical reduction imaging.

    c. Magnetic resonance imaging.

    d. Master radiological imagery.

1. Jonelle Graybar, a 37-year-old female, is pregnant for the first time and is approximately 12 weeks' gestation. She is brought into the diagnostic center for a fetal biophysical profile with nonstress testing.

   _____

2. Max Wellington, a 15-year-old male, is brought into Dr. Eller's office with severe right leg pain. Dr. Eller takes x-rays of his right femur, AP and PA, to determine whether or not Max's leg is fractured.

   _____

3. Brandy Sorenna, a 75-year-old female, was brought into Dr. Appleton's office by her daughter because Brandy was complaining of a sharp pain in her chest. After a negative EKG, Dr. Appleton had a pulmonary quantitative differential function study taken, which confirmed a pulmonary embolism. Brandy was taken immediately by ambulance to the hospital. Code the pulmonary differential study only.

   _____

4. Dr. Zeigleman saw Vernon Unger, a 31-year-old male, with a swollen right eye and loss of vision. Dr. Zeigleman ordered a CT with contrast of the right eye and area, which revealed marked proptosis of the right orbit, thrombosis, and enlargement of the right superior ophthalmic vein.

   _____

5. Xavier Pollack, a 51-year-old male, was diagnosed with intrinsic laryngeal cancer, supraglottic T1 tumor. With the tumor confined to one subsite in the supraglottis, Dr. Westerman provided radiation treatment delivery, with a single port, simple block, of 4.5 MeV.

   _____

6. Carol-Ann Springer, a 22-year-old female, came into the Diagnostic Imaging Center for her annual screening mammogram. Due to her family history of malignant neoplasms of the breast (both her mother and sister have been diagnosed), the mammogram was ordered with computer-aided detection (CAD).

   _____

7. Conrad Michaelson, a 29-year-old male, is brought into Dr. Culverwell's office with sharp pains in his lower right abdomen, shooting across to the left side. Dr. Culverwell ordered some blood work and a magnetic resonance angiography to confirm the suspected diagnosis of acute appendicitis. Code the MRA.

   _____

8. Alden Roberts, a 33-year-old male, was in training at Cape Canaveral when he hit his head in a weightlessness simulator, causing him to lose consciousness for three minutes. Dr. Astrone, the on-call physician, took a skull x-ray, three views, and did an MRI without contrast of Alden's brain.

   _____

9. Olivia Kane, a 61-year-old female, was experiencing pain in her back that radiated around her trunk. She was also suffering with spastic muscle weakness. Dr. Neumours ordered a radioisotope bone scan of Olivia's lumbar spinal area. The scan identified a metastatic invasion of L1–L3.

   _____

10. Olivia Kane, newly diagnosed with metastatic lumbar spinal tumors, has been referred to Dr. Duncan for the creation of a simple radiation therapy plan.

   _____

11. Jason Miolo had been diagnosed with a malignancy and came today for intravenous radiopharmaceutical therapy.

   _____

12. Before beginning a series of treatments, Brianna Logan came to the Diagnostic Imaging Center for a metabolic evaluation PET scan of her brain.

   _____

13. Carl Gadsden, a 13-month-old male, was brought to radiology for a real-time, limited, static ultrasound of his hips.

   _____

14. Miriam Lightfoot, a 55-year-old female, arrived at the Barton Imaging Center to have a SPECT performed on her left kidney.

   _____

15. Dr. Morrison performed a complete ultrasound evaluation of Eliot Shapin's pelvis. The procedure included evaluation and measurement of Eliot's urinary bladder, evaluation of his prostate and seminal vesicles, and pathology of his enlarged prostate.

   _____

Below and on the following pages you will find the procedure notes for radiologic services. You may recognize the patient's name or the case scenario. Find the best, most appropriate codes from the Radiology section of the CPT book for each of these reports. You are coding for the radiologist.

CIPHER, VICTORS, & ASSOCIATES
A Complete Health Care Facility
234 MAIN STREET • ANYTOWN, FL 32711 • 407-555-1234

PATIENT: WHITE, SIERRA
MRN: WHITSI001
Date: 17 September 2008

Procedure Performed: X-rays, front/lat, chest
                             X-rays, AP, shoulder
                             C-spine AP/lat
                             MRI, shoulder joint

Radiologist: Keith Robbins, MD
Referring Physician: James I. Cipher, MD

Indications: R/O torn ligament, shoulder after MVA

Impressions: X-rays of all areas are unremarkable
                             C-spine, negative for fracture or trauma
                             MRI indicates a torn coracohumeral ligament, right side

---

Keith Robbins, MD

KR/mg   D: 9/17/08 09:50:16   T: 9/20/08 12:55:01

Find the best, most appropriate code(s).

_____

_____

_____

CIPHER, VICTORS, & ASSOCIATES
A Complete Health Care Facility
234 MAIN STREET • ANYTOWN, FL 32711 • 407-555-1234

PATIENT: PARKER, PETER
MRN: PARKPE001
Date: 1 October 2008

Procedure Performed: X-rays, skull, two views
                                 CT, soft tissue of neck, with contrast
                                 MRI, brain stem

Radiologist: Keith Robbins, MD
Referring Physician: Valerie R. Victors, MD

Indications: Concussion, after fall from ladder

Impressions: X-rays negative for fracture
                                 CT negative
                                 MRI indicates subdural hematoma

---

Keith Robbins, MD

KR/mg   D: 10/1/08 09:50:16   T: 10/2/08 12:55:01

Find the best, most appropriate code(s).

_____

_____

_____

CIPHER, VICTORS, & ASSOCIATES
A Complete Health Care Facility
234 MAIN STREET • ANYTOWN, FL 32711 • 407-555-1234

PATIENT: FRANKLIN, FRANCES
MRN: FRANFR001
Date: 17 October 2008

Procedure Performed: Screening mammogram, bilateral, two views each breast

Radiologist: Keith Robbins, MD
Referring Physician: Valerie R. Victors, MD

Indications: Routine annual assessment

Impressions: Mammogram unremarkable

Keith Robbins, MD

KR/mg   D: 10/17/08 09:50:16   T: 10/20/08 12:55:01

Find the best, most appropriate code(s).

_____

_____

_____

CIPHER, VICTORS, & ASSOCIATES
A Complete Health Care Facility
234 MAIN STREET • ANYTOWN, FL 32711 • 407-555-1234

PATIENT: TREADWELL, TRACY
MRN: TREATR001
Date: 5 November 2008

Procedure Performed: Radiation treatment delivery

Radiologist: Keith Robbins, MD
Referring Physician: James I. Cipher, MD

Indications: Kaposi's sarcoma, extracutaneous, lungs, and GI tract (esophagus)

Impressions: 15 MEV, two separate treatment areas

_____

Keith Robbins, MD

KR/mg   D: 11/5/08 09:50:16   T: 11/7/08 12:55:01

Find the best, most appropriate code(s).

_____

_____

_____

CIPHER, VICTORS, & ASSOCIATES
A Complete Health Care Facility
234 MAIN STREET • ANYTOWN, FL 32711 • 407-555-1234

PATIENT: BUSCH, JAKE
MRN: BUSCJA001
Date: 29 September 2008

Procedure Performed: CT scan of the head

Radiologist: Keith Robbins, MD
Referring Physician: James I. Cipher, MD

Indications: Left CVA

Impressions:
The current study is compared to the previous one of 9-25-07.

Compared to the previous study, there is a focal area of hypodensity present in the right posterior cerebral arterial distribution adjacent to the falx, a finding suspicious for a small acute infarction, nonhemorrhagic, most likely the parieto-occipital branch.

No other abnormality detected. There is no intra or extra-axial hemorrhages. There is no significant midline shift or hydrocephalus.

Small new area as described above is suspicious for an area of acute infarction in the right posterior cerebral arterial distribution, likely the occipital branch. Please clinically correlate.

_____

Keith Robbins, MD

KR/mg   D: 9/29/08 09:50:16   T: 9/30/08 12:55:01

Find the best, most appropriate code(s).

_____

_____

_____

10

Pathology and Laboratory Coding

KEY TERMS

Cytology

Etiology

Gross examination

Laboratory

Microscopic examination

Pathology

Qualitative

Quantitative

Specimen

Surgical pathology

LEARNING OUTCOMES

- Interpret the guidelines for accurately coding pathology procedures.
- Translate the guidelines for accurately coding laboratory procedures.
- Apply the guidelines regarding panels to avoid unbundling.
- Distinguish between gross and microscopic examination for surgical specimens.
- Discern between quantitative and qualitative test results.
- Determine how and when to use modifiers.

EMPLOYMENT OPPORTUNITIES

Diagnostic laboratories

Infectious disease specialists

Endocrinologists

Pathologists

Hematologists

Diagnostic imaging centers

Clinics

Hospitals

Portable x-ray suppliers

Multispecialty clinics

As physicians and health care professionals work to help their patients, very often they need medical science to guide them. The guidance frequently comes from tests performed by professionals working in a **laboratory,** studying the evolution of a patient's disease. Such study is called **pathology,** which includes **etiology.**

Pathology and lab testing help detect the early presence of disease, rule out or in, con-

ditions that might have similar symptoms yet need to be treated differently, and predict the occurrence of disease in the future. You probably already know from your own experiences the importance of such work. Your annual physical has certainly included blood tests to measure your cholesterol. Physicians order blood work to confirm pregnancy or a urinalysis to determine if a symptom could be the result of an infection. Testing takes time and

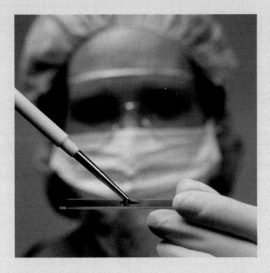

the expertise of professionals educated in interpreting the results. It also takes materials and resources.

As a coding specialist, you may work for a health care organization that has a lab within its facilities, a billing company that codes everything, or a lab—an independent facility that does nothing other than taking and analyzing the **specimen.** In any case, you should understand the different aspects of pathology and lab testing and procedures, as well as the guidelines involved in coding the services.

The specimen sent to the laboratory for testing may be from any number of different sources. A sample can be taken of a patient's blood, urine, other bodily fluids; tissue; or other part of the body.

PANELS

When you turn to the Pathology and Laboratory section of the CPT book, you will notice that many codes include a long list of elements within the code's description. These groupings of tests commonly performed at the same time are called *panels.*

EXAMPLE

80051 Electrolyte panel

This panel must include the following: Carbon dioxide (82374); Chloride (82435); Potassium (84132); and Sodium (84295)

The example shows you that in order for code 80051 to be the most accurate code, the lab must have performed all four tests: carbon dioxide, chloride, potassium, and sodium.

If the lab performs fewer than *all* the tests listed in a panel, you must code the tests separately: You are *not* permitted to use the panel code.

Again, the CPT book will help you. Should you have to code any of the tests separately, the individual test code is given, in parentheses, right next to the name of the test listed there. From our example, next to carbon dioxide, you will notice the number 82374. Turn to code 82374, and you will see that it is the code for testing carbon dioxide alone.

Let's say, instead of doing fewer tests than those listed in a panel, the lab performs more. The guidelines state that you are to code those additional tests separately and additionally.

Concerned that Anna Donner, a 43-year-old female, might be suffering from hypercholesterolemia, Dr. Raider ordered some blood work including a total cholesterol serum test, lipoprotein (direct measurement of high-density lipoprotein), and triglycerides. He also added a potassium serum test to the order.

Let's Code It!

The lab performed four tests: *total cholesterol serum test, lipoprotein (direct measurement of high-density lipoprotein), triglycerides,* and *potassium serum.* When you look up the tests individually, you are directed to codes for each. However, when it comes to pathology and laboratory coding, you must take an extra step. Turn to the numeric listings, to the beginning of the Pathology and Laboratory section, where you find the standardized panels listed. Review the list of tests included in each of the panels, and match it with the list of tests Dr. Raider ordered. You see that the code "80061 Lipid Panel" includes three of the four tests performed. Since none of the panels includes all four tests, you use the lipid panel code and code the potassium test additionally, code 84132.

> 84132 Potassium; serum

Therefore, you have two codes for the lab work's claim: 80061, 84132. Good job!

Remember: Experience and practice will help you learn the elements easily. After working at a lab or for a facility with a lab, you will recognize the lab tests that are typically performed together and, consequently, probably have a panel code grouping them. Should that not be the case, the alphabetic index will direct you to the correct individual code for that test.

TESTING METHODOLOGY AND SOURCES

Quantitative

The counting or measurement of something.

Qualitative

The determination of character or essential element(s).

While no one expects you, as the coding specialist, to be completely knowledgeable about the details of laboratory and pathological testing, you will need certain information regarding the performance of the tests in order to code them correctly. This may begin with exactly what is being tested, going beyond just the name of the test itself.

One aspect of the testing performed will be whether or not the test is **quantitative** or **qualitative.**

EXAMPLE

> 82355 Calculus; qualitative analysis
> 82360   quantitative analysis, chemical

The guidelines tell you that if the documentation does not specify, you may assume that the examination performed was quantitative. However, remember that documentation is absolute in our industry. Therefore, it is recommended that you query the lab technician or pathologist and request that the paperwork include this important detail.

All the details regarding the specimen and the testing are important. There are times when the code descriptions use the type of test, the type of specimen, or both.

Let's look back at Anna Donner's cholesterol test. Go to the alphabetic index and look up *cholesterol.*

EXAMPLE

Cholesterol

Measurement	83721
Serum	82465
Testing	83718–83719

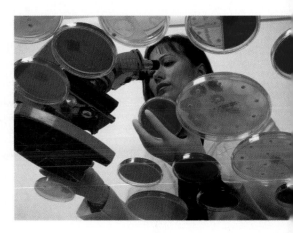

You can see that the fact that Dr. Raider ordered a total cholesterol *serum* test makes a difference in which code is best. In addition, *cholesterol, serum* (82465) is the test included in the lipid panel code we used for reporting Anna's tests. If Dr. Raider had ordered a cholesterol *measurement* test instead of the serum test, you would not be able to use the 80061 lipid panel test code. Then, you would have to code each of Anna's tests separately. Our example highlights the importance of reading the details of the testing beyond the element or category.

In addition to how the test is performed, you must also know the type of specimen involved in the testing and, sometimes, how many specimens or sources were involved.

First, the type of specimen being tested may change the code. Let's look again at Anna Donner's case, specifically at her potassium test. Let's go to the alphabetic index for *potassium.*

EXAMPLE

Potassium	84132
Urine	84133

The first code, listed next to the word *potassium,* guides us to code 84132, but does not contain any additional descriptors. However, the second code, listed under potassium indicates that it would be the code used if the potassium were tested from Anna's urine rather than her blood (serum). When you look at the codes' complete descriptions in the numeric listing, you see the details shown.

EXAMPLE

84132 Potassium; serum	
84133	urine

The listings clearly show that there is a difference in which code is correct based on the source of the specimen.

In certain circumstances, an analysis may be performed on multiple specimens collected at different times or from different sources. In such cases, the guidelines tell you to code each source and each specimen separately. However, be certain to always read the code descriptions carefully. Some codes already include multiple tests and/or multiple sources.

CLINICAL CHEMISTRY

The most common types of lab tests performed in everyday health care use chemical processes to distinguish qualities and quantities of elements in specimens provided. Typically, the specimens provided are samples of a patient's blood or urine. Other elements with which you might be familiar include:

- *Blood glucose* (sugar) is used to diagnose conditions such as diabetes mellitus (hyperglycemia) or hypoglycemia.
- *Electrolytes* are used to diagnose metabolic or kidney disorders.
- *Enzymes* can be released into the blood stream by a damaged or diseased organ. The presence of creatine kinase can indicate damage after a heart attack, or amylase and lipase elevations may be a sign of cancer of the pancreas and/or pancreatitis.
- *Hormones,* such as cortisol, in quantities too high or too low might indicate the malfunction of the patient's adrenal glands.
- *Lipids* (fatty substances) can signal coronary heart disease or liver disease.
- *Metabolic substances,* such as uric acid at incorrect levels, can identify the presence of gout.
- *Proteins* identified at the wrong levels on electrophoresis can point to malnutrition or certain infections.

Many tests can be easily performed in the physician's office with a small amount of blood or urine. Companies have created kits that make measuring such elements as simple as dipping a little slip of special paper into the patient's specimen. It means that you have a much greater opportunity to code any number of tests.

YOU CODE IT! CASE STUDY

Jeffrey Farthington, a 27-year-old male, is an up-and-coming stockbroker who does not pay much attention to a proper diet. He came to see his physician, Dr. Stanley, because he has been experiencing episodes of light-headedness. Dr. Stanley asks his assistant, Marlene Fleet, to do a quantitative blood glucose test using a reagent strip. Marlene takes a capillary stick (on Jeff's fingertip), goes to the back, and checks the specimen. The results indicate that Jeff has hypoglycemia.

You Code It!

Go through the steps of coding, and determine the codes that should be reported for this encounter between Dr. Stanley and Jeffrey Farthington.

Step 1: Read the case completely.

Step 2: Abstract the notes: Which key words can you identify relating to the procedures performed?

_____

Step 3: Query the provider, if necessary.

Step 4: Diagnosis: Hypoglycemia.

Step 5: Code the procedure(s).

_____

Step 6: Link the procedure codes to at least one diagnosis code.

Step 7: Back code to double-check your choices.

Answer

Did you find the correct code to be:

82948 Glucose; blood, reagent strip

Good work!

MOLECULAR DIAGNOSTICS

Molecular diagnostic tests investigate infectious disease, oncology concerns (malignant neoplasms), hematology (the study of blood and its disorders), neurology, and inherited disorders (genetics).

For genetics tests, you must include the appropriate modifier from the special list of genetic testing code modifiers found in Appendix I. These modifiers are to be used with both CPT and HCPCS Level II codes, as appropriate, to specify the probe type or the condition being tested. By using special modifiers, more detailed information can be gathered for statistical and other important data without requiring the rewriting of any of the existing code descriptions. The genetic testing code modifiers consist of two characters: the first a number (0 through 9) and the second a letter (A through Z).

YOU CODE IT! CASE STUDY

Marcus Angelli, a 3-year-old male, has a cousin who had been diagnosed with cystic fibrosis last year. Recently, he has been wheezing and has a dry, nonproductive cough. The fact that his cousin has cystic fibrosis means that Marcus has a 25% chance of carrying the disease. Therefore, Dr. Cauldwell ordered a molecular diagnostic test for the mutation of delta F 508 deletion in his DNA by sequencing, single segment.

You Code It!

Go through the steps of coding, and determine the codes that should be reported for this encounter between Dr. Cauldwell and Marcus Angelli.

CPT © 2007 American Medical Association. All Rights Reserved.

Step 1: Read the case completely.

Step 2: Abstract the notes: Which key words can you identify relating to the procedures performed?

_____

Step 3: Query the provider, if necessary.

Step 4: Diagnosis: Family history of cystic fibrosis.

Step 5: Code the procedure(s).

_____

Step 6: Link the procedure codes to at least one diagnosis code.

Step 7: Back code to double-check your choices.

Answer

Did you find the correct code to be:

> 83904-8A Molecular diagnostics; mutation identification by sequencing, single segment, each segment; CFTR (Cystic fibrosis)

Good job!

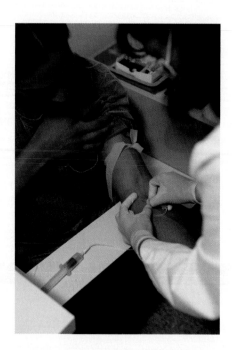

HEMATOLOGY AND COAGULATION

The study of blood and its disorders is called *hematology*. Hematologic tests can help diagnose such conditions and diseases as anemia, hemophilia, and leukemia. Very often, these tests are referred to by their initials, so let's go over the most common tests and their acronyms:

- CBC = Complete blood count, which includes the following tests:
- WBC = White blood cell count
- RBC = Red blood cell count
- Platelet count, which is used to diagnose or monitor bleeding and clotting disorders
- HCT = Hematocrit
- HB = Hemoglobin concentration, which is the oxygen-carrying pigment in red blood cells
- Differential blood count

In addition, one other test is used frequently:

- PT = Prothrombin time, which is used to evaluate bleeding and clotting disorders

Abbreviations for pathology and laboratory tests are used in reports from labs all over the country. Some of the most common are shown in Table 10-1.

CODING TIP »»

Remember that the CBC includes the WBC, RBC, HCT, HB, platelet count, and differential count. Therefore, you are not to code those tests separately.

TABLE 10-1 Abbreviations and Acronyms for Most Common Diagnostic and Laboratory Tests

ABG	Arterial blood gases	DIFF	Differential	PH	Hydrogen ion concentration
ACE	Angiotensin-converting enzyme	EIA	Enzyme immunoassay	PLT	Platelet
ACT	Activated clotting time	EOS	Eosinophil count	PSA	Prostate-specific antigen
AFP	Fetoprotein	ESR	Erythrocyte sedimentation rate	PT	Prothrombin time
A/G	Albumin/globulin ratio	FBS	Fasting blood sugar	PTT	Partial thromboplastin time
AIT	Agglutination inhibition test	GTT	Glucose tolerance test	RBC	Red blood cells
ALT	Alanine aminotransferase	HCT	Hematocrit	RDW	Red cell distribution width
ALP	Alkaline phosphatase	HDL	High-density lipoprotein	RPR	Rapid plasma reagin test
AMA	Antimitochondrial antibody	HGB	Hemoglobin	SEGS	Segmented neutrophils
ANA	Antinuclear antibody	HPF	High power field	SGOT	Serum glutamic-oxaloacetic transaminase
APTT	Activated partial thromboplastin time	INR	International normalization ratio	SGPT	Serum glutamic-pyruvic transaminase
AST	Aspartate aminotransferase	LD	Lactic dehydrogenase	SMA	Sequential multiple analyzer
BMC	Bone mineral content	LDL	Low-density lipoprotein	SP GRAV	Specific gravity
BMD	Bone marrow density	LFT	Liver function tests	STS	Serologic test for syphilis
BASO	Basophiles	LPF	Low power field	T&C	Type and crossmatch
BST	Blood serologic test	LYMPHS	Lymphocytes	TSH	Thyroid-stimulating hormone
BUN	Blood urea nitrogen	MCH	Mean corpuscular hemoglobin	UA	Urinalysis
CBC	Complete blood count	MCHC	Mean corpuscular hemoglobin concentration	WBC	White blood cell
CEA	Carcinoembryonic antigen	MCV	Mean corpuscular volume		
CK	Creatine kinase	MONO	Monocyte count		
CMV	Cytomegalovirus	MPV	Mean platelet volume		
CO_2	Carbon dioxide	NEUT	Neutrophils		
CPK	Creatine phosphokinase	PAP	Prostatic acid phosphatase		
DIC	Disseminated intravascular coagulation				

IMMUNOLOGY

Immunology is the study of the body's immune system—how it works and what can go wrong. Immunologic tests identify problems that may occur when a disease causes the body's defense system to attack itself (called an *autoimmune disease*) or when a disease causes a malfunction of the body's immune system (called an *immunodeficiency disorder*). The tests can also evaluate the compatibility of tissues and organs for transplantation.

Conditions and diseases that you may be familiar with, which fall into this category, include rheumatoid arthritis, allergies, and, of course, HIV (human immunodeficiency virus).

LET'S CODE IT! SCENARIO

Alfred Manning, a 49-year-old male, was diagnosed with hemophilia many years ago. As a result of a blood transfusion, he contracted HIV. He has come today for lab work to check on his T cell count, an indicator of whether or not the HIV is progressing.

Let's Code It!

Alfred is having a test to determine the *count* of *T cells* in his blood. Turn to the alphabetic index to the letter *T*. Are you surprised at the many listings with T cell in the heading? Read through them all carefully. Remember that Alfred does not have leukemia; he has HIV. Keep going down the list to T cells, under which you see *count,* with the suggested code 86359.

The complete code description in the numeric listing shows us:

86359 T cells; total count

Good job!

MICROBIOLOGY

Microbiologic tests use many different methods to study bacteria, fungi, parasites, and viruses. The specimens used in the tests might be blood, urine, sputum (mucous, also called phlegm), feces (stool), cerebrospinal fluid (CSF), and other body fluids. Blood cultures are used to diagnose bacterial infections of the blood, sputum cultures can identify respiratory infections like pneumonia, and stool cultures can confirm the presence of pinworms and other parasites.

27340-00
HUMAN
BLOOD
SMEAR

LET'S CODE IT! SCENARIO

Veronica Adderson, a five-year-old female, went to a picnic at the park with her playgroup and had a rare hamburger. Later that evening, her parents rushed her to the hospital because she was vomiting and had severe diarrhea. Dr. Calvinelli ordered an infectious agent antigen enzyme immunoassay for E. coli 0157. Fortunately, the test was negative and it turned out that she just ate too much ice cream and milk.

Let's Code It!

Dr. Calvinelli ordered "an infectious agent antigen enzyme immunoassay" for Veronica to determine if she was suffering from *Escherichia coli (E coli).* Let's go to the alphabetic index to *immunoassay* and find *infectious agent* below it, with the suggested codes 86317–86318, 87449–87451. Let's go to the numeric listings and read the complete code descriptions.

> 86317 Immunoassay for infectious agent antibody, quantitative, not otherwise specified (For immunoassay techniques for antigens, see 83516, 83518, 83519, 83520, 87301–87450, 87810–87899.)

The code description states *antibody,* but the notes say *antigen.* Luckily, the CPT book is guiding you via the parenthetical notation below the code description, which directs us to a long list of codes. The descriptions for 83516, 83518, 83519, and 83520 do not come any closer to Dr. Calvinelli's notes. Let's turn to the next set of suggested codes:

> 87301 Infectious agent antigen detection by enzyme immunoassay technique, qualitative or semiquantitative, multiple step method; adenovirus enteric types 40/41

Come down the list a little farther:

> 87335   Escherichia coli 0157

When you read the complete description, you get the following:

> 87335 Infectious agent antigen detection by enzyme immunoassay technique, qualitative or semiquantitative, multiple step method; Escherichia coli 0157

Sometimes, even with the CPT book pointing at codes, it may take a lot of reading to be certain you have the best, most appropriate code.

CYTOPATHOLOGY AND CYTOGENETIC STUDIES

Cytology studies one cell at a time to discover abnormal cells present in tissue or bodily fluids. Cytological testing is used to detect cancer cells and infectious organisms and to screen for fetal abnormalities.

Specimens used in cytopathological testing are obtained by fine-needle aspirations (as in amniocentesis), scraping of tissue surfaces (as in pap smears), and collecting bodily fluids (as with sputum or seminal fluid, or sperm).

Cytology

The investigation and identification of cells.

LET'S CODE IT! SCENARIO

Barbara Rosen, a 51-year-old female, came to see Dr. Farber for her annual well-woman checkup. In addition to the examination, Dr. Farber took a pap smear, to be done using the Bethesda reporting system with manual screening. Barbara's examination showed she was completely healthy.

Dr. Farber took a *smear* of tissue for a *cytopathological* examination of Barbara's *cervical cells using the Bethesda system.* Let's go to the alphabetic index to *cytopathology, smears, cervical or vaginal,* with the suggested codes 88141–88167, 88174–88175. However, we want to point out that, in this case, you can also go to *pap smears* and see the suggested codes 88141–88155, 88164–88167, and 88174–88175. Note that there is a difference: Codes 88160, 88161, and 88162 are not included in the listing under pap smears. Let's go to the numeric listings and read the complete code descriptions.

Before you begin reading all the code descriptions, read the paragraph of instructions directly before code 88141. You will note that these instructions tell you to "Use codes 88164–88167 to report Pap smears that are examined using the Bethesda System of reporting." That saves you quite a lot of time.

88164 Cytopathology, slides, cervical or vaginal (the Bethesda System); manual screening under physician supervision

Reading that one small paragraph directed you to the three best codes. Great job!

SURGICAL PATHOLOGY

Surgical pathology

The study of tissues removed from a living patient during a surgical procedure.

When a biopsy is taken during a surgical procedure (or is the surgical procedure itself), the specimen is sent to the lab for testing. The testing, typically performed immediately upon receipt from the OR, is called **surgical pathology.** Its purpose, much like other testing and studies, is to provide the information necessary to diagnose a disease or condition and to set forth a treatment plan. In such cases, all the steps (taking the specimen, testing, diagnosis, and treatment) may occur during one surgical session. The benefit of this quick and immediate process is that there is less trauma for the patient, having to undergo anesthesia and an invasive procedure only once. In addition, it saves money for the patient, the facility, and the third-party payer.

Codes 88300 through 88309 represent six levels of surgical pathological testing.

The codes include accession, the testing itself, and the written report from the pathologist. The codes (with the exception of 88300) also include both **gross examination** (also known as macroscopic examination) of the specimen and **microscopic examination.**

Gross examination

The visual study of a specimen (with the naked eye).

The first level, code 88300, is applicable for any and all specimens that are only examined by visual, or gross, examination. It means that the sample has not been looked at under a microscope.

88300 Level I—Surgical pathology, gross examination only

Microscopic examination

The study of a specimen using a microscope (under magnification).

Codes 88302 through 88309 recognize the various amounts of work required by the pathologist, or physician doing the examination, in order to determine the accurate condition of the specimen. Don't worry—you don't have to study pathology to decide which level to use properly to represent the work done. Each code level is determined by the anatomical site from where the specimen was taken. Under each, the sites are listed in alphabetic order. However, you have to know what had happened in the OR to find the correct code, because that will change the level involved.

YOU CODE IT! CASE STUDY

Trent Bingham, an 11-year-old male, was taken to the OR to have his tonsils removed. However, due to additional symptoms, Dr. Ellendale did a biopsy and sent a specimen of Trent's tonsil to the lab for surgical pathology examination. The report came back from the lab that Trent had a malignant neoplasm of his tonsils. Dr. Ellendale surgically removed additional sections to be certain that the entire tumor had been removed. Trent tolerated the procedure well and was taken to the recovery room.

You Code It!

Go through the steps of coding and determine the codes that should be reported for this encounter between Dr. Ellendale and Trent Bingham.

Step 1: Read the case completely.

Step 2: Abstract the notes: Which key words can you identify relating to the procedures performed?

_____

Step 3: Query the provider, if necessary.

Step 4: Diagnosis: Malignant neoplasm, tonsil.

Step 5: Code the procedure(s).

_____

Step 6: Link the procedure codes to at least one diagnosis code.

Step 7: Back code to double-check your choices.

Answer

Did you find the correct code to be:

88305 Level IV; Tonsil, Biopsy

Good work!

After the listings for the six levels of surgical pathological examinations, there are other codes and descriptions for services that may be performed in addition to the gross and microscopic examinations of the specimen. Should any of those services be performed instead of, or in addition to, the surgical pathological examination, it should be coded separately.

MODIFIERS FOR LABORATORY CODING

If your health care facility uses an outside laboratory that bills your office, you include the charges for the lab work on the claim form that you file. In such instances, you must append the CPT code for the lab test with modifier 90. If the outside lab bills the patient's insurance directly, you will not include the test code or modifier on the claim form that you submit.

> 90 **Reference (Outside) Laboratory:** When laboratory procedures are performed by a party other than the treating or reporting physician, the procedure may be identified by adding modifier 90 to the usual procedure number.

Also on occasion, you may find that a lab test has to be repeated, on the same day for the same patient, in order to get several readings of a level or measurement.

> 91 **Repeat Clinical Diagnostic Laboratory Test:** In the course of treatment of the patient, it may be necessary to repeat the same laboratory test on the same day to obtain subsequent (multiple) test results. Under these circumstances, the laboratory test performed can be identified by its usual procedure number and the addition of modifier 91. *Note:* This modifier may not be used when tests are rerun to confirm initial results; due to testing problems with specimens or equipment; or for any other reason when a normal, one-time, reportable results is all that is required. This modifier may not be used when other code(s) describe a series of test results (e.g., glucose tolerance tests, evocative/suppression testing). This modifier may only be used for laboratory test(s) performed more than once on the same day on the same patient.

The usage of testing kits is increasing in health care facilities because they make it easier to obtain fast, accurate results. When this is the case, append the modifier.

> 92 **Alternative Laboratory Platform Testing:** When laboratory testing is being performed using a kit or transportable instrument that wholly or in part consists of a single use, disposable analytical chamber, the service may be identified by adding modifier 92 to the usual laboratory procedure code.

CHAPTER SUMMARY

Pathology and laboratory tests provide health care professionals with definitive evidence as to the condition that may be interfering with a patient's good health. That proof will help direct the physician toward a more accurate diagnosis and a beneficial treatment plan. Lab tests are an invaluable part of the health care toolbox, and must be coded accurately.

Chapter 10 Review
Pathology and Laboratory Coding

1. Laboratory tests can be performed
   a. In a free-standing lab.
   b. In a hospital.
   c. At a physician's office.
   d. All of the above.

2. Most often, the coding specialist responsible for reporting the lab work works for
   a. The physician who ordered the tests.
   b. The facility that performed the tests.
   c. The hospital.
   d. The third-party payer.

3. A specimen can be
   a. Blood.
   b. Urine.
   c. Sputum.
   d. All of the above.

4. When not all of the tests listed in a panel are performed, you should
   a. Code the panel with modifier 52.
   b. Code the panel alone.
   c. Code the tests individually.
   d. Code the panel with modifier 53.

5. When more tests are performed including all those listed in a panel, you should
   a. Code the panel with modifier 21.
   b. Code the panel alone.
   c. Code the panel, plus the additional tests performed.
   d. Code all the tests individually.

6. Genetic testing code modifiers are used when reporting
   a. Clinical chemistry.
   b. Molecular diagnostics.
   c. Hematology.
   d. Immunology.

7. CBC stands for
   a. Comprehensive blood cytology.
   b. Concentration blood count.
   c. Cellular blind concentration.
   d. Complete blood count.

8. CBC includes
   a. WBC.
   b. RBC.
   c. HCT.
   d. All of the above.

9. Surgical pathology may include
   a. Gross examination.
   b. Microbiology.
   c. Genetic testing.
   d. Nuclear medicine.

10. Quantitative testing is
    a. The determination of essential elements.
    b. The listing of all components.
    c. The measurement of an element.
    d. The total assessment.

1. Leroy Matheson, a 39-year-old male, was feeling rundown and tired all the time. So, Dr. Lowe, thinking that Leroy may have anemia, ordered a complete CBC, automated with an automated differential WBC count.

   _____

2. Tiffany Deloach, an 18-year-old female, has been living on the street and in shelters, and comes to the free clinic for a checkup because she is five months' pregnant. Dr. Jacobs orders a complete CBC; automated and appropriate manual differential WBC count; hepatitis B surface antigen, rubella antibody, qualitative syphilis test, RBC antibody screening, blood typing ABO, and Rh factor.

   _____

3. Caitlyn Calhoun, a 2-year-old female, is at her pediatrician's office, Dr. Childers, for her regular checkup. Dr. Childers notices that Caitlyn is very small for her age and orders a growth hormone stimulation panel to be done.

   _____

4. Sean McCully, a 27-year-old male, went to the shore with his friends and feasted on raw oysters and beer. About five hours later, after getting home, he began to cough and vomit, and he found blood in his stool. He went to the walk-in clinic where Dr. Ferguson ran a smear test for ova and parasites, particularly *Anisakis.*

   _____

5. Chad Tanger, a 33-year-old male, was diagnosed with prostate cancer last week. Before beginning radiation treatments, which would make him unable to have children, he comes today to submit his sperm for cryopreservation.

   _____

6. Rulon Porter, a 67-year-old male, has a history of gastrointestinal problems, including intestinal polyps. After taking a special kit home, he submits fecal specimens for an occult blood test by immunoassay.

   _____

7. Margaret Kahlil, a 29-year-old female, just got a new job with the space industry. As a condition of her employment, she came to the lab today for a qualitative drug screening for alcohol, amphet-

amines, and barbiturates. The procedure was then confirmed to be negative for all drugs.

_____

8. Reyna Cutler, a 23-year-old female, was found unconscious by her roommate and brought into the ED by ambulance. The roommate stated that Reyna was very depressed, and she feared that Reyna might have taken an overdose of her medication. Dr. Farmer ordered a therapeutic drug assay for phenobarbital.

_____

9. Edward Stuart, a 15-year-old male, is overweight, bordering on obese, and Dr. Swenson is concerned that he may be developing diabetes, so he orders an insulin tolerance panel for adrenocorticotropic hormone (ACTH) insufficiency.

_____

10. Georgia Olin, a 44-year-old female, goes to her physician, Dr. Rodriquez, for her annual checkup, which includes a nonautomated urinalysis with microscopy for glucose, ketones, and leukocytes. Dr. Rodriquez's assistant Tracy performed the test, by dipstick, in the office. The results were normal.

_____

11. Jolene Abernathy, a 19-year-old female, got drunk at a party and had unprotected sex. She came into the clinic today for an HIV-1 and HIV-2 single assay test.

_____

12. At the doctor's suggestion, Jolene was also tested for syphilis, qualitative (VDRL).

_____

13. Vivian Zeeman, a 41-year-old female, is pregnant for the first time. Dr. Lanahan performed an amniocentesis to do a chromosome analysis, count 15 cells, 1 karyotype, with banding. The results showed that the baby is fine.

_____

14. Jay Winegarten, a 53-year-old male, was in the OR for Dr. Ashley to perform a subtotal resection of his pancreas. Surgical pathology showed no malignancy.

_____

15. Walter Praxis, a 15-day-old male, was born at 33 weeks' gestation, and there is concern that he may have hyperbilirubinemia. Therefore, Dr. Stevenson performed a total transcutaneous bilirubin.

_____

Below and on the following pages you will find the procedure notes for pathology and laboratory services, including some of those ordered for cases from earlier chapters of this text. You may recognize the patient's name or the case scenario. Find the best, most appropriate codes from the Pathology and Laboratory section of the CPT book for each of these reports. Remember, you are coding for the pathologist.

CIPHER, VICTORS, & ASSOCIATES
A Complete Health Care Facility
234 MAIN STREET • ANYTOWN, FL 32711 • 407-555-1234

PATIENT: FRANKLIN, FRANCES
MRN: FRANFR001
Date: 17 October 2008

Procedure Performed: Comprehensive metabolic panel

Pathologist: Caryn Simonson, MD

Referring Physician: Valerie R. Victors, MD

Indications: Routine physical exam

Impressions:

Albumin	3.9
Bilirubin	Small*
Calcium	8.9
Carbon dioxide (CO_2)	28
Chloride	96 L
Creatinine	1.2
Glucose	102
Phosphatase, alkaline	90
Potassium	3.9
Protein, total	30*
Sodium	138
Transferase, alanine amino (ALT)(SGPT)	30
Transferase, aspartate amino (AST)(SGOT)	29
Urea nitrogen (BUN)	18

* = Abnormal, L = Low, H = High

Caryn Simonson, MD

CS/mg   D: 10/17/08 09:50:16   T: 10/20/08 12:55:01

Find the best, most appropriate code(s).

CIPHER, VICTORS, & ASSOCIATES
A Complete Health Care Facility
234 MAIN STREET • ANYTOWN, FL 32711 • 407-555-1234

PATIENT: TRANSIL, BRENT
MRN: TRANBR001
Date: 29 September 2008

Procedure Performed: Tissue, skin, head, mutation identification

Pathologist: Caryn Simonson, MD

Referring Physician: James I. Cipher, MD

Indications: Suspected melanoma

Impressions: Abnormal cells present
                                Molecular diagnostics; mutation identification by sequencing, single
                                segment

Caryn Simonson, MD

CS/mg   D: 9/29/08 09:50:16   T: 9/30/08 12:55:01

Find the best, most appropriate code(s).

_____

_____

_____

PATIENT: HAVERSTROM, OLIVIA
MRN: HAVEOL001
Date: 15 November 2008

Procedure Performed: Surgical pathology, gallbladder, gross and microscopic examination

Pathologist: Caryn Simonson, MD

Referring Physician: Valerie R. Victors, MD

Indications: R/O malignancy

Impressions: All tissues unremarkable
                              Surgical pathology, gross and microscopic examination of gallbladder

Caryn Simonson, MD

CS/mg   D: 11/15/08 09:50:16   T: 11/20/08 12:55:01

Find the best, most appropriate code(s).

_____

_____

_____

CIPHER, VICTORS, & ASSOCIATES
A Complete Health Care Facility
234 MAIN STREET • ANYTOWN, FL 32711 • 407-555-1234

PATIENT: FRIEDMAN, DORIS
MRN: FRIEDO001
Date: 23 September 2008

Procedure Performed: Rectal biopsies, gross and microscopic examination

Pathologist: Caryn Simonson, MD

Referring Physician: Matthew Appellet, MD

Indications: Inflammatory bowel disease

Impressions: All tissues normal
            Surgical pathology, gross and microscopic examination, colon biopsy

---

Caryn Simonson, MD

CS/mg D: 9/23/08 09:50:16 T: 9/25/08 12:55:01

Find the best, most appropriate code(s).

_____

_____

_____

CIPHER, VICTORS, & ASSOCIATES
A Complete Health Care Facility
234 MAIN STREET • ANYTOWN, FL 32711 • 407-555-1234

PATIENT: FRANKS, ELMER
MRN: FRANEL001
Date: 17 June 2008

Procedure Performed: Mass (fat tissue), upper eyelid gross and microscopic examination

Pathologist: Caryn Simonson, MD

Referring Physician: Mark C. Welby, MD

Indications: Herniated orbital fat pad, OD

Impressions: Carcinoma in situ
                       Surgical pathology, gross and microscopic examination, soft tissue tumor,
                       extensive resection

Caryn Simonson, MD

CS/mg   D: 6/17/08 09:50:16   T: 6/20/08 12:55:01

Find the best, most appropriate code(s).

_____

_____

_____

Medicine Coding

LEARNING OUTCOMES

- Interpret the guidelines for coding the administration of vaccines and toxoids.
- Apply the guidelines to determine the best, most appropriate code(s).
- Abstract physician's notes to accurately describe cardiovascular services.
- Determine the correct coding parameters for reporting psychiatric services.
- Identify specifics to correctly report osteopathic, chiropractic, and acupuncture services.
- Determine how and when to use modifiers.

EMPLOYMENT OPPORTUNITIES

General practices

Family practices

Internal medicine specialists

Allergy/immunologists

Multispecialty clinics

Chiropractor offices

Physical therapy practices

Ophthalmologists

Opticians

The Medicine section of the CPT book has codes for other services that are supplied by health care professionals but not represented in the other sections of the CPT book. Services reported using codes from the Medicine section include:

- Flu shots
- Vaccinations for the kids to go back to school
- Allergy shots
- Chiropractic services
- Psychotherapy
- Dialysis
- Hearing evaluations
- Vision checks
- Chemotherapy
- Acupuncture

Wherever you work as a coding specialist, there is an excellent chance you will be using this section. Let's go through it together.

IMMUNIZATIONS

Immunization

To make someone resistant to a particular disease by vaccination.

When a patient receives an **immunization**, there are actually two parts to the process: the medication itself and the administration of the medication. Each part is coded separately.

The medication may be an immune globulin, an antitoxin, a vaccine, or a toxoid. Codes 90281 through 90399 and 90476 through 90749 are available for you to identify the specific drug.

Medications can be given, or administered, to the patient in several different ways: percutaneous, intradermal, subcutaneous, or intramuscular injections; intranasal or oral; intra-arterial or intravenous. The method of administration will help guide you to the correct administration codes 90465–90474 and 90765–90779.

Additionally, many vaccinations and immunizations are given in a series. In such cases, use the add-on codes for the administration of the additional injections. You will find that most of the codes are offered in sets: the first injection, administration, or hour and then the add-on code for each additional injection, administration, or hour.

LET'S CODE IT! SCENARIO

Carlton Travella, a 5-year-old male, came to Dr. Quon for his MMR vaccine so Carlton could start kindergarten next month. Dr. Quon administers an injection, subcutaneously. Dr. Quon met face to face with Carlton's mother and discussed the importance of the vaccine, as well as indications of a reaction that she should watch for. Carlton chose a red balloon as his prize for being a good patient.

Let's Code It!

Dr. Quon gave Carlton *one subcutaneous injection* of the *MMR vaccine*. Do you know what *MMR* stands for? Even if you don't know that it is an acronym for measles, mumps, and rubella, you can look it up in the alphabetic index under MMR shots. The suggested code is 90707. The numeric listing confirms that:

> 90707 Measles, mumps, and rubella virus vaccine (MMR), live, for subcutaneous use.

The description matches Dr. Quon's notes exactly. However, the code will only reimburse Dr. Quon's office for the drug itself, not Dr. Quon's time and expertise in administering the injection and counseling the family. You could go back to the alphabetic index, or you could read the instructional paragraph at the beginning of the Vaccines, Toxoids

CODING TIP » »

To use codes 90704 Mumps virus vaccine + 90705 Measles virus vaccine + 90706 Rubella virus vaccine instead of code 90707 Measles, mumps and rubella virus vaccine is an example of "unbundling" and is not permitted.

subsection (where you found the code 90707). You will see that this paragraph tells you that you must use these codes "in addition to an immunization administration code(s) 90465–90474." Let's turn to the first code 90465 and read the description:

> 90465 Immunization administration under 8 years of age (includes percutaneous, intradermal, subcutaneous, or intramuscular injections) when the physician counsels the patient/family; first injection (single or combination vaccine/toxoid), per day

Now, you have the codes to reimburse Dr. Quon for the drug, as well as his time and expertise administering the injection and talking with Carlton's mother.

EXAMPLE

If Dr. Quon had not spent time face to face with Carlton and his mother, 90465 would not be used. Instead you would use code 90471, which does not include the phrase "when the physician counsels the patient/family" in the code description.

INJECTIONS AND INFUSIONS

The administration of fluids (such as saline solution to hydrate a patient suffering from dehydration), pharmaceuticals (such as medications for treatment or preventive purposes), or dyes (such as those used for diagnostic testing) are coded from the Injections and Infusions subsection, which include codes 90760–90779.

The **infusion** and **injection** codes include certain standard parts involved in administering liquids. Services included but not reported separately are:

- The administration of a local anesthetic
- The initiation of the intravenous
- Accessing an indwelling intravenous, subcutaneous catheter or port
- Flushing the line at the completion of the infusion
- The appropriate supplies: tubing, syringes, etc.

The guidelines for coding injections and infusions provide further direction when coding these services:

- When more than one infusion is provided into one intravenous site, report only the first service.
- Should more than one intravenous site be used, report the appropriate services for each site.
- Report different drugs or materials and that service separately.
- Report infusion time as the actual time the fluid is provided.

Infusion

Introduction of a fluid into a blood vessel.

Injection

Compelling a fluid into tissue or cavity.

››› CODING TIP

The administration of chemotherapy drugs is not coded from the Injections and Infusions subsection, but from the Chemotherapy Administration subsection, codes 96401–96549.

Allison Bradley, a 45-year-old female, postmastectomy for malignant neoplasm of the breast, has been having chemotherapy treatments. She is seen today for nausea and vomiting as a result of this therapy. Dr. Eider orders an antiemetic 10 mg IV push and another antiemetic IV infusion over 30 minutes.

Let's Code It!

Allison received two medications via two different routes of administration: *intravenous push* and *intravenous infusion*. Therefore, you need two codes.

The notes report that an intravenous push was given, which is an injection given intravenously. Turn to the alphabetic index and look up *injection, intravenous.*

> Injection
>
> > Intravenous   90779

Keep reading below that, and you will see:

> Injection
>
> > Intravenous push   90774–90776

That looks perfect. Turn to the numeric listing, and read the complete descriptions. You see that 90774 matches the notes:

> 90774 Therapeutic, prophylactic or diagnostic injection (specify substance or drug); intravenous push, single or initial substance/drug

You also know that Allison was given an *infusion, intravenously,* and that it was for *therapeutic* reasons—to eliminate her nausea and vomiting. Let's go to the alphabetic index and look up *infusion, intravenous, therapeutic.*

> Infusion
>
> > Intravenous
>
> > > Therapeutic   90760–90768

When you turn to the numeric listing to check the code descriptions, you see that codes 90760–90761 are for hydration only. Look through the complete descriptions for the next grouping, 90765–90768, and you see that the best, most accurate code is:

> 90767 Intravenous infusion, for therapy, prophylaxis, or diagnosis (specify substance or drug); additional sequential infusion, up to one hour.

The notes indicate that Allison was given the infusion after the first (sequentially) for 30 minutes. Excellent!

Therefore, the claim form for this encounter with Allison will show 90774, 90767. Great job!

PSYCHIATRY, PSYCHOTHERAPY, AND BIOFEEDBACK

Sometimes we become so focused on physical health care issues that we forget the health care professionals who treat mental health concerns. The area is a great opportunity for coding specialists, because more and more health care plans cover psychotherapy and psychiatric services. Codes 90801 through 90911 provide details on such services.

When coding psychotherapy services, the best, most appropriate code is determined first by the location (where the therapeutic services were provided, similar to when you code evaluation and management services):

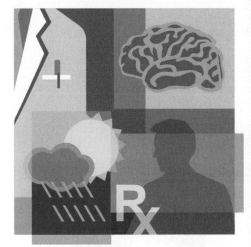

- Office or other outpatient facility
- Inpatient hospital or residential care facility

Next, review the documentation to determine the type of therapy provided:

- Insight oriented/behavior modification/supportive
- Interactive using play equipment, physical devices, language interpreter, or other mechanisms of nonverbal communication

Once the type of therapy is determined, the next factor to consider is how much time the provider spent face to face with the patient.

Last, you must find out from the documentation if the physician or therapist provided medical evaluation and management services in addition to the therapy session at the same time or on the same day. If such services were provided but not at the same time or on the same day, then a code from the Evaluation and Management section of the CPT book may be appropriate.

LET'S CODE IT! SCENARIO

Rick Springer, a 29-year-old male, was sent to Dr. Wheeler for behavior modification because of anger management issues. Dr. Wheeler spent 45 minutes with Rick in her office and then worked on her evaluation report.

Let's Code It!

Rick saw Dr. Wheeler in *her office,* for *behavior modification therapy,* for *45 minutes.* Let's look in the alphabetic index under *psychotherapy,* beneath which you see *family* or *group* as choices. The notes indicate that Rick had an individual psychotherapy session. That does not match. Let's look at *psychiatric treatment,* which does have an individual listing. Indented below *individual* is *insight-oriented,* and then *office or outpatient,* with the suggested codes 90804–90809. Let's look at the numeric listing and see if this matches Dr. Wheeler's notes.

90806 Individual psychotherapy, insight oriented, behavior modifying and/or supportive, in an office or outpatient facility, approximately 45 to 50 minutes face-to-face with the patient

90807   with medical evaluation and management services

The next issue to consider is whether or not Dr. Wheeler provided medical evaluation and management services at the same time. According to her notes, she did. This leads us directly to code 90807. Great job!

DIALYSIS

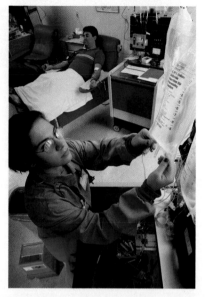

In addition to hospitals providing dialysis, independent centers help patients receive treatment. Almost always, the services are covered by a form of health insurance. Patients with end-stage renal disease (ESRD) are eligible for Medicare coverage, regardless of age.

Due to the regularity of dialysis for those with ESRD, codes 90918, 90919, 90920, and 90921—chosen on the basis of a patient's age—represent a full month of outpatient dialysis services and, therefore, are only reported once a month. If a facility does not provide a full month of services to a patient, for whatever reason, then the coder should use codes 90922–90925, accordingly, multiplied by each day of service.

For ESRD patients who receive dialysis as an inpatient, code 90935 or 90937 for hemodialysis or 90945 or 90947 for dialysis other than hemodialysis during the hospitalization.

For patients who receive dialysis but are not diagnosed with ESRD, code their treatments using 90935, 90937, 90945, or 90947, whether the services are provided on an outpatient or inpatient basis.

LET'S CODE IT! SCENARIO

Verna Abernathy, a 63-year-old female, was diagnosed with ESRD six months ago. She has just moved to Mayfield to be closer to her daughter, and began her daily dialysis on June 20 at the Mayfield Dialysis Center. Prepare the claim for dialysis services for June.

Let's Code It!

Verna has *ESRD* and has received *dialysis* as an *outpatient* from Mayfield Dialysis Center. When you look up *dialysis* in the alphabetic index, you see the listing for *end-stage renal disease* with the suggested code range of 90918–90925. When you turn to the numeric listing, you remember that codes 90918–90921 are only for a full month of treatment. Verna received *11 days* of treatment from the facility (June 20 through June 30 is 11 days). So you have to find the code to report each day of service to Verna. Codes 90922–90925 are chosen by the patient's age. Verna is *63 years old,* bringing us to the following code:

> 90925 End stage renal disease (ESRD) related services (less than full month), per day; for patients twenty years of age and over

Great! So on the claim form for Verna's June services, the code will read 90925 × 11.

GASTROENTEROLOGY

A limited number of tests and services for the gastroenterological system—from the patient's mouth down their esophagus to the stomach through the intestinal tract to the rectum—are included in the Medicine section of the CPT book. The alphabetic index will guide you to the best, most appropriate code in the best section, depending upon the service provided.

YOU CODE IT! CASE STUDY

Sabrina Gentry, a 2-year-old female, was playing in the bedroom at her grandmother's house while her Nana was cooking dinner. No one realized until later that she had gotten into the bottle on the nightstand and eaten its contents: five Premarin tablets. They called 911 and rushed Sabrina to the emergency department, where Dr. Michaels immediately performed a gastric intubation (commonly known as pumping her stomach).

You Code It!

Go through the steps of coding, and determine the codes that should be reported for this encounter between Dr. Michaels and Sabrina Gentry.

Step 1: Read the case completely.

Step 2: Abstract the notes: Which key words can you identify relating to the procedures performed?

_____

Step 3: Query the provider, if necessary.

Step 4: Diagnosis: Poisoning, hormones, accidental.

Step 5: Code the procedure(s).

_____

Step 6: Link the procedure codes to at least one diagnosis code.

Step 7: Back code to double-check your choices.

Answer

Did you find the correct code to be:

91105 Gastric intubation, and aspiration or lavage for treatment (e.g., for ingested poisons)

That's perfect!

OPHTHALMOLOGY

Ophthalmologists are commonly called *eye doctors* or *vision specialists.* However, be careful not to confuse them with **optometrists,** who are eyeglass specialists.

Ophthalmologist

A physician qualified to diagnose and treat eye disease and conditions with drugs, surgery, and corrective measures.

Optometrist

A professional qualified to carry out eye examinations and to prescribe and supply eyeglasses and contact lenses.

CODING TIP »»

Codes for ophthalmologic services include attention to both eyes. Therefore, if only one eye is addressed by the physician, you have to include modifier 52 Reduced Services with the code.

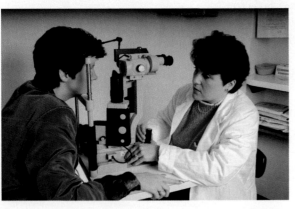

The Ophthalmology subsection of the CPT book deals with the services of an ophthalmologist. General services, codes 92002–92014, are divided in two ways:

1. *The relationship between the patient and the physician: new patient or established patient.* Remember this from E/M coding? As a reminder, a new patient is one who has not received any services or treatments from the ophthalmologist (or any other physician with the same specialty in the same group practice) within the last three years.

2. *The level of service: intermediate or comprehensive.* An intermediate service is similar to a problem-focused evaluation. That is, the patient has a new or existing specific condition to be addressed by the physician. The comprehensive service is more of a general evaluation of the patient's entire visual system.

It is important to remember that these general services include both technical examinations and medical decision-making services. Therefore, it is not appropriate to code any of those services separately.

However, special services may be coded separately if provided at the same time as general services, or evaluation and management services. The documentation must be specific in its identification of the additional services. (Of course, special services can be provided alone and coded as such.)

LET'S CODE IT! SCENARIO

Raymond Nailer, a 55-year-old male, has been having a problem with blurred vision and pain in his eyes. His father has glaucoma, which makes Raymond a high risk for the disease. Therefore, Dr. Roberts is going to perform a bilateral visual field examination and a serial tonometry with multiple measurements. None of these services is done as a part of a general ophthalmologic service provided to Raymond.

Let's Code It!

Dr. Roberts is giving Raymond a "bilateral visual field examination and a serial tonometry" today. Let's go to the alphabetic index and look at *visual field exam.* The index suggests codes 92081–92083. Let's take a look at the numeric listing's code description.

> 92081 Visual field examination, unilateral or bilateral, with interpretation and report; limited examination (e.g., tangent screen, Autoplot, arc perimeter, or single stimulus level automated test, such as Octopus 3 or 7 equivalent)

It matches the notes. Now, you need to code the second test, the tonometry. You see that the alphabetic index shows *tonometry, serial* and suggests code 92100. Let's take a look at the complete code description:

92100 Serial tonometry (separate procedure) with multiple measurements of intraocular pressure over an extended time period with interpretation and report, same day (e.g., diurnal curve or medical treatment of acute elevation of intraocular pressure)

That's great! You are ready to create the claim form for Raymond's tests: codes 92081, 92100. Good job!

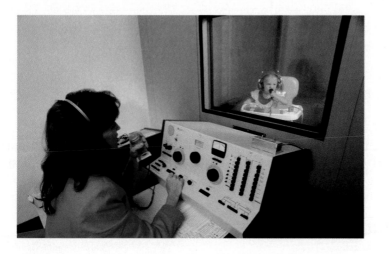

OTORHINOLARYNGOLOGIC SERVICES

In the otorhinolaryngologic services portion of the Medicine section are codes for special services that are not usually included in an office visit or evaluation encounter in the field of **otorhinolaryngology.**

Throughout the listings for codes 92502 through 92700, you will see all types of tests and services that can help health care professionals diagnose and treat conditions relating to a patient's ears, nose, and throat and their functions.

Otorhinolaryngology

The study of the human ears, nose, and throat systems.

YOU CODE IT! CASE STUDY

Kim Whirlon came with her husband, Arlen, to see Dr. Dean because of the problems Arlen has been having sleeping. Kim noticed that Arlen snores terribly during the night and has, at times, abruptly stopped. She is concerned that he may actually stop breathing during one of his episodes. Dr. Dean performed a nasopharyngoscopy with an endoscope to check Arlen's adenoids and lingual tonsils. The results of the exam indicated that Arlen is suffering from sleep apnea.

You Code It!

Go through the steps of coding, and determine the codes that should be reported for this encounter between Dr. Dean and Arlen Whirlon.

Step 1: Read the case completely.

Step 2: Abstract the notes: Which key words can you identify relating to the procedures performed?

_____

Step 3: Query the provider, if necessary.

Step 4: Diagnosis: Sleep apnea.

Step 5: Code the procedure(s).

_____

Step 6: Link the procedure codes to at least one diagnosis code.

Step 7: Back code to double-check your choices.

Answer

Did you find the correct code to be:

92511 Nasopharyngoscopy with endoscope (separate procedure)

That is exactly what Dr. Dean did. In addition, he did not perform it as a part of any other service, so it was a separate procedure. Excellent!

CARDIOVASCULAR SERVICES

In cardiovascular services you will find both diagnostic and therapeutic services for conditions of the heart and its vessels. As you look through the descriptions of the codes in this section, you might think that some appear to be surgical in nature, such as an atherectomy, and others appear to be imaging (radiologic), such as an echocardiogram. Regardless of what we think, the CPT book is structured the way it is, and it is your job as a coding specialist to find the best, most appropriate code to represent the service or treatment provided by the physician or health care professional for whom you are reporting. Again, this is why it is so very important that you take nothing for granted, read all notations and instructions carefully, and use the alphabetic index to guide you through the numeric listings.

Cardiovascular Therapeutic Services: 92950–92998

A variety of procedures relating to the heart are included in the Cardiovascular Therapeutic Services subsection that might seem more appropriate for other places in the CPT book. For example, intravascular ultrasound or percutaneous transluminal coronary balloon angioplasty illustrates the importance of using the alphabetic index to locate the correct range of codes for the procedures performed.

YOU CODE IT! CASE STUDY

Josiah Moore was in Dr. Toller's office when Josiah went into cardiac arrest. Dr. Toller immediately performed CPR. The nurse called 911, and Josiah was taken to the hospital after regaining consciousness and being stabilized.

Go through the steps of coding, and determine codes that should be reported for this encounter between Dr. Toller and Josiah Moore.

Step 1: Read the case completely.

Step 2: Abstract the notes: Which key words can you identify relating to the procedures performed?

_____

Step 3: Query the provider, if necessary.

Step 4: Diagnosis: Cardiac arrest.

Step 5: Code the procedure(s).

_____

Step 6: Link the procedure codes to at least one diagnosis code.

Step 7: Back code to double-check your choices.

Answer

Did you find the correct code to be:

92950 Cardiopulmonary resuscitation (e.g., in cardiac arrest)

It matches the notes perfectly. Good work!

Cardiography: 93000-93278

The electronic measurement of heart rhythms very often uses an electrocardiograph (ECG, also called an EKG, machine). Services involving an electrocardiogram are coded from the Cardiography subsection.

EXAMPLE

Mary Alice Fallon experienced a rapid heartbeat and mild pain in her chest. Dr. Jacobson took a 12-lead routine ECG to rule out a heart attack. He interpreted the tracing and wrote a report for the file. The code is:

93000 Electrocardiogram, routine ECG with at least 12 leads; with interpretation and report

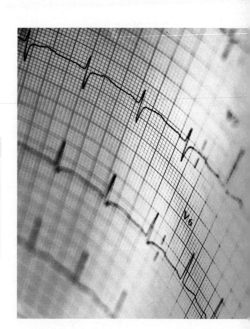

Echocardiography: 93303-93350

Echocardiography is different from an electrocardiography. As the name indicates, the echocardiography uses ultrasound (sound waves to produce an echo), rather than the measurement by electronic impulses, as with the ECG.

When coding echocardiography, the codes already include:

- The exam (the recording of the images of the organ or anatomical areas being studied)

- The interpretation and report of the findings

⟨⟨⟨ CODING TIP

If your physician only performed the interpretation and report, append modifier 26 Professional Component to the correct echocardiography code.

You are not permitted to use these codes for echocardiograms that have been taken when no interpretation or report has been done.

Cardiac Catheterization: 93501-93572

The codes available for reporting cardiac catheterization include the following:

- The introduction of the **catheter**(s)
- The positioning and repositioning of the catheter(s)
- Recording of the intracardiac and intravascular pressure
- Obtaining blood samples for the measurement of blood gases, dilution curves, and/or cardiac output with or without electrode catheter placement
- Final evaluation and report of the procedure

Catheter

A thin flexible tube, inserted into a body part, used to inject fluid, empty fluid, or to keep a passage open.

CODING TIP »»

Injection procedures (93539, 93540, 93544, and/or 93545) may be reported, as appropriate, along with 93508.

LET'S CODE IT! SCENARIO

Vladimir Susnow, a 5-month-old male, has been experiencing cyanotic episodes, known as "blue" spells. Dr. Isaacson, his pediatrician, performs a transthoracic echocardiogram, which identified a ventricular septal defect and hypertrophied walls of the right ventricle. He then performed a right cardiac catheterization that confirmed a diagnosis of a tetralogy of Fallot.

Let's Code It!

Dr. Isaacson performed two tests on little Vladimir: first, a *transthoracic echocardiogram* and, second, a *right cardiac catheterization*. Let's go to the alphabetic index and look for the *echocardiogram*. Beneath it, you see *transthoracic* with a series of suggested codes. But before you go on, take a look at the indented listing below transthoracic for *congenital anomalies*. Vladimir is only 5 months old, and his heart problems are congenital; therefore, those are likely the more accurate codes. Let's take a look at the complete descriptions in the numeric listing for the suggested codes 93303–93304.

93303 Transthoracic echocardiography for congenital cardiac anomalies; complete

This matches the notes. Now, we must code the catheterization. In the alphabetic index, under *catheterization,* you find *cardiac,* and indented below that you find *right heart*. And look what is indented below that for congenital cardiac anomalies. Let's take a look at the complete description:

93530 Right heart catheterization, for congenital cardiac anomalies

CODING TIP »»

There may be times when the physician must repeat a catheterization because it wasn't the correct size or wasn't placed properly the first time. You will only code it once to represent the one completed, correct procedure.

Excellent. Now, you can see how terms you learned from coding the first procedure—congenital cardiac anomalies—made coding the second procedure easier. It is a small example of how practice and experience will make the entire coding process go more smoothly for you.

Electrophysiological Procedures: 93600-93662

Intracardiac electrophysiologic studies (EPS) codes include:

- The insertion of the electrode catheters (usually performed with two or more catheters)
- The repositioning of the catheters
- Recording of electrograms both before and during the pacing or programmed stimulation of multiple locations of the heart
- Analysis of the recorded electrograms
- Report of the procedure and the findings

There are cases when a diagnostic EPS is followed by treatment (**ablation**) of the problem at the same encounter. When ablation is done at the same time as an EPS, you must code it separately.

NONINVASIVE VASCULAR STUDIES

Codes 93875–93990 are provided for reporting noninvasive vascular studies of the arteries and veins of a patient and include the following:

- Preparation of the patient for the testing
- Supervision of the performance of the tests
- Recording of the study
- Interpretation and report of the findings

Codes are chosen by the type of study done: noninvasive physiologic; transcranial Doppler (TCD); or **duplex scan.**

««« **CODING TIP**

Pacing, or programmed stimulation, may include **arrhythmia** induction, which means that the heart is actually caused to misfire during the procedure. When mapping is done at the same session, it has to be coded additionally.

Arrhythmia

An irregular heartbeat.

Ablation

Destruction or eradication of tissue.

««« **CODING TIP**

If the device used does *not* record the test, then you may not use a separate code for the service.

Duplex scan

Ultrasonic scanning procedure to determine blood flow and pattern.

YOU CODE IT! CASE STUDY

Dr. Unger was giving Itzel Malaga her annual physical examination. She had a low-grade fever, and swelling and cyanosis was evident on her lower right leg. Concerned that she might have deep-vein thrombophlebitis, he performed a duplex Doppler ultrasonogram to study the arteries in her leg.

You Code It!

Go through the steps of coding, and determine the codes that should be reported for this encounter between Dr. Unger and Itzel Malaga.

Step 1: Read the case completely.

CPT © 2007 American Medical Association. All Rights Reserved.

Step 2: Abstract the notes: Which key words can you identify relating to the procedures performed?

_____

Step 3: Query the provider, if necessary.

Step 4: Diagnosis: Cyanosis of lower limb, swelling of lower limb, fever.

Step 5: Code the procedure(s).

_____

Step 6: Link the procedure codes to at least one diagnosis code.

Step 7: Back code to double-check your choices.

Answer

Did you find the correct code to be:

93926 Duplex scan of lower extremity arteries or arterial bypass grafts; unilateral or limited study

Good job!

PULMONARY _____

Codes 94002–94799 in the Pulmonary subsection of the CPT book identify procedures and tests on the pulmonary system and include:

- The exam and/or laboratory procedure
- Interpretation of the findings

YOU CODE IT! CASE STUDY

Cahlil Cabel, a 2-day-old male, was born at 35 weeks' gestation, with a birthweight of 1,450 g. After exhibiting hypotension, peripheral edema, and oliguria, Dr. Redmon diagnosed him with respiratory distress syndrome and performed the initiation of continuous positive airway pressure ventilation (CPAP).

You Code It!

Go through the steps of coding, and determine the codes that should be reported for this encounter between Dr. Redmon and Cahlil Cabel.

Step 1: Read the case completely.

Step 2: Abstract the notes: Which key words can you identify relating to the procedures performed?

_____

Step 3: Query the provider, if necessary.

Step 4: Diagnosis: Respiratory distress syndrome.

Step 5: Code the procedure(s).

Step 6: Link the procedure codes to at least one diagnosis code.

Step 7: Back code to double-check your choices.

Answer

Did you find the correct code to be:

94660 Continuous positive airway pressure ventilation (CPAP) initiation and management

Excellent!

ALLERGY AND CLINICAL IMMUNOLOGY

Codes 95004–95199 cover allergy and clinical immunology procedures. Allergies can be responsible for many different reactions in the human body. Beyond the typical sneezing and watery eyes, outcomes can cause anything from hives and rashes to behavioral problems, sleeplessness, and even death. Often, when there is concern or suspicion that a patient may be suffering from an allergic reaction, the physician will begin with allergy sensitivity tests. In these cases, small, yet potent, samples of the suspected allergen are given to the patient in one of a number of methods: percutaneously (scratch, puncture, or prick), intracutaneously (intradermal), inhalation, and ingestion. Then the patient is watched, and the body's reaction to the allergen is documented. The results of the tests tell the physician to which elements the patient is considered allergic.

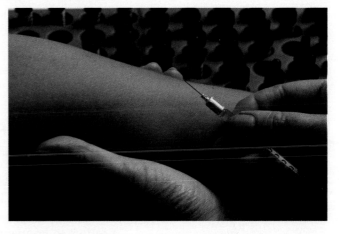

Once an allergy is identified, immunotherapy may be provided. The therapy is a way of retraining the patient's immune system, or desensitizing it, so that the body no longer views the particles as a threat.

《《 **CODING TIP**

The process of desensitizing can take weeks or months, so watch dates of service carefully.

EXAMPLE

Dr. Baylord conducted percutaneous scratch testing with immediate reactions on Laura to identify what may be causing her asthma. He tested her for one dozen common allergens. This would be coded 95004 . . . 12 tests.

NEUROLOGY AND NEUROMUSCULAR PROCEDURES

As with so many other headings in this section, the neurology and neuromuscular procedure codes (95805–96004) include the recording of the test, as well as the physician's interpretation and report of the findings.

Acronyms often seen in this arena of health care services include:

EEG	Electroencephalogram	EMG	Electromyogram
EOG	Electrooculogram	MEG	Magnetoencephalography

《《 **CODING TIP**

For physician interpretation and report only, append modifier 26 Professional Component to the correct procedure code from the Neurology and Neuromuscular subsection.

Alberto Hernandez, a 37-year-old male, was having a hard time staying awake during the day and asleep during the night. Dr. Hartford sent him down the hall to have a polysomnography, with three additional parameters, to rule out sleep apnea.

Let's Code It!

Dr. Hartford performed a *polysomnography* on Alberto to see if he has sleep apnea. Turn to the alphabetic index, and find:

Polysomnography   95808–95811

As you read through the complete code descriptions in the numeric listing, you will see that because Dr. Hartford ordered *three additional parameters*, the best code is:

95808 Polysomnography; sleep staging with 1–3 additional parameters of sleep, attended by a technologist

Excellent!

CENTRAL NERVOUS SYSTEM ASSESSMENTS _____

When a patient exhibits problems with cognitive processes, generally testing evaluates the extent of the condition so that a treatment plan can be established. It is expected that the results of the tests in the Central Nervous System subsection (codes 96101–96125) will be formulated into a report to be used in the creation of the treatment plan.

YOU CODE IT! CASE STUDY

Chase Baltich, a 3-year-old male, does not appear to be developing appropriately for his age. Dr. Reese performed an Early Language Milestone Screening. Once he interpreted the results, he sent his report to a speech therapist to consult on a treatment plan.

You Code It!

Go through the steps of coding, and determine the codes that should be reported for this encounter between Dr. Reese and Chase Baltich.

Step 1: Read the case completely.

Step 2: Abstract the notes: Which key words can you identify relating to the procedures performed?

_____

Step 3: Query the provider, if necessary.

Part 1   CPT

Step 4: Diagnosis: Delayed development of speech.

Step 5: Code the procedure(s).

_____

Step 6: Link the procedure codes to at least one diagnosis code.

Step 7: Back code to double-check your choices.

Answer

Did you find the correct code to be:

96110 Developmental testing; limited (e.g., Developmental Screening Test II, Early Language Milestone Screen), with interpretation and report

Good work!

CHEMOTHERAPY ADMINISTRATION _____

Codes 96401–96549 cover the different methods of chemotherapy dispensation that may be used with one patient. Each method (such as steroidal agents and biological agents) and/or each technique (such as infusion or intravenous push) should be coded separately. The codes include the following services:

- The administration of a local anesthetic
- The initiation of the intravenous
- Accessing an indwelling intravenous, subcutaneous catheter, or port
- Flushing the line at the completion of the infusion
- The appropriate supplies: tubing, syringes, etc.
- The preparation of the chemotherapy agent(s)

YOU CODE IT! CASE STUDY

Gary Whitworth is admitted today for his chemotherapy that consists of an antineoplastic drug, 500 mg IV infusion over three hours. Dr. Thatcher is in attendance during Gary's treatment.

You Code It!

Go through the steps of coding, and determine the codes that should be reported for this encounter between Dr. Thatcher and Gary Whitworth.

Step 1: Read the case completely.

Step 2: Abstract the notes: Which key words can you identify relating to the procedures performed?

_____

Step 3: Query the provider, if necessary.

Step 4: Diagnosis: Chemotherapy.

Step 5: Code the procedure(s).

Step 6: Link the procedure codes to at least one diagnosis code.

Step 7: Back code to double-check your choices.

Answer

Did you find the correct code to be:

96413 Chemotherapy administration, intravenous infusion technique; up to 1 hour, single or initial substance/drug

+96415   each additional hour, 1 to 8 hours (for second hour)

+96415   each additional hour, 1 to 8 hours (for third hour)

PHYSICAL MEDICINE AND REHABILITATION

Throughout the Physical Medicine and Rehabilitation heading and its subheadings, read codes 97001–97799 carefully because some groups of codes require the provider to have direct (face-to-face) contact with the patient during the course of the treatment and others do not.

EXAMPLE

Codes 97010-97028, "Application of a modality to one or more areas," *do not* require provider-patient contact during the treatment; however, codes 97597-97606 *do* require a personal encounter.

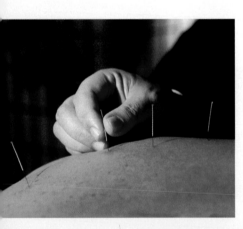

ACUPUNCTURE

The health care industry is always evolving and incorporating new techniques into its accepted methods for helping patients. In this case, the techniques of acupuncture (codes 97810–97814) are thousands of years old.

Acupuncture services are measured in 15-minute increments of direct provider-patient contact. While the needles may be in place for a longer period of time, you are only permitted to report the time actually spent with the patient.

LET'S CODE IT! SCENARIO

Charlene Brown, a 55-year-old female, was having a real problem with menopause. Because of the reported concerns about hormone replacement therapy (HRT), she decided to try acupuncture. After discussing

her symptoms and discussing a treatment plan, Dr. Kini inserted several needles. The needles were removed 20 minutes later. Dr. Kini reviewed the follow-up plan and made an appointment for Charlene's next visit. Dr. Kini spent 30 minutes in total, face to face with Charlene, who reported marked improvement.

Let's Code It!

Dr. Kini's treatment of Charlene included *30 minutes' face-to-face time* and *several needles* during the *acupuncture* treatment. Turn to the alphabetic index, and look up *acupuncture*.

Acupuncture

| With Electrical Stimulation | 97813–97814 |
| Without Electrical Stimulation | 97810–97811 |

There is no mention of electrical stimulation being used in Charlene's treatment, so turn to the codes recommended for *without electrical stimulation*.

97810 Acupuncture, 1 or more needles; without electrical stimulation, initial 15 minutes of personal one-on-one contact with the patient

+97811 without electrical stimulation, each additional 15 minutes of personal one-on-one contact with the patient, with re-insertion of needles(s) (List separately in addition to code for primary procedure.)

The first code, 97810, reports Dr. Kini's services, but only for the first 15 minutes. You have to add the second code, 97811, to report the remainder of the time so the doctor can be reimbursed for the total 30 minutes for the session.

OSTEOPATHIC MANIPULATIVE TREATMENTS

Codes 98925–98929, to report osteopathic manipulative treatments (OMT), are defined by the number of body regions involved in the encounter. Ten regions are identified with the codes:

- Head
- Cervical
- Thoracic
- Rib cage
- Upper extremities
- Lumbar
- Sacral
- Abdominal/visceral
- Pelvic
- Lower extremities

CHIROPRACTIC MANIPULATIVE TREATMENT _____

Similar to the osteopathic treatment codes, chiropractic manipulative treatment (CMT) codes 98940–98943 are measured by the number of regions treated during an encounter. The codes use spinal or extraspinal descriptions and are identified as follows:

Spinal Regions

- Cervical, including atlanto-occipital joint
- Thoracic, including costovertebral and costotransverse joints
- Lumbar
- Sacral
- Pelvic, including the sacroiliac joint

Extraspinal Regions

- Head, including temporomandibular joint (but not the atlanto-occipital)
- Upper extremities
- Rib cage, excluding costotransverse and costovertebral joints
- Abdomen
- Lower extremities

YOU CODE IT! CASE STUDY

Ivan Lampkin, a 23-year-old male who is 6 ft 6 in. tall, has problems with pain in his neck and spine. Dr. Turner treats his cervical, thoracic, lumbar, sacral, and pelvic regions to alleviate Ivan's pain.

You Code It!

Go through the steps of coding, and determine the codes that should be reported for this encounter between Dr. Turner and Ivan Lampkin.

Step 1: Read the case completely.

Step 2: Abstract the notes: Which key words can you identify relating to the procedures performed?

_____

Step 3: Query the provider, if necessary.

Step 4: Diagnosis: Pain, neck and spine.

Step 5: Code the procedure(s).

_____

Step 6: Link the procedure codes to at least one diagnosis code.

Step 7: Back code to double-check your choices.

EDUCATION AND TRAINING FOR PATIENT SELF-MANAGEMENT

Technology and other health care treatment and pharmaceutical advancements have made it easier for the average patient to care for him or herself or for a caregiver to administer treatments, formerly provided exclusively by a physician. Of course, this is not something that should be done without guidance, so it is important that the patient or caregiver is taught how to administer it properly. Education and training for patient self-management training is reported using codes 98960–98962.

EXAMPLE

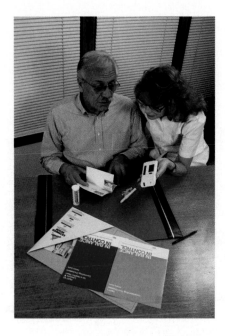

- Teaching a diabetic patient how to self-administer insulin injections
- Teaching a caregiver how to change a dressing

NON-FACE-TO-FACE NONPHYSICIAN SERVICES

Nurses and allied health care professionals extend the ability of a physician to communicate with patients. When a qualified nonphysician member of the health care team provides an assessment and management service to an established patient via telephone or on-line electronic contact, this service is reported with the most accurate of codes 98966–98969.

When telephone or on-line evaluations are performed by the physician, use the most accurate choice from codes 99441–99444.

SPECIAL SERVICES, PROCEDURES, AND REPORTS

There are times when a health care professional is required to provide a service or write a report that is outside the normal realm of his or her responsibilities or outside of the scope of other codes in the CPT book. In those cases, match the circumstance to one of the descriptions in the Special Services, Procedures, and Reports subsection (codes 99000–99091). Each code identifies a different special situation.

EXAMPLE

Dr. Jocamona comes into the office to meet Drew Larson on Thanksgiving because Drew was bitten by his nephew's pet snake and Dr. Jocamona has the only antidote for that species. You would use the following code:

99050 Services provided in the office at times other than regularly scheduled office hours, or days when the office is normally closed (e.g., holidays, Saturday or Sunday), in addition to basic service

QUALIFYING CIRCUMSTANCES FOR ANESTHESIA

You should remember the qualifying circumstances codes from Chap. 6, "Anesthesia Coding." The codes are not only shown in the guidelines pages directly in front of the Anesthesia section of the CPT book but also repeated in the Qualifying Circumstances for Anesthesia subsection of the Medicine section, in their numerical order, for your reference. The codes are added to the claim form when an anesthesiologist provides services to a patient with any of four complications:

- Extreme age
- Total body hypothermia
- Controlled hypotension
- Emergency conditions

CODING TIP »»

Minimal sedation–also known as anxiolysis, deep sedation, or MAC–services are not coded from the Moderate (Conscious) Sedation subsection. Use codes from the Anesthesia section.

MODERATE (CONSCIOUS) SEDATION

Also in Chap. 6, "Anesthesia Coding," as well as in Chaps. 7 and 8 on surgery, we reviewed the details of moderate (conscious) sedation (codes 99143–99150). The codes are to be used when a patient is given medication to reduce anxiety and possibly cause sleepiness but not unconsciousness. The codes may only be used when conscious sedation is not already included in the procedure code, as indicated by the bull's eye (⊙) symbol shown to the left of that procedure code.

HOME HEALTH PROCEDURES/SERVICES

In Chap. 5, "Evaluation and Management Codes, Part 2," we studied codes 99341–99350 for services provided by a physician at the patient's home. However, occasionally a health care professional in your facility other than the physician provides services to a patient at their home. The person may be a nurse or therapist, for example. For such professionals, you must use the codes 99500–99602 from the home health procedures/services in the Medicine section.

EXAMPLE

Margaret Sanders, RN, stopped by Terrell Anderson's home to give him an injection of morphine sulfate, 10 mg, IM for pain management. You would code Nurse Sanders's visit with 99506.

MODIFIERS

There are many codes in the Medicine section of the CPT book that include interpretation and the report along with the particular service or exam, such as neurological and nonvascular studies. You may remember the details of modifier 26 from Chap. 9, "Radiology Coding," but a little reminding never hurt anyone. Therefore, when you are using any of the codes from the Medicine section and your health care professional is interpreting the findings and writing the report but has not performed the test or procedure, you must append the procedure code with modifier 26.

26 **Professional Component:** Certain procedures are a combination of a physician component and a technical component. When the physician component is reported separately, the service may be identified by adding modifier 26 to the usual procedure number.

CHAPTER SUMMARY

Many services provided by physicians, therapists, chiropractors, and other trained health care professionals must receive reimbursement. So much like the other sections of the CPT book, the Medicine section holds much information about the services. The variety of services included in the Medicine section emphasizes the fact that finding the correct code begins in the alphabetic index and culminates in the numeric listings.

1. When an immunization is given, you will need

   a. One code for administering the immunization.

   b. Two codes: one for the administration and one for the drug.

   c. One code for the medication or drug.

   d. HCPCS Level II codes.

2. Vaccinations and immunizations can be administered

   a. Percutaneous.

   b. Intradermally.

   c. Subcutaneously.

   d. All of the above.

3. When a patient receives infusion therapy via more than one site, code

   a. Only the first site.

   b. All appropriate sites.

   c. Report infusion time instead of number of sites.

   d. Only when chemotherapy is infused.

4. Psychotherapy services are coded first by

   a. Location.

   b. Relationship of the patient.

   c. Type of therapy.

   d. Qualifications of the treating health care professional.

5. Dialysis codes are reported

   a. By patient age.

   b. Number of days treated.

   c. Location of treatment (inpatient or outpatient).

   d. All of the above.

6. An optometrist is qualified to

   a. Diagnose and treat eye diseases.

   b. Supply glasses and contact lenses.

   c. Write prescriptions for the treatment of eye diseases.

   d. Perform surgery.

7. An otorhinolaryngologist treats all except

   a. Ear.

   b. Nose.

   c. Throat.

   d. Stomach.

8. Duplex scans are

   a. Ultrasonic.

   b. Noninvasive.

   c. Records of blood patterns and flow.

   d. All of the above.

9. Acupuncture codes are determined by

   a. Age of the patient.

   b. Time spent face to face with patient.

   c. Electrical stimulation used or not.

   d. Both (b) and (c).

10. Chiropractic treatment codes are chosen by

    a. Time spent face to face with the patient.

    b. The total number of treatments in a month.

    c. The number of regions treated.

    d. The age of the patient.

1. Roberta Crushey, a 71-year-old female, has been suffering from bronchitis off and on for two years. Dr. Martin has ordered a pulmonary stress test for her. Dr. Martin notes that he wants her CO_2 measured during the test, O_2 uptake, and an electrocardiogram to be recorded.

   _____

2. David Pinchot, a 61-year-old male, has uncontrolled diabetes and comes into the emergency department complaining of signs of hyperglycemia. Dr. Tennison gives him insulin subcutaneous and intravenous push to bring his blood sugar down.

   _____

3. After finding relief nowhere else, Felicia Heath, a 39-year-old female, goes to Dr. Kini, an acupuncturist, for treatment of her osteoarthritic knee. Dr. Kini spends 15 minutes with the patient reviewing history and symptoms, palpating and locating the points to treat, and inserts the needles and applies electrical stimulation. Felicia is asked to rest. Dr. Kini comes back in about 10 minutes and spends 5 minutes monitoring the patient and restimulating the needles. Ten minutes later, Dr. Kini sees that the pain and swelling in Felicia's knee has reduced, removes the needles, and instructs Felicia on home care measures. Dr. Kini spent a total of 30 minutes in direct contact with Felicia.

   _____

4. Alice Gardener, a 6-year-old female, is brought to Dr. Kaplan by her mother after a referral from the school counselor and her pediatrician. Alice is having difficulties with class work. Mrs. Gardener also tells Dr. Kaplan that Alice has a problem understanding speech in noisy environments. Alice may have a hearing deficiency that has not shown up in hearing tests before, and it may account for her declining work in class. Dr. Kaplan performs a central auditory function evaluation, which takes one hour with report.

   _____

5. Jalel Covington, a 15-year-old male, suffered from a severe asthma attack while at the playground. He was rushed to the clinic where he was given a nebulizer treatment (nonpressurized inhalation).

   _____

6. Rubina Kalish, a 35-year-old female, broke out in a rash, which would not go away. After trying multiple over-the-counter treatments, she went to Dr. Brown who did a series of 11 allergenic extract scratch tests to see if he could identify an allergen. The tests pointed to an allergy to her new kitten.

_____

7. Rubina didn't want to give away her new kitten, so Dr. Brown prepared the allergenic extract and began immunotherapy injections. She received the first injection today.

_____

8. Elijah Gersten, a 44-year-old male, is beginning chemotherapy today with the administration of methotrexate, via intravenous push.

_____

9. Paul Cantrel, a 21-year-old male, is a lifeguard at the beach and came into the emergency clinic with uncontrolled nausea and vomiting. Paul told Dr. Guerva that he was on the beach for 12 hours straight with no breaks, because his replacement didn't show up. Dr. Guerva diagnosed him with severe dehydration and ordered 20 minutes of Zofran, intravenous infusion, and then saline for four hours.

_____

10. Zena Eggerton, a 27-year-old female, comes to Patricia Tallman, a licensed massage therapist, as prescribed by Dr. Ulverton. Zena is pregnant and has been suffering from acute lower back pain for over a month. Patricia performs therapeutic massage with effleurage on the left side and kneading on the iliac band, nerve stroking, and light compression on the gluteus.

_____

11. Kenya Kensington, a 7-day-old male, was born prematurely, and Dr. Valentine is concerned about Kenya's heart. He performs a combined right heart catheterization and transseptal left heart catheterization through the intact septum, in order to measure the blood gases and record Kenya's intracardiac pressure. Dr. Valentine provides conscious sedation to Kenya before beginning the procedure.

_____

12. Darlene Conner, a 6-year-old female, comes to see Dr. Beech for an evaluation of her cochlear implant. Dr. Beech reprograms the implant to improve Darlene's reception.

_____

Part 1   CPT

13. Rasheem Overton, a 66-year-old male, came to see Dr. Macinaw, his ophthalmologist, for an annual checkup of his eyes. Dr. Macinaw does a general evaluation of Rasheem's complete visual system.

   _____

14. Grant Johnston, a 55-year-old male, came to see Dr. Hawkins because he was having chest pain. Dr. Hawkins performed a routine ECG with 15 leads. After talking with Grant and reviewing the ECG results, Dr. Hawkins determined that Grant was having a bout of indigestion.

   _____

15. Marlene Smith, a 20-year-old female, is a professional gymnast who pulled a muscle in her shoulder. Today, Dr. Tunner is measuring her range of motion in the shoulder to confirm that the area has healed completely. Dr. Tunner then wrote and signed the report.

   _____

YOU CODE IT! Simulation
Chapter 11. Medicine Coding

On the following pages, you will see physicians' notes documenting encounters with patients at our textbook's health care facility, Cipher, Victors, & Associates. Carefully read through the notes, and find the best code or codes from the Medicine section for each of the cases.

CIPHER, VICTORS, & ASSOCIATES
A Complete Health Care Facility
234 MAIN STREET • ANYTOWN, FL 32711 • 407-555-1234

PATIENT: KRAUS, MAYNARD
ACCOUNT/EHR #:   KRAUMA001
Date: 10/13/08

Attending Physician: James I. Cipher, MD

S: This new Pt is a 35-year-old male who works in a mattress factory. He states that he has had a piercing ring-ing sound in his left ear that began six months ago. He noticed the ringing sound in his ear upon awakening one morning, and it remains a considerable annoyance all day long, interfering with his ability to enjoy television, movies, and even conversation. Pt states he has trouble sleeping, as well.

O: Pt taken to testing suite for a bilateral tinnitus assessment: pitch (frequency) matching; loudness matching; and masking procedures are included. Findings of the testing indicate a positive determination of tinnitus. Patient is informed of the outcome, along with the recommendations for remediation therapy.

A: Acute tinnitus

P: Follow-up with masking therapy treatment plan

James I. Cipher, MD

JIC/mg   D: 10/13/08 09:50:16   T: 10/15/08 12:55:01

Find the best, most appropriate code from the Medicine section.

_____

_____

_____

CIPHER, VICTORS, & ASSOCIATES
A Complete Health Care Facility
234 MAIN STREET • ANYTOWN, FL 32711 • 407-555-1234

PATIENT: MCDANIEL, CICI
ACCOUNT/EHR #:   MCDACI001
Date: 10/21/08

Attending Physician: Sigmund Freund, MD

Pt is a 16-year-old female recently released from a residential drug rehabilitation program and has moved back into the family home. Her therapy plan calls for a combination of individual counseling and family psychotherapy to help all members of the household understand the circumstances of her addiction and how to help her maintain a healthy, drug-free lifestyle.

    Today is the first family psychotherapy session. Present are Helen McDaniel, the patient's mother; Raul Esponoza, the patient's stepbrother; Jake Esponoza, the patient's stepfather; and Lucy McDaniel, the patient's paternal grandmother. The patient, Cici McDaniel, is also present.

    The group talks openly and shows genuine concern for the patient. The session lasts 50 minutes.

P: 1. Individual session: scheduled next Monday
      2. Next family session; two weeks

___

Sigmund Freund, MD

SF/mg   D: 10/21/08 09:50:16   T: 10/25/08 12:55:01

Find the best, most appropriate code from the Medicine section.

___

___

___

CIPHER, VICTORS, & ASSOCIATES
A Complete Health Care Facility
234 MAIN STREET • ANYTOWN, FL 32711 • 407-555-1234

PATIENT: BEETER, KYLE
ACCOUNT/EHR #:   BEETKY001
Date: 9/30/08

Attending Physician: Laverne Aspiras, MD

Indications: This new Pt is a 9-year-old male with end-stage renal disease, here for
                                 dialysis, monitoring, assessment, and counseling with parents

Procedure: Dialysis services for month of September—30 days

_____

Laverne Aspiras, MD

LA/mg   D: 9/30/08 09:50:16   T: 9/30/08 12:55:01

Find the best, most appropriate code from the Medicine section.

_____

_____

_____

CIPHER, VICTORS, & ASSOCIATES
A Complete Health Care Facility
234 MAIN STREET • ANYTOWN, FL 32711 • 407-555-1234

PATIENT: ROBINET, RENAY
ACCOUNT/EHR #:   ROBIRE001
Date: 10/7/08

Attending Physician: Walter P. Henricks, DC
Referring Physician: Valerie Victors, MD

This new Pt is a 36-year-old female who was in a car accident one month ago. She is diagnosed with whiplash.
    She presents today for chiropractic manipulative treatment of her cervical spine.
    Treatment plan calls for one treatment a week for two months, at which point her status will be reevaluated.

Walter P. Henricks, MD

WPH/mg   D: 10/7/08 09:50:16   T: 10/9/08 12:55:01

Find the best, most appropriate code from the Medicine section.

_____

_____

_____

CIPHER, VICTORS, & ASSOCIATES
A Complete Health Care Facility
234 MAIN STREET • ANYTOWN, FL 32711 • 407-555-1234

PATIENT: WILLIAMSON, BELINDA
ACCOUNT/EHR #:   WILLIBE001
Date: 10/15/08

Attending Physician: Rhonda E. Beardall, MD
Referring Physician: James I. Cipher, MD

Pt is a 75-year-old female who recently had a stroke. She is here on referral from Dr. Cipher for an assessment of her aphasia.

     Assessment of expressive and receptive speech and language function; language comprehension, speech production ability, reading, spelling, writing, using Boston Diagnostic Aphasia Examination.

Interpretation and report to follow.

Total time: 60 minutes

_____

Rhonda E. Beardall, MD

REB/mg   D: 10/15/08 09:50:16   T: 10/17/08 12:55:01

Find the best, most appropriate code from the Medicine section.

_____

_____

_____

Part 1   CPT

Category II and Category III Coding

12

KEY TERMS

Category I codes
Category II codes
Category III codes
Customary clinical documentation
Experimental
Intervention
Medical exclusion criteria
Patient population
Performance measure
Unlisted codes

LEARNING OUTCOMES

- Interpret the guidelines for using Category II codes.
- Identify the guidelines for using Category III codes.
- Apply the guidelines to determine the best, most appropriate Category II code(s).
- Utilize the guidelines to ascertain the best, most appropriate Category III code(s).
- Correctly use Category II code modifiers.
- Correctly follow notational instructions with Category III codes.

EMPLOYMENT OPPORTUNITIES

Nuclear medicine offices
Cardiology offices
Obstetrics/gynecology offices
Osteopathic physicians offices
Podiatric offices
Optometric offices
Oral surgeons' offices
Dental offices

Chiropractic offices
Psychologists' offices
Registered dieticians and nutrionists' offices
Physical therapy offices
Occupational therapy offices
Speech-language therapy offices

Category II codes are used for statistical purposes, to track and measure performance and the quality of care in a health care facility. They are not used as part of the reimbursement process and may not be used in substitution for a Category I code (a code from the main text of the CPT book). Category II codes are optional, so it is possible that you may never use them. However, they are important to the growth of the health information management industry.

The Physician Quality Reporting Initiative (PQRI), signed into law on December 20, 2006 by the President as a part of the Tax Relief and

289

Health Care Act of 2006 (TRHCA), instructs eligible professionals to report on designated sets of quality measures using CPT Category II codes.

Category III codes offer the opportunity to collect detailed information on the use of new technological advancements, services, and procedures at their entry point into health care practices throughout the United States. Each code identifies an innovative procedure that is at the forefront of services, but not yet widely used or accepted as a standard of care. It is why the codes in this section of the CPT book are considered temporary.

Category II codes

Codes for performance measurement and tracking.

Category III codes

Codes for emerging technology.

CODING TIP »»

Category II codes do not replace Category I (CPT) codes and are not a part of proper coding for reimbursement purposes. While they will be placed on the CMS-1500 claim form, they must be shown with a charge of $0.00.

CATEGORY II CODES

Category II codes are listed directly after the Medicine section of the CPT book. The listing is used in conjunction with the CPT Appendix H, "Alphabetic Index of Performance Measure by Clinical Condition or Topic."

While the number of Category II codes is small, the codes identify services and test results that physicians should provide to their patients, that is, specific services that have been proved to be connected to quality patient care.

Each code's description explains clinical fundamentals (such as vital signs), lab test results, patient education, or other facets that might be provided within a typical office visit. However, individually, these component services do not have any billable value and, therefore, are not assigned a code from Category I CPT codes. Assigning Category II codes simply is a way for the industry and the government to specifically calculate how often these services are being given.

The Centers for Medicare and Medicaid Services (CMS), in response to the TRHCA's mandate for a physician quality reporting system, created the PQRI. This program provides for a bonus payment of up to 1.5% to those eligible professionals who meet the criteria for successful reporting.

Category II codes have five characters: four numbers followed by the letter *F*.

EXAMPLE

0001F

3006F

They are compiled into eight categories:

- Composite measures
- Patient management
- Patient history
- Patient examination
- Diagnostic/screening processes or results
- Therapeutic, preventive or other interventions

- Follow-up or other outcomes
- Patient safety

The categories were taken from **customary clinical documentation** formatting.

Appendix H

As a coding specialist, you must refer to the additional data included in the chart in Appendix H. The chart shows specific details regarding the following:

- Complete explanation of what is being measured within the component
- Characteristics of patients that would make them eligible for this report
- Factors that would automatically include or exclude a particular patient

Turn to Appendix H in your CPT book, and let's look at one example.

Brief Description of Performance Measure & Source and Reporting Instructions	CPT Code(s)	Brief Code Descriptor
Hypertension (HTN)		
Blood Pressure Measurement[1]—Number of visits with blood pressure measurement recorded per number of visits **Numerator:** Patient visits with blood pressure measurement recorded **Denominator:** All patient visits for patients aged ≥18 years with hypertension **Percentage** of patient visits with blood pressure recorded for patients aged ≥18 years **Reporting Instructions:** There are no exclusions for this measure; modifiers 1P, 2P, and 3P may not be used.	**2000F**	Blood pressure measured

[1]Physician Consortium for Performance Improvement, www.physicianconsortium.org

Right after the phrase "Blood Pressure Measurement," you will notice a superscript number one. It directs you to footnote 1, which references the Physician Consortium for Performance Improvement, www.physicianconsortium.org.

Other items in the appendix show a superscript number two that directs you to the National Committee on Quality Assurance (NCQA), Health Employer Data Information Set, www.ncqa.org. Superscript number three refers to the Joint Commission, ORYX Initiative Performance Measures, www.jointcommission.org/PerformanceMeasurement.

Superscript number four refers to National Diabetes Quality Improvement Alliance (NDQIA) performance measures, www.nationaldiabetesalliance.org. Superscripts five and six have been added to identify measures from the Physician Consortium and NCQA, as well as the Society of Thoracic Surgeons and the National Quality Forum.

Many clinical measurement sets focus on specific **patient populations,** such as those 18 years of age or older or patients diagnosed with

CPT © 2007 American Medical Association. All Rights Reserved.

Intervention

Action taken to change or prevent something that is happening; most often to stop or prevent something undesirable.

coronary artery disease (CAD). The reason for this is the large amount of scientific evidence that exists that indicates a particular **intervention** is important to the health or continued health of that type of patient.

EXAMPLE

- The Tobacco Use measurement set covers patients aged 18 years and older.
- The Adult Influenza Immunization measurement set focuses on patients 50 years and older.

  Dr. Pinnati's practice is located near a large university. Most of his patients are in their twenties. Actually, statistically, 75% of his established patients (his patient population) are between the ages of 18 and 34.

  Dr. Seng's practice is located in a neighborhood where most of the residents have been living for 20 years or more. About 70% of Dr. Seng's patient population is aged 50 and older.

  Therefore, in terms of Category II coding, it would make sense for Dr. Pinnati's coding specialist to include data related to the tobacco use performance measurement and for Dr. Seng's coding specialist to include data about patient flu shots. The guidelines recommend that health care facilities do just this—pick the individual measurement sets that make the most sense for their circumstances. No one wants anyone wasting time. That is not productive.

The health care professional will be reimbursed for the evaluation and discussion with the patient, most often by reporting an E/M code. However, an E/M code does not provide the specific details in a manner that will enable statistical research. This is the reason for Category II codes—to enable calculation and evaluation of individual health care services.

Category II Modifiers

Performance measurement modifiers are used *only* with Category II codes and explain that the specific service indicated by the code was *not* actually provided. You might look at this as coding a service that was not performed, and you would be correct. In such cases, the research wants to quantify how often the physician recommends a service, even if the patient does not accept the recommendation. When you think about it, how else can researchers learn these facts? They may know if a patient agrees to smoking-cessation therapy, for example, by tracking the prescription for the medication. However, if the patient refuses the physician's urging to quit, without these codes the information is restricted to the patient's chart.

The fact that the physician made the recommendation, along with the reasons the service might not be performed, must be documented. The reasons may be medical circumstances or personal issues vocalized by the patient and will be reported by you using one of the modifiers in this section.

Category II Code modifiers include the following:

- **1P.** Performance measure exclusion modifier due to medical reasons
  - **Includes:**
    - Not indicated (absences of organ/limb, already received/preformed, other)

Part 1   CPT

- Contraindicated (patient allergic history, potential adverse drug interaction, other)
- Other medical reasons

- **2P.** Performance measure exclusion modifier due to patient reasons
  - **Includes:**
    - patient declined
    - economic, social, or religious reasons
    - Other patient reasons

- **3P.** Performance measure exclusion modifier due to system reasons
  - **Includes:**
    - Resources to perform the services not available
    - Insurance coverage/payor-related limitations
    - Other reasons attributable to health care delivery system

- **8P.** Performance measure reporting modifier—action not performed, reason not otherwise specified

Certain Category II codes are exempt from these modifiers. In such cases, a notation is included below the code description.

Take a look at the following code:

4015F Persistent asthma, preferred long term control medication or an acceptable alternative treatment, prescribed (Asthma)[1]

[Note: There are no **medical exclusion criteria.**]

(Do not report modifier 1P with 4015F.)

(To report patient reasons for not prescribing, use modifier 2P.)

You can see that the CPT book, once again, reminds you of the guidelines, as they relate to the use of these modifiers.

Medical exclusion criteria

A medical reason why a patient's data should not be reported with a certain code.

《《《 **CODING TIP**

The superscript number one shown after the word (*Asthma*) in the description of code 4015F refers to the same footnoted websites as noted in Appendix H.

LET'S CODE IT! SCENARIO

Candace Sheridan, a 69-year-old female, comes to see Dr. Devin for her annual checkup. After the examination, Dr. Devin discusses smoking. He offers Candace, a smoker for over 20 years, a prescription for a nicotine patch to help her quit. She thanks him but says no.

Let's Code It!

Of course, you know that you will use an E/M code for the encounter, along with any specific tests or exams that Dr. Devin ordered as a part of Candace's regular physical to make certain Dr. Devin is properly reimbursed for his work. If Candace had accepted his offer for the prescription, a diagnosis code for long-term tobacco use could support the writing of the prescription. However, there is no place in the standard reporting codes of the CPT book to document that Dr. Devin *offered pharmacological therapy* to a patient who is a *known tobacco user,* because she turned him down. This is an excellent example of the benefits of Category II codes. Turn to the Category II code section.

Under the heading, "Patient History," find the code that identifies this patient is a current tobacco user (smoker). You will see code:

1034F Current tobacco smoker (CAD, CAP, COPD, PV)[1] (DM)[4]

NOTE: PV stands for Preventive.

You know from the notes that Dr. Devin offered Candace a prescription, so that would lead us to

4001F Tobacco use cessation intervention, pharmacologic therapy (COPD, CAD, CAP, PV)[1] (DM)[4]

Next, you must reference Appendix H and look through the qualifiers for these two codes. You will see that the chart, under the heading Preventive Care & Screening (PV) shows

Tobacco Use Intervention[1]—whether or not patient identified as a tobacco user received cessation intervention

Numerator: Patients identified as tobacco users who received cessation intervention

Denominator: All patients >18 years at the beginning of the two-year measurement period identified as tobacco users

Percentage of patients identified as tobacco users who received cessation intervention during the two-year measurement period

Reporting Instructions: Report 1034F, 1035F, or 1036F for each patient. If patient is a tobacco user (1034F or 1035F) and received cessation intervention, report 4000F or 4001F or both.

There are no exclusions for this measure; modifiers 1P, 2P, and 3P may not be used.

This is in direct agreement with the physician's notes, and there is nothing in the patient's chart that would exclude her from the measurement set. There is just one more step.

You'll remember that Category II codes require a modifier if the service was not, in fact, provided. The notes indicate that the patient *says no.* Go to the list in the beginning of the Category II section, and review the definitions of the modifiers. You see that the modifier 2P matches perfectly.

2P Performance measure exclusion modifier due to patient choice; including patient refusal

So your report for this encounter includes the Category II code 1034F, 4001F-2P.

PQRI Participation

A health care provider who participates in the PQRI program may receive bonus monies when meeting all of the criteria. CMS has outlined four steps to properly report quality measurement data:

1. Eligible clinicians must identify Medicare-covered patients who are qualified for one or more reportable quality measures.

2. The provider must document the fulfillment of the measure or measures in the notes for the encounter.

3. Assign the appropriate Category II codes to accurately report the documented service, in addition to the proper CPT Category I codes for the visit. If appropriate Category II codes are not available, HCPCS Level II G-codes may be used.

4. Submit the claim form showing the appropriate diagnosis and procedure codes for normal billing, as well as the performance measurement codes that will show a charge of $0.00.

The bonus payments are based on the "successful reporting" of designated quality data. CMS defines the term "successful reporting" as the submission of correctly presented data for at least 80% of the eligible cases for at least three quality measures. This percentage is evaluated for each individual provider, based on the national provider identifier (NPI) shown on each submitted claim.

The bonus payment is calculated at 1.5% of the total "allowed amounts" for services provided during the designated time frame paid for by Medicare. The first block was set to cover dates of service from July 1 through December 31, 2007. Each bonus is subject to a Bonus Incentive Payment Cap, and validation by CMS.

Each year, the PQRI quality measures must be:

- Adopted by a consensus organization such as the National Quality Forum (NQF)

- Include measures that have been submitted by a physician specialty

- Identified by CMS as having used a consensus-based process for development

- Include structural measures, such as the use of electronic health records and electronic prescribing technology

Proposed quality measures for the year are expected to be published in the Federal Register in August, and the final set to be published by November of each year. More information can be found at www.cms.hhs .gov/pqri.

Category II codes are updated twice a year with new codes, deletions, and other changes on January 1 and June 1. The most current listing, along with guidelines, can be found at www.ama-assn.org/go/cpt.

CATEGORY III CODES

Newspapers and television are always mentioning new drugs, cures, and procedures that allow a longer, better quality of life than ever before. Whether a new use for a laser or the latest surgical method, it must go through continued evaluation in the health care industry before becoming an accepted component of the standard of care.

Category III codes are the internship for potential Category I codes (the codes in the main text of the CPT book). New procedures and services are assigned a Category III code so that actual usage can be accurately measured. They are placed in this special section of the CPT book and given a code that has five characters: four numbers followed by the letter *T* (for temporary) in the fifth position.

EXAMPLE

0017T Destruction of macular drusen, photocoagulation

0031T Speculoscopy

Category I codes

The codes listed in the main text of the CPT book, also known as CPT codes.

Unlisted codes

Codes shown at the end of each subsection of the CPT used as a catchall for any procedure not represented by an existing code.

The use of Category III codes is mandatory, as appropriate, according the physician's documentation. If there isn't any accurate **Category I code** in the CPT book to report the physician's services, you must check the Category III section for an appropriate code *before* you are permitted to use a Category I **unlisted code.** The good news is that the CPT book will continue to help you. Category III codes are included in the alphabetic index. In addition, there are notations throughout the main text (numeric) listings that will direct you to a Category III code, if applicable.

EXAMPLE

In the Medicine section of the CPT book, under the subheading Neurology and Neuromuscular Procedures, you will see a notation:

> (For repetitive transcranial magnetic stimulation for treatment of clinical depression, see Category III codes 0160T, 0161T.)

LET'S CODE IT! SCENARIO

Allen Jamison, a 58-year-old male, is a computer technology fanatic. He also has a family history of colon cancer. When he comes to Dr. Goodman for his screening colonoscopy, Allen asks about the new virtual colonoscopy that he saw on television. The patient swallows a large pill that is actually a camera that records the entire passage through the body by using computed tomography. Dr. Goodman agrees to run the procedure.

Let's Code It!

You can see by the notes that Allen had a *screening colonoscopy,* done *virtually* using *computed tomography.* Let's go to the alphabetic index and look this up the way you would normally, under *colonoscopy.* Beneath the heading, you find the listing for:

Colonoscopy

   Virtual   0066T, 0067T

Now, you know that the *T* indicates that this code will be found not in the main numeric listing but in the Category III code section, after the Medicine section.

Turn to Category III codes, and find the complete code description:

0066T Computed tomographic (CT) colonography (i.e., virtual colonoscopy); screening

0067T   diagnostic

Allen had a screening colonoscopy, so 0066T is the best code. That's just like coding from the rest of the book.

CODING TIP »»»

Use a Category III code when both the following conditions are true:

1. A regular CPT code *is not* appropriate.
2. A Category III code *is* appropriate.

Use an unlisted code when both the following conditions are true:

1. A regular CPT *is not* appropriate.
2. A Category III code *is not* appropriate.

Category III Notations

Once a procedure or service has been accepted by health care professionals and is found to be effective, safe, and beneficial in clinical prac-

Part 1   CPT

tice, the code will be "promoted" to a Category I code. At that time, the T code is deleted, and the procedure is given a five-digit code and placed into the appropriate section of the main text of the CPT book. A notation is placed in the Category III section that states the T code has been deleted and provides the new five-digit code for reference.

EXAMPLE

(0023T has been deleted. To report, use 87900.)

As a new coder, this will not affect you very much. Such notations will be helpful once you have been coding for a while, in a particular health care facility that might use such codes frequently. If a code used in your office changes, you need the notation to direct you to the new code. Remember, your claim form may be rejected or denied if it includes a deleted code.

Similar to notations in the main text of CPT, you may see the direction to use a specific Category III code along with a CPT code. This will help you properly report the addition of new technology being used along with a standard procedure.

EXAMPLE

+0164T Removal of total disc arthroplasty, anterior approach, lumbar, each additional interspace

(Use 0164T in conjunction with 22865.)

Notations in this section will also highlight mutually exclusive codes—those codes that cannot be reported on the same claim form as another.

EXAMPLE

0137T Biopsy, prostate, needle, saturation sampling for prostate mapping

(Do not report 0137T in conjunction with 76942.)

0096T Revision of total disc arthroplasty, anterior approach cervical; single interspace

(Do not report 0096T in conjunction with 0093T.)

Sometimes, the notation explains that if an alternative to the code description is performed, another code is correct.

EXAMPLE

0058T Cryopreservation; reproductive tissue, ovarian

0059T   oocyte(s)

(For cryopreservation of embryo(s), sperm, and testicular reproductive tissue, see 89258, 89259, 89335.)

It is important that you are aware of the fact that Category III codes represent up-and-coming technology. Because of this, the third-party

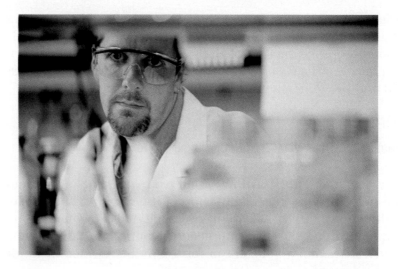

Experimental

A procedure or treatment that has not yet been accepted by the health care industry as the standard of care.

payers from whom you seek reimbursement may consider some services **experimental**. When you work in a health care facility that uses any procedures or services identified by a Category III code, it is critical that you determine the carrier's rules and coverage with regard to the treatment or test. Should the carrier exclude it and refuse to pay, the patient and your office are better off knowing it as soon as possible. You may be able to petition the payer, convince it of the medical necessity and the cost efficiency of the new technology, and receive an approval after all. Waiting for the denial notice is not the efficient way to handle the situation. That is also not respectful to the patient.

A particular Category III code, once assigned, is reserved for five years, whether the code is upgraded to a Category I code or deleted altogether. It allows for the fact that certain technologies or procedures may take time to find acceptance and prevents confusion.

YOU CODE IT! CASE STUDY

Henry Battsmann, a 47-year-old male, had a heart transplant two months ago. He has not been feeling well, so Dr. Rufani performs a breath test for heart transplant rejection. This is a new experimental test, but it is noninvasive.

You Code It!

Go through the steps of coding, and determine the codes that should be reported for this encounter between Dr. Rufani and Henry Battsmann.

Step 1: Read the case completely.

Step 2: Abstract the notes: Which key words can you identify relating to the procedures performed?

_____

Step 3: Query the provider, if necessary.

Step 4: Diagnosis: Heart transplant follow-up.

Step 5: Code the procedure(s).

Step 6: Link the procedure codes to at least one diagnosis code.

Step 7: Back code to double-check your choices.

Answer

Did you find the correct code to be:

0085T Breath test for heart transplant rejection

Good work!

CHAPTER SUMMARY

Category III codes, like Category II codes, are updated twice a year. The latest adjustments are released on January 1 and June 1. So if you are working as a coding specialist for a health care facility that uses any Category III codes, you will be responsible for staying on top of the changes. The most current listing, along with guidelines, can be found at www.ama-assn.org/go/cpt.

1. Category I codes are also known as

   a. Temporary codes.

   b. Experimental codes.

   c. CPT codes.

   d. Modifiers.

2. Category II codes are used for reporting

   a. Emerging technology.

   b. Experimental procedures.

   c. Performance measurement.

   d. Neurological procedures.

3. When coding Category II codes, you have to also reference

   a. Appendix H.

   b. Appendix A.

   c. Appendix C.

   d. Appendix G.

4. The modifiers 1P and 2P are used with

   a. CPT codes.

   b. Category II codes.

   c. Category III codes.

   d. All of the above.

5. An example of a Category II code is

   a. 11111.

   b. 1111T.

   c. 1111F.

   d. H1111.

6. Category III codes should be used

   a. Only if no unlisted codes are appropriate.

   b. Only if no Category I codes are appropriate.

   c. First.

   d. Only if no Category II codes are appropriate.

7. An unlisted code should only be used when

   a. An accurate Category I code is not available.

   b. An accurate Category III code is not available.

   c. (a) and (b).

   d. (a) or (b).

8. Category III codes are updated

   a. Once a year.

   b. Twice a year.

   c. Once every two years.

   d. Quarterly.

9. The use of Category II codes is

   a. Optional.

   b. Mandatory for reimbursement.

   c. Determined by each individual third-party payer.

   d. None of the above.

10. Coding for reimbursement properly may include all except

    a. CPT codes.

    b. Category II codes.

    c. Category III codes.

    d. HCPCS Level II codes.

YOU CODE IT! Practice
Chapter 12. Category II and Category III Coding

Find the best, most appropriate code or codes from the Category II and Category III sections.

1. Dr. Mendelsohn inserted a temporary prostatic urethral stent into Bart Garrity to help diminish the symptoms of his benign prostatic hyperplasia.

   _____

2. Arlene Register, a 25-year-old female, came for her first prenatal care visit. She enrolled in a managed care organization just 10 days before she conceived. She is now two months pregnant.

   _____

3. Ellis Felton, a 37-year-old male, and his wife have been trying to have a baby for a long time. At Dr. Zelna's recommendation, Ellis is here today to have a hyaluronan binding assay sperm evaluation.

   _____

4. Ann Hovenarian, a 69-year-old female, has been having a problem with incontinence. Today she is here for a pulsed magnetic neuro-modulation treatment.

   _____

5. Bernard Hodges, a 61-year-old male, had an artificial heart implanted three months ago. Today, Dr. Yamagucci replaced the thoracic unit of Bernard's heart.

   _____

6. Shirley Kiley, a 73-year-old female, was diagnosed with coronary artery disease (CAD) last year. During her regular checkup with Dr. Pauli, her blood pressure was measured.

   _____

7. Dr. Spevack has an office in downtown Manhattan. In order to care for his patients more efficiently and effectively, he has created a special online service to enable communication electronically. Patients requesting to participate receive a special password. Rona Calendar signed up and e-mailed Dr. Spevack about a concern she had. He responded with an answer.

   _____

8. Fonda Gold, a 27-year-old female, is here today to have reproductive tissue from her ovary cryopreserved before she begins chemotherapy for a malignant tumor of the patella.

_____

9. Trudy Summerlin, a 23-year-old female, has a grandmother, mother, and sister who have all been diagnosed with breast cancer. Dr. Forrest performs an electrical impedance scan of both of Trudy's breasts to assess her risk for the disease.

_____

10. Patrick McNeil, a 37-year-old male, has a family history of melanoma. He is very concerned, so Dr. Francetti requested that whole body integumentary photography be taken to monitor him.

_____

11. Ava Vitasek, a 66-year-old female, had a myocardial infarction (MI) last year, and has also been diagnosed with coronary artery disease (CAD). Dr. Loreneta prescribed beta-blocker therapy for her at this visit.

_____

12. Frank Milotti, a 43-year-old male, had a heart transplant five months ago. He is beginning to show signs that he may be rejecting the heart, so Dr. Yuan gives him a breath test.

_____

13. Kelly Scotcia, a 24-year-old female, is the first person in this area to have an artificial heart implanted. She also had a cardiectomy.

_____

14. Edward Rotan, a 79-year-old male, received a new prescription from his cardiologist today. His daughter was worried about possible problems with the new medication reacting with his other medications. She and her father went to the pharmacy and sat down with the pharmacist for a 30-minute assessment of all of Edward's drugs.

_____

15. Maria Vasquez, a 71-year-old female, has type I diabetes and was diagnosed with coronary artery disease (CAD). Dr. Willimina prescribed an angiotensin-converting enzyme (ACE) inhibitor for her.

_____

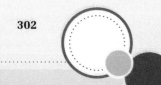

Part 1   CPT

Below and on the following pages, you will see physicians' notes documenting encounters with patients at our textbook's health care facility, Cipher, Victors, & Associates. Carefully read through the notes, and find the best code, or codes, from the Category III sections. Code for the attending physician services.

CIPHER, VICTORS, & ASSOCIATES
A Complete Health Care Facility
234 MAIN STREET • ANYTOWN, FL 32711 • 407-555-1234

PATIENT: PYLE, CARTER
ACCOUNT/EHR #:   PYLECA001
Date: 11/13/08

Diagnosis: Discogenic back pain

Procedure: Annuloplasty, percutaneous intradiscal, unilateral

Physician: Marion M. March, MD

Anesthesia: Local

Procedure: Patient is a 39-year-old male, with chronic back pain. The patient is positioned on the table, prepped and draped in a sterile fashion. Anesthetic is injected, and fluoroscopy is used to localize the area. A spinal needle is placed adjacent to the L4–5 disc, the depth is measured, and local anesthetic is injected. An introducer needle is placed into the disc and advanced obliquely into the anterolateral quadrant of the disc space. This position is confirmed by fluoroscopy. The annuloplasty catheter is checked for any defects and to ensure proper working condition. The catheter is advanced through the introducer needle and navigated into the area of disc pathology. Final positioning is again confirmed by fluoroscopy. The catheter is connected to the generator and the disc is treated.

   The patient is monitored during the procedure by the physician for a pain response that may require adjusting treatment intensity of increasing the level of sedation. The patient is also monitored for any radicular symptoms that would indicate impending nerve injury and that would necessitate repositioning the catheter.

   Antibiotic solution is injected into the disc. The catheter and needle are removed. Dressings are applied. Patient tolerated the procedure well and is taken to the recovery room.

Marion M. March, MD

MMM/mg   D: 11/13/08 09:50:16   T: 11/13/08 12:55:01

Find the best, most appropriate code(s) from the Category III section.

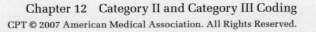

CIPHER, VICTORS, & ASSOCIATES
A Complete Health Care Facility
234 MAIN STREET • ANYTOWN, FL 32711 • 407-555-1234

PATIENT: DEKALB, CYRUS
ACCOUNT/EHR #:   DEKACY001
Date: 10/20/08

Attending Physician: James I. Cipher, MD

S: Pt is a 5-year-old male, with a history of respiratory illnesses. He is brought in today by his mother for a spectroscopy.

O: Pt taken to testing suite for a spectroscopic measure of his exhaled breath. The laser spectroscope is put in place, and the boy exhales into the device. Carbon dioxide levels showed the sample was in correct quantity. The nitric oxide (NO) levels measured greater than 20 ppb indicating a lower airway inflammation.

A: Bronchial Asthma

P: 1. Rx corticosteroid inhaler
     2. Follow-up in one month

James I. Cipher, MD

JIC/mg   D: 10/20/08 09:50:16   T: 10/23/08 12:55:01

Find the best, most appropriate code(s) from the Category III section.

_____

_____

_____

CIPHER, VICTORS, & ASSOCIATES
A Complete Health Care Facility
234 MAIN STREET • ANYTOWN, FL 32711 • 407-555-1234

PATIENT: CHEN, REBECCA
ACCOUNT/EHR #:   CHENRE001
Date: 11/15/08

Diagnosis: Malignant neoplasm, urinary bladder

Procedure: Compensator-based beam modulation treatment

Physician: Marion M. March, MD

Anesthesia: Local

Procedure: Patient is a 47-year-old female, brought in to undergo external beam radiation to the bladder with dose escalation to 32 Gy. A fluence map was generated for a 5-field compensator-based beam modulation technique to treat this patient while meeting the required constraints. Once this was approved, the final plan was generated using a single compensator for each beam of varying thickness throughout its area to generate the required fluence map. The compensator was milled according to specifications. The treatment was delivered to a film phantom using these compensators and images overlaid well with the dose distributions. The treatments were delivered as prescribed: daily for 5 days.

Marion M. March, MD

MMM/mg   D: 11/15/08 09:50:16   T: 11/21/08 12:55:01

Find the best, most appropriate code(s) from the Category III section.

_____

_____

_____

PATIENT: WYNDHAM, MAXWELL
MRN: WYNDMA001
Date: 15 November 2008

Procedure performed: Cerebral perfusion analysis, CT scan

Radiologist: Keith Robbins, MD

Referring Physician: James I. Cipher, MD

Indications: R/o vascular obstruction

Impressions: With contrast administration. Postprocessing of parametric maps with determination of cerebral blood flow, cerebral blood volume and mean transit time

Keith Robbins, MD

KR/mg   D: 11/15/08 09:50:16   T: 11/17/08 12:55:01

Find the best, most appropriate code(s) from the Category III section.

_____

_____

_____

CIPHER, VICTORS, & ASSOCIATES
A Complete Health Care Facility
234 MAIN STREET • ANYTOWN, FL 32711 • 407-555-1234

PATIENT: COLLIER, ANITA

ACCOUNT/EHR #:   COLLAN001

Date: 11/11/08

Diagnosis: Septal blockage

Procedure: Implantation, VAD, extracorporeal, percutaneous

Physician: Marion M. March, MD

Anesthesia: General

Procedure: Patient is a 51-year-old female, brought into the OR and placed on the table in the supine position. The patient is draped in a sterile fashion. A ventricular assist device is inserted, extracorporeally, using percutaneous transseptal access with single cannulation.

Marion M. March, MD

MMM/mg   D: 11/11/08 09:50:16   T: 11/12/08 12:55:01

Find the best, most appropriate code(s) from the Category III section.

_____

_____

_____

_____

PART TWO

HCPCS LEVEL II

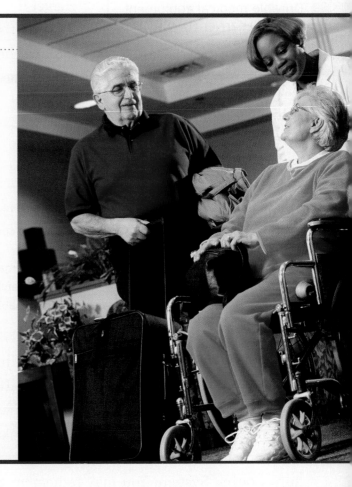

13

HCPCS Level II Coding: Introduction and Guidelines

LEARNING OUTCOMES

- Abstract physician's notes to identify the need for reporting HCPCS Level II codes.
- Correctly use the rules and guidelines for reporting HCPCS Level II codes.
- Distinguish between CPT and HCPCS Level II codes.
- Follow the directions supplied by the notations and symbols.
- Apply the instructions for properly coding with HCPCS Level II codes.

EMPLOYMENT OPPORTUNITIES

Skilled nursing facilities

Assisted living communities

Dental offices

Hospice care organizations

Long-term rehabilitation

Short-term rehabilitation

Home health care companies

Orthotic specialists

Prosthetic specialists

Ambulance service providers

Health and charitable agencies

There is another portion to the procedure coding system that professional coding specialists use to report services and treatments. HCPCS (pronounced "hick-picks") is the acronym for Healthcare Common Procedure Coding System. You may remember the following from Chap. 2:

- HCPCS Level I codes are referred to as CPT codes.

- HCPCS Level II codes are referred to as HCPCS codes.

HCPCS LEVEL II CATEGORIES

HCPCS Level II codes and modifiers are listed in their own book and are used to report a service, procedure, and supplies that are not properly described in the CPT book. There are almost 5,000 HCPCS codes, each represented by five-characters: one letter followed by four numbers.

EXAMPLE

C1715 Brachytherapy needle

M0075 Cellular therapy

HCPCS Level II codes cover specific aspects of health care services, including:

- Durable medical equipment (e.g., a wheelchair or a humidifier)
- Pharmaceuticals administered by a health care provider (e.g., a saline solution or a chemotherapy drug)
- Medical supplies provided for the patient's own use (e.g., an eye patch or gradient compression stockings)
- Dental services (e.g., all services provided by a dental professional)
- Transportation services (e.g., ambulance services)
- Vision and hearing services (e.g., trifocal spectacles or a hearing screening)
- **Orthotic** and **prosthetic** procedures (e.g., scoliosis braces or post-surgical fitting)

Not all insurance carriers accept HCPCS Level II codes, but Medicare and Medicaid want you to use them. It is your responsibility as a coding specialist to find out whether a third-party payer, with which your facility works, accepts HCPCS Level II codes. If not, you have to ask for its policies on reporting the services and supplies covered by HCPCS Level II.

Orthotic

A device used to correct or improve an orthopedic concern.

Prosthetic

Fabricated artificial replacement for a damaged or missing part of the body.

EXAMPLE

Medicare accepts HCPCS Level II codes and therefore requires you to code an injection of tetracycline, 200 mg, with two codes (for giving the shot and the drug inside the syringe).

90772 Therapeutic, prophylactic or diagnostic injection (specify material injected); subcutaneous or intramuscular

J0120   Injection, tetracycline, up to 250 mg

Barton Health Insurance does not accept HCPCS Level II codes. This payor includes reimbursement for the drug in the CPT code for the actual injection. Therefore, you would only report the one code to get paid for both the service (the giving of the shot) and the material (the drug inside the syringe).

90772 Therapeutic, prophylactic or diagnostic injection (specify material injected); subcutaneous or intramuscular

The process for using HCPCS Level II codes is the same as you have learned throughout this book for coding from the CPT book. You abstract the key words from the physician's notes regarding the services and procedures, look those key words up in the alphabetic index of the appropriate book (CPT or HCPCS), confirm the code in the numeric listing, and report the service using that code. You know how to do this already!

However, there are specific elements unique to HCPCS Level II coding that you need to know, which you will learn here and the following two chapters.

Understanding how to use HCPCS codes accurately will open new employment opportunities for you. In addition to hospitals, physician's offices, and outpatient clinics, nursing homes, home health care agencies, health care equipment and supply companies, and other facilities use the codes quite extensively.

THE ALPHABETIC INDEX

CODING TIP »»

Never, never, never, never, never code from the alphabetic index. Always confirm the code in the alphanumeric listing before deciding which code to report.

Like the other coding books, the HCPCS book has an alphabetic index, as well as an alphanumeric listing.

The index lists the Level II code descriptions in alphabetical order from A to Z. After abstracting the key terms from the provider's notes, you can look up key words in the index using the following:

- Brand name of the drug
- Generic name of the drug
- Medical supply item
- Orthotic
- Prosthetic
- Service
- Surgical supply

The index will recommend a code or a range of codes, similar to CPT's alphabetic index. Then as you have done before, you look the suggestions up in the alphanumeric listing, read the complete description(s), and determine the best, most appropriate code. *Note:* The alphabetic index in the HCPCS Level II book does not list all the codes included in the alphanumeric listing. So if you can't find what you are looking for in the index, you might want to find something closely related to get you to the appropriate section of the book and then look around.

This index includes many alternate terms identified by notations in the alphanumeric listings.

EXAMPLE

In the alphabetic index, you will see:

    Abarelix, J0128

    Plenaxis, J0128

In the alphanumeric listing, you will see:

    J0128 Injection, abarelix, 10 mg

Use this code for Plenaxis.

Deleted code descriptions are not included in the alphabetic index. However, the new codes that are to be used instead of the deleted code are listed.

When the alphanumeric listing shows a notation to use one code with another code, the alphabetic index provides you with the same direction.

HCPCS Level II codes are listed in sections, grouped by the type of service, the type of supply item, or the type of equipment they represent. However, you should not assume that a particular item or service is located in a specific section. Use the alphabetic index to direct you to the correct category in the alphanumeric listing of the book. One type of service or procedure might be located under several different categories depending upon the details.

THE ALPHANUMERIC LISTING

The alphanumeric listing presents the codes in alphabetical order by the first letter and then numerical order beginning with the first number of that code.

Let's go through all the sections together so you can get a clearer understanding of what procedures, services, and supplies are reported using these codes.

A0000-A0999 Transportation Services Including Ambulance

You will learn more about reporting transportation services in Chap. 14.

EXAMPLE

A0021 Ambulance service, outside state per mile, transport

A0420 Ambulance waiting time (**ALS** or **BLS**), one-half hour increments

A4000-A8999 Medical Supplies

The codes cover medical supplies, surgical supplies, and some services and supplies related to **durable medical equipment (DME).**

EXAMPLE

A4245 Alcohol wipes, per box

A4452 Tape, waterproof, per 18 sq in.

A4490 Surgical stocking above knee length, each

A4637 Replacement, tip, cane, crutch, walker, each

A9000-A9999 Administrative, Miscellaneous, and Investigational

You will find codes in this section for:

- Nonprescription drugs (also known as over-the-counter drugs)
- Exercise equipment
- Radiopharmaceutical diagnostic imaging agents
- Noncovered items and services

Note: An item or service may be non-covered with regard to national standards but covered by your state or other third-party carrier. Never take anything for granted, always ask!

EXAMPLE

A9280 Alert or alarm device, not otherwise classified

A9505 Supply of radiopharmaceutical diagnostic imaging agent, thallous chloride TI-201, per millicurie

---

Advanced life support (ALS)

Life-sustaining, emergency care is provided, such as airway management, defibrillation, and/or the administration of drugs.

Basic life support (BLS)

The provision of emergency CPR, stabilization of the patient, first aid, control of bleeding, and/or the treatment of shock.

Durable medical equipment (DME)

Apparatus and tools that help individuals accommodate physical frailties, deliver pharmaceuticals, and provide other assistance that will last for a long time and/or be used to assist multiple patients over time.

Part 2   HCPCS Level II

Anabelle Simpson, a 67-year-old female, has been diagnosed with malignant neoplasm of the liver. She has lost all her hair because of the chemotherapy and radiation treatments. Dr. Tippin prescribed a wig to help lift her spirits and self-esteem.

Let's Code It!

You have to submit a claim to Medicare for the *wig*. Let's go to the alphabetic index of the HCPCS Level II book and find the *W* section. Beneath this, find:

> Wig, A9282

Go to the alphanumeric listing to confirm it is the best code.

> A9282 Wig, any type, each

B4000-B9999 Enteral-Parenteral Therapy

The codes cover supplies, formulas, nutritional solutions, and infusion pumps for **enteral-parenteral** therapy.

EXAMPLE

> B4083 Stomach tube–Levine type
>
> B9006 Parenteral nutrition infusion pump, portable

C1000-C9999 Outpatient PPS

Codes from this category are used to report drugs, biologicals, devices for transitional pass-through payments for hospitals, and items classified in new technology ambulatory payment classifications.

EXAMPLE

> C1724 Catheter, transluminal atherectomy, rotational
>
> C2636 Brachytherapy linear source, palladium 103, per 1 mm
>
> C9428 Mesna, 200 mg, brand name

D0000-D9999 Dental Procedures

This category is the Current Dental Terminology (CDT) code set, copyrighted by the American Dental Association. The codes are used to report dental services.

EXAMPLE

> D0240 Intraoral–occlusal film
>
> D1110 Prophylaxis–adult
>
> D3310 Anterior (excluding final restoration)

Enteral

Within, or by way of, the gastrointestinal tract.

Parenteral

By way of anything other than the gastrointestinal tract, such as intravenous, intramuscular, intramedullary, or subcutaneous.

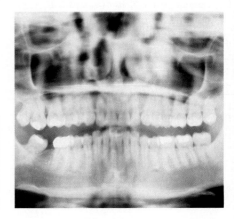

Prophylaxis is also known as a dental cleaning, and *anterior (excluding final restoration)* is one of the codes that can be used to report root canal therapy.

LET'S CODE IT! SCENARIO

Daniel Roseman, a 73-year-old male, came to Dr. Franks for a complete maxillary denture. His old one was broken beyond repair, so Daniel needed something immediately.

Let's Code It!

CODING TIP »»

Should you choose to code for a dental office, the CDT code set is published as an individual book but includes the same codes given here.

Dr. Franks provided Daniel with a *complete maxillary denture*. Let's go to the HCPCS Level II alphabetic index:

Dentures (removable)
  Adjustments, D5410–D5422
    Complete, D5110–D5140

As you read the full list, you see that the reference matches Dr. Franks's notes. Next, turn to the alphanumeric listing to see which code is the most accurate.

D5110   Complete denture–maxillary

D5120   Complete denture–mandibular

D5130   Immediate denture–maxillary

D5140   Immediate denture–mandibular

Is there additional information in the notes that will help us determine the best code? They state that Daniel needed the denture *immediately*. It leads us directly to:

D5130   Immediate denture–maxillary

Excellent!

CODING TIP »»

Be careful not to confuse the E codes with ICD-9-CM E codes which report how and where an injury occurred.

E0980 Safety vest, wheelchair: Letter followed by four numbers (from HCPCS)

E980.0 Poisoning, unknown, analgesics: Letter followed by three numbers, a period, and, possibly additional numbers (from ICD-9-CM)

E0100–E9999 Durable Medical Equipment

The E codes are used to identify certain pieces of durable medical equipment (DME) provided to a patient.

EXAMPLE

E0105   Cane, quad, or three-prong, includes canes of all materials, adjustable or fixed, with tips

E0156   Seat attachment, walker

E0242   Bathtub rail, floor base

More information about durable medical equipment codes is in Chap. 14.

G0000-G9999 Procedures/Professional Services (Temporary)

Codes from this section are used to report services and procedures that do not have an accurate code description in the main portion of the CPT book.

EXAMPLE

G0102 Prostate cancer screening; digital rectal examination

G0151 Services of physical therapist in home health setting, each 15 minutes

G0266 Thawing and expansion of frozen cells for therapeutic use, each cell line

H0001-H2037 Alcohol and Drug Abuse Treatment Services

When alcohol and drug treatment, as well as some other mental health services are provided, some state Medicaid agencies will have you use codes from this category.

EXAMPLE

H0006 Alcohol and/or drug services; group counseling by a clinician

H0038 Self-help/peer services, per 15 minutes

H2020 Therapeutic behavioral services, per diem

J0000-J9999 Drugs Administered Other Than Oral Method

As the title so clearly states, this category provides you with codes to identify drugs that are given to the patient, by a health care professional in any way other than by mouth. This includes chemotherapy drugs, immunosuppressive drugs, inhalation solutions, and other miscellaneous drugs and solutions.

EXAMPLE

J0207 Injection, amifostine, 500 mg

J7100 Infusion, dextran 40, 500 ml

J7613 Albuterol, inhalation solution, administered through DME, unit dose, 1 mg

You will find that drugs identified in the code descriptions are most often the chemical, or generic, name of the pharmaceutical. At times the brand, or trade, name is listed in the alphabetic index and/or in the table of drugs in Appendix 1. If your provider notes refer to a name that you cannot find in this book, you might need to look in the *Physician's Desk Reference* (PDR) to find an alternate name for the drug. Chap. 14 of this text will go into more detail.

Remember that a coding specialist's job is to report with the greatest specificity. There will be times when you will need a code from this section because it provides more specificity than a code from the CPT.

K0000-K9999 Temporary Codes

The K codes were developed for **DMERC**s to report services that are not currently identified by other codes.

EXAMPLE

K0001   Standard wheelchair

K0462   Temporary replacement for patient owned equipment being repaired, any type

L0000-L4999 Orthotic Procedures and L5000-L9999 Prosthetic Procedures

The codes included in these categories identify orthotic devices, orthopedic shoes, prosthetic devices, prosthetic implants, and scoliosis equipment.

EXAMPLE

L0170   Cervical, collar, molded to patient model

L0984   Protective body sock, each

L5050   Ankle, Symes, molded socket, SACH foot

M0000-M0301 Medical Services

The codes in this category cover cellular therapy, prolotherapy, intragastric hypothermia, intravenous **chelation therapy,** and fabric wrapping of an abdominal aneurysm (MNP).

EXAMPLE

M0075 Cellular therapy

M0301 Fabric wrapping of abdominal aneurysm

P0000-P9999 Pathology and Laboratory

For lab and pathology services not listed in the CPT book, HCPCS codes in this category include chemistry, toxicology, microbiology, screening Papanicolaou (Pap) procedures, and numerous blood products.

Durable medical equipment regional carrier (DMERC)

A company designated by the state or region to act as the fiscal intermediary for all DME claims.

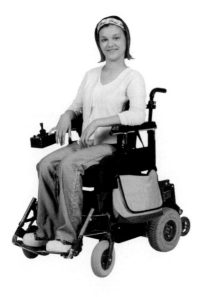

Chelation therapy

The use of a chemical compound that binds with metal in the body so that the metal will lose its toxic effect. It might be done when a metal disc or prosthetic is implanted in a patient, eliminating adverse reactions to the metal itself as a foreign body.

P2031   Hair analysis (excluding arsenic)

P7001   Culture, bacterial, urine; quantitative, sensitivity study

P9051   White blood or red blood cells, leukocytes reduced, CMV-negative, each unit

Q0000-Q9999 Q Codes (Temporary)

The Q codes replace the less specific codes that you may find elsewhere in the coding process for casting and splinting supplies when a health care professional cares for a patient with a fracture. The section also includes codes for certain drugs and services having nothing to do with the management of a fracture.

Q0113   Pinworm examination

Q2017   Injection, teniposide, 50 mg

Q4049   Finger splint, static

«« **CODING TIP**

Remember that you must always choose the code with the greatest specificity.

R0000-R5999 Diagnostic Radiology Services

The codes in this category are used to report the hauling of portable radiological equipment.

R0070   Transportation of portable x-ray equipment and personnel to home or nursing home, per trip to facility or location, one patient seen

R0076   Transportation of portable EKG to facility or location, per patient

S0000-S9999 Temporary National Codes (Non-Medicare)

This category of codes was developed by the Health Insurance Association of America (HIAA) and the Blue Cross Blue Shield Association (BCBSA) for use by the Medicaid program and other third-party payers. The codes cover supplies, services, and drugs for which there are no other codes.

S0081   Injection, piperacillin sodium, 500 mg

S0317   Disease management program; per diem

S2060   Lobar lung transplantation

S9015   Automated EEG monitoring

T1000-T9999 National T Codes Established for State Medicaid Agencies

Planned for use by state agencies that administer Medicaid programs, these codes are used to report services not otherwise described by a code. Services represented in this category include nursing and home health–related services, substance abuse treatment, and training-related procedures.

EXAMPLE

T1013   Sign language or oral interpretive services, per 15 minutes

T2022   Case management, per month

T2045   Hospice general inpatient care; per diem

V0000-V2999 Vision Services

Ophthalmic and optometric services and supplies may be coded from this category, if not represented by any other codes, including contact lenses, intraocular lenses, miscellaneous lenses, prostheses, spectacles, and other vision-related supplies.

EXAMPLE

V2118   Aniseikonic lens, single vision

V2321   Lenticular lens, per lens, trifocal

V2530   Contact lens, scleral, gas impermeable, per lens

V5000-V5999 Hearing Services

Services related to hearing and speech-language pathology are included in this category and cover hearing tests, repair of augmentative communicative system, speech-language pathology screenings, and other hearing test related supplies and equipment.

EXAMPLE

V5008   Hearing screening

V5100   Hearing aid, bilateral, body worn

V5364   Dysphagia screening

YOU CODE IT! CASE STUDY

Eric Ziambi, a 17-year-old male, lost his eye in a skiing accident and has come to see Dr. Voltain to receive his prosthetic eye. It is a custom-made, plastic prosthesis. Code for the prosthesis only.

You Code It!

Go through the steps of coding, and determine the codes that should be reported for this encounter between Dr. Voltain and Eric Ziambi.

Step 1: Read the case completely.

Step 2: Abstract the notes: Which key words can you identify relating to the item provided?

_____

Step 3: Query the provider, if necessary.

Step 4: Diagnosis: Acquired absence of eye.

Step 5: Code the item(s).

_____

Step 6: Link the item code(s) to at least one diagnosis code.

Step 7: Back code to double-check your choices.

Answer

Did you find the correct code to be:

V2623 Prosthetic eye, plastic, custom

SYMBOLS AND NOTATIONS _____

Throughout the HCPCS Level II book, you will see notations that will help you use the codes correctly and determine the best, most appropriate code available.

Symbols

●

A large bullet, or black circle, shown next to a code indicates that it is the first year that the code is included in the book.

▲

A black triangle shown next to a code lets you know that the code's description has been changed or adjusted since last year or that a rule or guideline regarding the code has changed.

○

An open circle next to a code identifies that the code had been deleted but now has been restored (reinstated).

⊘

The circle with a slash through it, in the HCPCS book, identifies a code that is not covered under the skilled nursing facility prospective payment system (PPS).

☑

A check mark inside a square box marks a code description that identifies a specific quantity of material or supply. It is a reminder for you to

⟨⟨⟨ CODING TIP

In the CPT book, the symbol ⊘ means that the code may not be used with modifier 51. In HDPCS, it means not covered under SNFPPS.

Should the provider administer less than the indicated amount in the code descriptor, you are permitted to simply report the code as shown. For example, if the provider administered 3 mg of mitomycin, you would report C9432.

When more than the quantity shown in the code description is indicated in the provider's notes, report the appropriate code in the proper number. For example, if the provider gave the patient 2 mg of decitabine, you would report J0894 x2 to indicate two units.

check the detail in the notes and report the code not only for the item it represents but by the amount as well.

EXAMPLE

J0894   Injection, decitabine, 1 mg

K0073   Caster pin lock, each

♂

The male symbol is placed next to codes that identify procedures, services, and equipment that can *only* be performed or used on a male patient.

EXAMPLE

L3219   Orthopedic footwear, man's shoes, Oxford

L8330   Truss, addition to standard pad, scrotal pad

♀

The female symbol identifies codes used to report procedures, services, and equipment that can *only* be performed or used on a female patient.

EXAMPLE

A4286   Locking ring for breast pump, replacement

L8600   Implantable breast prosthesis, silicone or equal

A

The "A" symbol highlights the fact that a code is used only for procedures, services, and equipment that are performed or used on a patient of a certain age group. Read the code description carefully to ensure the age limitation of the code matches the patient.

M

The "M" symbol is used to remind you that the code describes maternity procedures, services, and equipment that are performed or used on a pregnant female, 12–55 years of age.

~~Z1111~~

When a code and its description are shown with a line through the center, it means that the code has been deleted and may no longer be used.

Notations

Just as in the CPT book, you will find notations (below code descriptions in the alphanumeric listing) that guide you as to how to use HCPCS codes correctly.

Always Report Concurrent to the xxx Procedure

The notation directs you to be certain to use the indicated code with another code—the code for the procedure. The notation is similar to the "code also" instruction found in CPT or ICD-9-CM.

EXAMPLE

A4263 Permanent, long-term, nondissolvable lacrimal duct implant, each

Always report concurrent to the implant procedure.

Here, the A code is for the implant itself, and the note reminds you that you have to code the physician's services for putting the implant into the patient.

See Also Code Z1111

The *see also code* notation cross-references the code with another code that may be similar in description. The notation serves as a reminder for you to double-check that you are using the most accurate code.

EXAMPLE

A4450 Tape, non-waterproof, per 18 sq. in.

See also code A4452

A4452 Tape, waterproof, per 18 sq. in.

See also code A4450

Clarifications of Coverage

Such notations are actually worded differently from code to code but serve the same purpose—to tell you when to use or *not* use the code.

EXAMPLE

A4565 Slings

Dressings applied by a physician are included as part of the professional service. Surgical dressings obtained by the patient to perform homecare as prescribed by the physician are covered.

Report in Addition to Code Z1111

There are times when codes are to be reported with other codes. The notation will identify those circumstances, and it not only tells you this but also tells you which code to use. You may notice that it is similar to an add-on code in CPT.

EXAMPLE

D2953 Each additional indirectly fabricated post–same tooth

Report in addition to code D2952

See Code Z1111

When a code has been deleted, you will often find a notation that directs you to another HCPCS Level II code that can be used instead.

EXAMPLE

E0180   Pressure pad, alternating with pump

See code(s) E0181, E0182

See Code(s): 00000

This notation refers you to a CPT code for a description that is *potentially* better and may be more specific for reporting what was actually done or given to the patient.

EXAMPLE

D6199   Unspecified implant procedure, by report

See code(s): 21299

Code 21299 Unlisted craniofacial and maxillofacial procedure

Determine if an Alternative HCPCS Level II or a CPT Code Better Describes . . .

Not otherwise specified (NOS)

Indicates that more detailed information is not available from the physician's notes.

You will see this notation beneath each miscellaneous, unlisted, unclassified, not otherwise classified (NOC), not otherwise listed, or **not otherwise specified (NOS)** code. The notation serves as warning to you to make certain that there is no better or more specific code in either the CPT or elsewhere in this HCPCS Level II book that correctly reports the services or procedures performed.

EXAMPLE

L0999   Addition to spinal orthosis, NOS

Determine if an alternative HCPCS Level II or a CPT code better describes the service being reported. This code should be used only if a more specific code is unavailable.

Use This Code For . . .

This notation provides you with alternative names, brand names, and other terms that are also represented by the code's description.

EXAMPLE

B4150   Enteral formula, nutritionally complete with intact nutrients, includes proteins, fats, carbohydrates, vitamins and minerals, may include fiber, administered through an enteral feeding tube, 100 calories = 1 unit

Use this code for Enrich, Ensure, Ensure HN, Ensure Powder, Isocal, Lonalac Powder, Meritene, Meritene Powder, Osmolite, Osmolite HN, Portagen Powder, Sustacal, Renu, Sustagen Powder, Travasorb.

Part 2   HCPCS Level II

Pertinent Documentation to Evaluate Medical Appropriateness Should Be . . .

Some procedures are not automatically accepted as being medically necessary. The notation warns you up-front that you should include the proper documentation along with the claim *the first time*, rather than wait to be asked by the third-party payer, which would delay payment.

EXAMPLE

D2980 Crown repair, by report

Pertinent documentation to evaluate medical appropriateness should be included when this code is reported.

Do Not Use This Code to Report . . .

Here, the notation warns you of circumstances when you are not permitted to use a code.

EXAMPLE

D3220 Therapeutic pulpotomy (excluding final restoration)—removal of pulp coronal to the dentinocemental junction and application of medicament

Do not use this code to report the first stage of root canal therapy.

Medicare Covers . . .

Throughout the HCPCS Level II book, you will see notations giving you information about coverage, particularly Medicare and Medicaid coverage. You should note that the book covers the entire nation and that both programs are state-administered. It means that you should still confirm the terms and policies of what is covered with your own state's fiscal intermediary (FI)—the agency or organization that is in charge of reimbursement for your state's program. Also check with other third-party payers to see if they will cover this item or service.

EXAMPLE

E0607 Home blood glucose monitor

Medicare covers home blood-testing devices for diabetic patients when the devices are prescribed by the patient's physicians. Many commercial payers provide this coverage to non-insulin dependent diabetics as well.

Code with Caution

When you see this notation beneath a code, you need to go back and double-check the provider's notes carefully. If this is what was actually done, then be certain to attach documentation explaining why that method was used instead of the newer technique, because it is surely going to be questioned.

EXAMPLE

P2028 Cephalin flocculation, blood

Code with caution: This test is considered obsolete. Submit documentation.

YOU CODE IT! CASE STUDY

Dr. Yawia modified Arthur Wassau's left orthopedic shoe by inserting a between sole metatarsal bar wedge to accommodate Arthur's shrinking Achilles tendon. Dr. Yawia checked off the code L3649 on the superbill. As the professional coding specialist, is this the best code available?

You Code It!

Go through the steps of coding, and determine the codes that should be reported for this encounter between Dr. Yawia and Arthur Wassau.

Step 1: Read the case completely.

Step 2: Abstract the notes: Which key words can you identify relating to the service performed?

_____

Step 3: Query the provider, if necessary.

Step 4: Diagnosis: Contracture of Achilles tendon (acquired).

Step 5: Code the procedure(s).

_____

Step 6: Link the procedure codes to at least one diagnosis code.

Step 7: Back code to double-check your choices.

Answer

Did you find the correct codes to be:

L3410   Metatarsal bar wedge, between sole

Now that's a much more specific code. Good job!

LET'S CODE IT! SCENARIO

Kim Whirlon came with her husband, Arlen, to see Dr. Dean because of the problems Arlen was having sleeping. You may remember their case from Chap. 11 in the text when you coded the nasopharyngoscopy with an endoscope that Dr. Dean performed to confirm that Arlen had sleep apnea. Dr. Dean supplied Arlen and Kim with an apnea monitor, complete with a recording feature, so Arlen's sleep could be monitored and Dr. Dean could further evaluate his condition.

Let's Code It!

In Chap. 11, you found the CPT code for the *nasopharynogoscopy with an endoscope*—code 92511. Now, you see that Dr. Dean supplied Arlen with an *apnea monitor with a recording feature*. It is considered durable medical equipment (DME). Arlen's insurance carrier accepts HCPCS Level II codes and modifiers. Therefore, we have to add another code to the claim form for the encounter, so that Dr. Dean can be reimbursed for the machine. Let's go to the alphabetic index and look up the word *monitor*, because that is the key word that best describes the item. Beneath the word *monitor*, indented slightly, you see the word *apnea*, with the suggestion for the code E0618. This seems to be exactly what Dr. Dean described in his notes, so let's turn to the alphanumeric listing to read the complete description of the code.

E0618   Apnea monitor, without recording feature

This matches the notes with one big exception. The code description specifically states *without* recording feature. You know that Dr. Dean documented giving Arlen a monitor *with* a recording feature. Keep reading, and you will find

E0619   Apnea monitor, with recording feature

Excellent! It matches perfectly.

LET'S CODE IT! SCENARIO

Dr. Porter provided Janine Matlock, a 73-year-old female, with a quad cane, after putting on a new handgrip. Code for the supply only.

Let's Code It!

When you pull out the key words that describe the items Dr. Porter should be reimbursed for, you see that Dr. Porter provided Janine with a *quad cane* and *new handgrip.*

It wouldn't be out of line to think that the codes are automatically going to be listed in the Durable Medical Equipment section, codes E0100–E9999. If you turned to that section directly, you would find the code for the quad cane rather quickly. It's right in the front. However, you could examine and search through the entire listing of 9,899 possible codes in the section and never find the correct code for the replacement handgrip. When you look these key words up in the alphabetic index first, you see very quickly, and more efficiently, that the codes you need are:

E0105   Cane, quad or three-prong, includes canes of all materials, adjustable or fixed, with tips

A4636   Replacement, handgrip, cane, crutch, or walker, each

It's great when the process works, isn't it? You bet!

APPENDIXES

The HCPCS Level II book provides you with additional information in the back of the book to help you code more accurately.

Appendix 1: Table of Drugs. Appendix 1 is an alphabetical listing of drug names, along with the standard unit of administration, a particular method of administration, and a reference to its HCPCS Level II code.

Appendix 2: Modifiers. This is an alphabetic list of all HCPCS Level II modifiers. You will learn more about these modifiers in Chap. 15 of this text.

Appendix 3: Abbreviations and Acronyms. Abbreviations and acronyms are used throughout the health care industry. Appendix 3 lists those used in HCPCS descriptions to help you better understand the meaning of the codes.

Appendix 4: PUB100 References. Certain components of the coding system change from time to time. Up-to-date manuals and information can be found online in the CMS manual system found at www.cms.hhs.gov/manuals. Included in each annual edition of the printed HCPCS Level II book are references to national coverage determinations made just prior to publication. As a student, this may be outside the scope of your studies. As you mature in your career, this reference will be very handy.

Appendix 5: New, Changed, Deleted, and Reinstated HCPCS Codes. This appendix lists all HCPCS Level II codes that have experienced a change since the previous year's printed book. As a student, this will have little relevance for you. But it serves as an excellent reference when the new book comes out for someone who may use the same code or codes over and over again.

Appendix 6: Place of Service and Type of Service Codes. Appendix 6 offers you a thorough explanation of each place of service (POS) and type of service (TOS) code required for boxes 24B and 24C of the CMS 1500 claim form.

CHAPTER SUMMARY

HCPCS Level II codes are updated quarterly and are officially effective January 1 of each year, with no grace period. Most printed versions of the book are published with those codes posted by the Centers for Medicare and Medicaid Services (CMS) as of November 1. Read the following notation in the introduction of the HCPCS Level II book:

> Because of the unstable nature of HCPCS Level II codes, everything has been done to include the latest information available at print time. Unfortunately, HCPCS Level II codes, their descriptions, and other related information change throughout the year. Consult the patient's payer and the CMS website to confirm the status of any HCPCS Level II code. The existence of a code does not imply coverage under any given payment plan.

Find the best answer regarding HCPCS Level II codes.

1. The symbol of a circle with a line through it ⊘ means

   a. A new code.

   b. A revised code.

   c. A code exempt from a particular modifier.

   d. A service not covered under the skilled nursing facility payment system.

2. The little box with a check mark in it ☑ indicates a code description that

   a. Includes a quantity measurement.

   b. Is always covered by Medicare.

   c. Is approved for reimbursement at a higher rate.

   d. Includes refills.

3. The J codes are used to bill insurance carriers for

   a. Prescription drugs patients get at the drug store.

   b. Drugs administered by a health care professional.

   c. Nothing. They are deleted codes.

   d. Items not accepted by Medicaid in any state for any reason.

4. HCPCS Level II codes are used, most often, to report all except

   a. Drugs used for treatment of a patient.

   b. Equipment provided to a patient.

   c. Anesthesia administered by an anesthesiologist.

   d. Dental services.

5. The acronym DME stands for

   a. Determination of medical effectiveness.

   b. Durable medical equipment.

   c. Donated medical equipment.

   d. Diluted drug equivalent.

6. HCPCS Level II codes are presented as

   a. Five numbers.

   b. One letter followed by four numbers.

   c. Four numbers followed by one letter.

   d. Five letters.

7. HCPCS is an acronym that stands for

   a. Health Care Professional Classification Systems.

   b. Health and Caretaker Providers Coding Series.

   c. Home Care Providers Coding System.

   d. Healthcare Common Procedure Coding System.

8. The code D1110 is an example of a

   a. HCPCS Level I code, also known as a CPT code.

   b. HCPCS Level II code.

   c. HCPCS Level III code.

   d. HCPCS Level IV code.

9. The D0000–D9999 codes are created and maintained by the

   a. American Medical Association.

   b. American Dental Association.

   c. Centers for Medicare and Medicaid Services.

   d. Department of Health and Human Services.

10. Gauze used by a physician as a surgical dressing is

    a. Not coded separately because they are included in the professional service.

    b. Coded separately when HCPCS Level II codes are accepted.

    c. Coded separately when a certain quantity is used.

    d. Not coded separately unless a CPT code is used.

11. The E codes shown in the HCPCS Level II book are

    a. An expansion of the E codes in the ICD-9-CM book.

    b. Used to identify DME provided to a patient.

    c. Not accepted by Medicaid.

    d. Always first listed on a claim form.

12. An example of DME is

    a. An injection of Demerol.

    b. A prosthetic ankle.

    c. A three-prong cane.

    d. Home infusion therapy.

13. A deleted code in the HCPCS Level II book means

    a. The procedure is obsolete.

    b. The service is no longer reimbursable.

    c. The code is reinstated.

    d. The code is no longer available to represent the service or item.

14. Alcohol intervention treatment might be coded from

    a. H0001–H2037.

    b. H5000–H9999.

    c. F1000–F9999.

    d. G0000–G9999.

15. A code with an **A** next to it means that

    a. A drug was administered intravenously.

    b. The machine can only be used for infusion therapy.

    c. The service is limited to a specific age group.

    d. The equipment is illegal in some states.

1. Oona Garrity, a 13-year-old female, has severe asthma. Dr. Summers ordered a nebulizer, with compressor for her to use at home. Code for the home health agency that supplied the equipment.

   _____

2. Leo Pennuzo, a 45-year-old male with ESRD, was fitted for a reciprocating peritoneal dialysis system. Code the supply of the equipment.

   _____

3. Next, due to his condition, Leo had to meet with his physician, face to face, twice a month. Code these professional services for one month.

   _____

4. Melissa Hallmark, a 19-year-old female with a history of bipolar disorder, was given an injection IM of Thorazine, 45 mg. Code for the drug.

   _____

5. Thomas Roberts, a 37-year-old male, was being prepared for his kidney transplant. The nurse administered 100 mg of Zenapax, IV, parenteral. Code the drug.

   _____

6. After Thomas received his kidney transplant, the nurse gave him an oral dose of 250 mg of CellCept (mycophenolate mofetil) in the hospital.

   _____

7. Latonya Terranzano, a 93-year-old female, was having trouble eating for such a long period of time that she was exhibiting signs of malnutrition. Therefore, Dr. Pollack ordered enteral formula (Ensure) to be administered through a feeding tube at 500 calories per day. Code for the nutritional supplement only.

   _____

8. Mandy Caulder, a 23-year-old male, came to see Dr. Kinder, his dentist, for an implant-supported porcelain crown on his back tooth.

   _____

9. Felicia Simon, a 13-year-old female, lost her retainer at camp. She is at Dr. York's office to get a replacement.

_____

10. Andrew Reynolds, a 10-year-old male, sat in poison ivy while camping in the woods. Dr. Storm prescribed a portable sitz bath for him to use at home.

_____

11. Gina Campbell, a 49-year-old female, was recuperating from surgery to repair a complex fracture of her tibia and a compound fracture of her ankle. To help her be more comfortable, Dr. Matson ordered a fixed-height hospital bed, without side rails and with a mattress, for her to use at home. Code for the DME only.

_____

12. Lawrence Tieborn, a 77-year-old male, was on complete bed rest while recuperating from surgery. Because his skin was very sensitive, he was particularly prone to decubitus ulcers. Dr. Ellington prescribed a lamb's wool sheepskin pad to help prevent any ulcers from forming.

_____

13. Dr. Rossini provided a complete set of dentures, maxillary and mandibular, for Allison Porter.

_____

14. Fred Plantman, a 55-year-old male, had surgery on his left foot. To enable him to take a shower safely, Dr. Porteous gave him a tub stool to sit on.

_____

15. Roger Madison came home from serving in the Marines a double-amputee, having had both legs damaged badly in a suicide bomber's attack. Dr. Leventhol supplied him with an amputee wheelchair, desk height, with detachable arms and no footrests or leg rests.

_____

YOU CODE IT! Simulation
Chapter 13. HCPCS Level II Coding

On the following pages, you will see physicians' notes documenting encounters with patients at our textbook's health care facility, Cipher, Victors, & Associates. Carefully read through the notes, and find the best code or codes from the *CPT and/or HCPCS* Level II books for each of the cases.

Note: All insurance carriers and third-party payers for the patients accept HCPCS Level II codes and modifiers.

CIPHER, VICTORS, & ASSOCIATES
A Complete Health Care Facility
234 MAIN STREET • ANYTOWN, FL 32711 • 407-555-1234

PATIENT: KELLER, ANDRIENNE
ACCOUNT/EHR #:   KELLAN001
Date: 12/21/08

Attending Physician: James I. Cipher, MD

S: This Pt is a 35-year-old female who was here six months ago for her annual physical. Today, she presents with a cut in the palm of her right hand. Pt states that she was hanging ornaments on her tree and a glass ball broke in her hand. She is otherwise healthy and has no other stated health concerns.

O: Pt lies back on the examination table and her right hand is draped in a sterile fashion. A topical antiseptic is applied and the superficial laceration, measuring 2.0 cm in length was checked for residual glass shards. None were found and the wound was cleansed, and a simple repair was accomplished with a tissue adhesive.

A: Superficial laceration of the right hand, 2.0 cm

P: Follow-up in 10 days.

James I. Cipher, MD

JIC/mg   D: 12/21/08 09:50:16   T: 12/22/08 12:55:01

Find the best, most appropriate CPT and HCPCS Level II code(s).

_____

_____

_____

CIPHER, VICTORS, & ASSOCIATES
A Complete Health Care Facility
234 MAIN STREET • ANYTOWN, FL 32711 • 407-555-1234

PATIENT: GRANT, AMOS
ACCOUNT/EHR #:   GRANAM001
Date: 11/05/08

Attending Physician: Valerie R. Victors, MD

S: This Pt is a 15-year-old male. I have not seen this patient since last July when he came in for a certificate to play sports in school. Today he is brought in by his father after being tackled during football practice and hurting his left wrist. He is complaining of pain upon flexing and is having difficulty moving his fingers.

O: Tenderness and swelling of the wrist is observed. Pt can move his fingers slightly indicating no fracture, however, AP/lat x-rays are taken to confirm. X-ray does confirm the wrist is sprained. A conforming, nonelastic (nonsterile) bandage, 2″ × 35″, is applied.

A: Sprain, radiocarpal ligament, wrist

P: Follow-up in one week.

_____

Valerie R. Victors, MD

VRV/mg   D: 11/05/08 09:50:16   T: 11/08/08 12:55:01

Find the best, most appropriate CPT and HCPCS Level II code(s).

_____

_____

_____

CIPHER, VICTORS, & ASSOCIATES
A Complete Health Care Facility
234 MAIN STREET • ANYTOWN, FL 32711 • 407-555-1234

PATIENT: WEINGARTEN, LEONORA
ACCOUNT/EHR #:   WEINLE001
Date: 10/26/08

Attending Physician: Valerie R. Victors, MD

S: Pt is a 71-year-old female who I diagnosed with type II diabetes mellitus two years ago. She comes in complaining of cramps and aching in her calves. Pt states that most times she can relieve the symptoms, but lately, the pain has not subsided during rest.

O: Ht. 5′ 2″, Wt 165 lb, comprehensive metabolic panel blood test taken. Each extremity is examined with special attention to lower leg, ankle, and feet. Lab results indicate that glucose levels are abnormal. Gradient compression stockings are applied to each leg, below knee, 18–30 mmHg. Patient is given instructions for proper use of these stockings.

A: Suspected peripheral arterial disease (PAD)
     Uncontrolled diabetes mellitus type II

P: 1. Order for computed tomographic scans of both legs, with contrast
     2. Follow-up after results of CT scans

Valerie R. Victors, MD

VRV/mg   D: 10/26/08 09:50:16   T: 10/27/08 12:55:01

Find the best, most appropriate CPT and HCPCS Level II code(s).

CIPHER, VICTORS, & ASSOCIATES
A Complete Health Care Facility
234 MAIN STREET • ANYTOWN, FL 32711 • 407-555-1234

PATIENT: ABERNATHY, CARTER
ACCOUNT/EHR #:   ABERCA001
Date: 10/15/08

Attending Physician: Valerie R. Victors, MD

S: Pt is a 45-year-old male diagnosed with carcinoma of the inner cheek three months ago. He has chewed tobacco for the last 20 years. Pt states he quit chewing 6 weeks ago. He presents today for his daily therapeutic injection.

O: Pt is brought into the examining room, and given an injection of Interferon Alfa-2a, 3 million units, IM.

A: Malignant carcinoma, cheek, internal

P: Series of injections to continue on daily basis

_____

Valerie R. Victors, MD

VRV/mg   D: 10/15/08 09:50:16   T: 10/17/08 12:55:01

Find the best, most appropriate CPT and HCPCS Level II code(s).

_____

_____

_____

CIPHER, VICTORS, & ASSOCIATES
A Complete Health Care Facility
234 MAIN STREET • ANYTOWN, FL 32711 • 407-555-1234

PATIENT: FISCHER, ELVIRA
ACCOUNT/EHR #:   FISCEL001
Date: 12/09/08

Attending Therapist: Stephen L. Brooks, MPT

Pt is a 37-year-old female hurt during a waterskiing accident. She was performing in a ski show at Water World Adventure Park when she came off the ski jump ramp at the wrong angle and hit the water unevenly, twisting her knee. Her physician, Dr. Cipher, ordered her to use a wheelchair for the next six weeks.

    I delivered a standard wheelchair with fixed full-length arms and swing-away, detachable footrests to the patient's home. I spent 15 minutes instructing the patient on the proper way to use the chair, transfer from the chair to standard furniture and back, and transfer to other function furniture including the toilet and the bed. She was instructed on how to stop and start the chair with the least amount of strain on her upper extremities, and how to apply the breaks. Patient stated she clearly understood all instructions.

    DX: Torn meniscus, lateral, knee

P: Patient given instruction booklet and technical support number

_____

Stephen L. Brooks, MPT

SLB/mg   D: 12/09/08 09:50:16   T: 12/11/08 12:55:01

Find the best, most appropriate CPT and HCPCS Level II code(s).

_____

_____

_____

14

Coding Medical Supplies, Durable Medical Equipment, Pharmaceutical, and Ambulance and Other Transportation Services

LEARNING OUTCOMES

- Interpret correctly the rules and guidelines for coding medical supplies.
- Apply the instructions for properly coding medical supplies with HCPCS Level II codes.
- Report the best, most appropriate HCPCS Level II codes for the supply of durable medical equipment.
- Determine the correct generic or brand name of drug.
- Utilize the guidelines for coding transportation services.
- Assign the best, most appropriate code for transportation services.

EMPLOYMENT OPPORTUNITIES

Hospitals

Physicians' offices

Clinics

Ambulatory care centers

Assisted living facilities

Nursing homes

Skilled nursing facilities

Short-term facilities

Long-term care facilities

Pharmacies

Medical supply companies

Ambulance companies

Taxi companies

Public transportation services

Air ambulance services

Nonprofit organizations

The most common items and services that are coded from the HCPCS Level II code set include medical supplies, durable medical equipment, pharmaceuticals administered by a health care professional, and transportation services. This chapter will review what you should know when coding these.

CODING MEDICAL SUPPLIES

In almost every health care encounter, materials and supplies are used. The paper used to cover the examination table and the disposable cover on the electric thermometer are good examples. Such medical supplies are used by the health care facility itself. However, they are *not* the types of medical and surgical supplies to which the HCPCS Level II book refers.

The codes in the HCPCS Level II book are for reporting supplies given to a patient to **self-administer** health care at home.

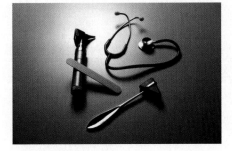

Self-administer

To give medication to oneself, such as a diabetic giving herself an insulin injection.

A Codes and B Codes

Let's begin by reviewing the subheadings throughout the A code and B code sections to get a good idea of which items are covered.

Miscellaneous Supplies A4206–A4290

The supplies used by a physician in the course of treatment (syringes, alcohol wipes, urine test strips, etc.) are included in the amount reimbursed for the provision of that treatment or service. The codes in miscellaneous supplies (HCPCS Level II) are to report, and be reimbursed for, supplies provided to patients for their own use at home. For example, if a diabetic patient requires a daily insulin shot at home, he would need to have syringes available.

EXAMPLE

A4207 Syringe with needle, sterile 2 cc, each

A4250 Urine test or reagent strips or tablets (100 tablets or strips)

Vascular Catheters A4300–A4306

In the subheading for vascular catheters, you will find codes to report the use of a disposable drug delivery system (DDS), as well as implantable access catheters. The codes are not for reporting the physician's work to implant the catheter, but for the facility to be reimbursed for the cost of the catheter itself.

EXAMPLE

A4300 Implantable access catheter, external access

A4306 Disposable drug delivery system, flow rate of 5 ml or less per hour

Incontinence Appliances and Care Supplies A4310–A4355

External Urinary Supplies A4356–A4359

The sections cover urinary supplies that a patient uses when they have been diagnosed with permanent, or chronic, **incontinence.**

Incontinence

The inability to control urination or fecal expulsion.

EXAMPLE

A4330 Perianal fecal collection pouch with adhesive, each

A4348 Male external catheter, with or without adhesive, disposable, each

Ostomy

Ostomy

An artificial opening made in the body surgically.

Ostomy Supplies A4361–A4434

Patients who have had surgery to create an **ostomy** need supplies every day to make their medical situation easier to deal with and to enable them to live their life more normally.

EXAMPLE

A4404 Ostomy ring, each

A4416 Ostomy pouch, closed, with barrier attached, with filter (one piece), each

Additional Miscellaneous Supplies A4450–A4608

Additional miscellaneous supplies represent a grouping of codes for other necessary items.

EXAMPLE

A4458 Enema bag with tubing, reusable

A4510 Surgical stocking full-length, each

YOU CODE IT! CASE STUDY

Carmella Sanfilippo, a 65-year-old female, was diagnosed with acute varicose veins in her legs. Dr. Bennett gave her a prescription for a pair of thigh-length surgical stockings. She received two pair from Thompson Health Care Supplies and Service.

You Code It!

Go through the steps of coding, and determine the codes that should be reported for this encounter between Dr. Bennett and Carmella Sanfilippo.

Step 1: Read the case completely.

Step 2: Abstract the notes: Which key words can you identify relating to the procedures performed?

_____

Step 3: Query the provider, if necessary.

Step 4: Diagnosis: Acute varicose veins.

Step 5: Code the for the provision of the stockings.

_____

Step 6: Link the procedure codes to at least one diagnosis code.

Step 7: Back code to double-check your choices.

Answer

Did you find the correct code to be:

A4495x4 Surgical stocking thigh length, each; four stockings

Good job!

Supplies for Oxygen and Related Respiratory Equipment A4611–A4629

Supplies for Other Durable Medical Equipment A4630–A4640

Here, and in other portions of this section, you will find the ancillary supplies and items used in conjunction with durable medical equipment, such as a **cannula** or a cleaning brush.

EXAMPLE

A4615 Cannula, nasal

A4626 Tracheostomy cleaning brush, each

A4637 Replacement, tip, cane, crutch, walker, each

Cannula

A tube that is inserted into the body to either deliver or extract fluid, such as a nasogastric tube.

YOU CODE IT! CASE STUDY

Benjamin Stiles, a 77-year-old male, diagnosed with acute emphysema, used a ventilator, purchased by him last year. Walter Synder, from Miller Medical Supplies, brought a new, heavy-duty replacement battery for the ventilator and installed it.

You Code It!

Go through the steps of coding, and determine the codes that should be reported for this encounter between Walter Synder and Benjamin Stiles.

Step 1: Read the case completely.

Step 2: Abstract the notes: Which key words can you identify relating to the procedures performed?

_____

Step 3: Query the provider, if necessary.

Step 4: Diagnosis: Acute emphysema.

Step 5: Code the replacement battery.

_____

Step 6: Link the procedure codes to at least one diagnosis code.

Step 7: Back code to double-check your choices.

Answer

Did you find the correct code to be:

A4611   Battery, heavy duty; replacement for patient-owned ventilator

Excellent!

Supplies for Radiologic Procedures A4641–A4932

Similar to other cases in this book, the codes for radiologic procedure supplies represent the ancillary items needed during and/or after some procedures—not the actual procedure itself.

EXAMPLE

A4644 Supply of low osmolar contrast material (100–199 mgs of iodine)

A4770 Blood collection tube, vacuum, for dialysis, per 50

A4931 Oral thermometer, reusable, any type, each

Additional Ostomy Supplies A5051–A5093

Additional Incontinence Appliances/Supplies A5102–A5114

Supplies for Either Incontinence or Ostomy Appliances A5119–A5200

These are additional codes for items needed by patients with medical situations.

EXAMPLE

A5055 Stoma cap

A5112 Urinary leg bag; latex

A5119 Skin barrier, wipes or swabs, per box 50

Diabetic Shoes, Fitting, and Modifications A5500–A5511

One thing you are certain to notice is that every one of the codes under this subheading begins with the same three words, "for diabetics only." Another detail you should notice is that each code specifies coverage of only one shoe. Therefore, if the patient gets a pair of shoes, you must report the appropriate code twice.

EXAMPLE

A5508 For diabetics only, deluxe feature of off-the-shelf depth-inlay shoe or custom-molded shoe, per shoe

Part 2   HCPCS Level II

Jerry Gaynor, a 71-year-old male, has diabetes mellitus with peripheral neuropathy with evidence of callus formation, particularly on his left foot. He came today so Marilyn Requin could do a fitting for a pair of custom-molded shoes.

You Code It!

Go through the steps of coding, and determine the codes that should be reported for this encounter between Jerry Gaynor and Marilyn Requin.

Step 1: Read the case completely.

Step 2: Abstract the notes: Which key words can you identify relating to the procedures performed?

_____

Step 3: Query the provider, if necessary.

Step 4: Diagnosis: Diabetic, peripheral neuropathy.

Step 5: Code for the shoes.

_____

Step 6: Link the procedure codes to at least one diagnosis code.

Step 7: Back code to double-check your choices.

Answer

Did you find the correct code to be:

A5501x2 For diabetics only, fitting (including follow-up) custom preparation and supply of shoe molded from cast(s) of patient's foot (custom-molded shoe), per shoe; two shoes

Great!

Dressings A6000–A7527

Wound care requires a lot of supplies, such as bandages that need to be changed frequently to ensure a clean and sterile environment for healing. Different wounds involve different dressings.

EXAMPLE

A6154 Wound pouch, each

A6215 Foam dressing, wound filer, per gram

A6410 Eye pad, sterile, each

Beverly Schuck, a 19-year-old female, was riding with her boyfriend on his motorcycle and burned her right calf on the tailpipe. Her friend told

her to put butter on the burn, and Beverly's calf became badly infected. After debriding the wound, Dr. Errol applied an alginate dressing 15 sq in., because it was oozing fluid. Dr. Errol provided Beverly with one additional dressing so she could change the wound cover in one week.

You Code It!

Go through the steps of coding, and determine the codes that should be reported for this encounter between Dr. Errol and Beverly Schuck.

Step 1: Read the case completely.

Step 2: Abstract the notes: Which key words can you identify relating to the procedures performed?

_____

Step 3: Query the provider, if necessary.

Step 4: Diagnosis: Infected burn, lower leg, right.

Step 5: Code for the alginate dressing.

_____

Step 6: Link the procedure codes to at least one diagnosis code.

Step 7: Back code to double-check your choices.

Answer

Did you find the correct code to be:

A6196 Alginate or other fiber gelling dressing, wound cover, pad size 16 sq in. or less, each dressing

You got it!

Administrative, Miscellaneous, and Investigational A9000–A9999

Administrative, miscellaneous, and investigational provide a catchall for items such as nonprescription medications, exercise equipment, and other supplies that may be provided for home care.

EXAMPLE

A9280 Alert or alarm device, not otherwise classified

A9504 Supply of radiopharmaceutical diagnostic imaging agent, technetium Tc 99m apcitide

Enteral Formulae and Enteral Medical Supplies B4034–B4162

Parenteral Nutrition Solutions and Supplies B4164–B5200

Enteral and Parenteral Pumps B9000–B9999

These codes report the supply of items related to providing nutrition to a patient by alternate means—other than by mouth and/or the digestive tract.

CODING TIP »»
....

Remember that even if a section in the HCPCS Level II book is named for a specific category of items, there may be codes elsewhere, such as S codes, that might be better and more appropriate. You should always consult the alphabetic index to ensure you are considering all code options.

LET'S CODE IT! SCENARIO

Jan Bagwell, a 71-year-old female, was diagnosed with a malignant neoplasm of the rectum. As a result, Dr. Garwood performed a colostomy on her last month. She is fitted with a drainable, rubber colostomy pouch with faceplate and drain along with a protective solid skin barrier, four by four.

Let's Code It!

The notes tell us that Dr. Garwood gave Jan a "drainable, rubber colostomy pouch with faceplate and drain," as well as a "protective solid skin barrier." Let's begin coding the pouch by going to the alphabetic index and looking up *pouch.* As you review the indented terms beneath, you notice immediately that there is no listing for *colostomy;* however, there are a few choice terms you can follow:

Pouch, drainable, A4388–A4389, A5061

Pouch, ostomy, A4375–A4378, A4387–A4391, A5051–A5054, A50061–A5063, A4416–A4420, A4423–A4434

Go to the alphanumeric listing, and read the complete description of each of the suggested codes. Did you find the one that matches the notes most accurately?

A4376 Ostomy pouch, drainable, with faceplate attached, rubber, each

Next, you want to code the skin barrier. Let's go back to the alphabetic index and look under *skin.* You find the suggested codes:

Skin, barrier, Ostomy, A4362, A4369, A4385

Check the complete code descriptions in the alphanumeric listing. While there is great similarity between A4362 and A4385, you notice that our physician's notes say nothing about it being an extended wear barrier. Therefore, A4362 is most accurate. Your claim form for the supplies Dr. Garwood provided to Jan shows:

A4376 Ostomy pouch, drainable, with faceplate attached, rubber, each

A4362 Skin barrier, solid, four by four or equivalent; each

Excellent! This matches perfectly.

CODING DURABLE MEDICAL EQUIPMENT

Science and technology have provided our society with great innovations that make life easier and more functional. Canes, walkers, and

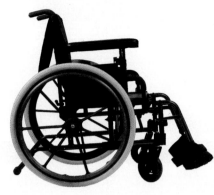

wheelchairs, among other items, help individuals move from one place to another without further assistance. Portable oxygen, humidifiers, vaporizers, and other equipment assist breathing, and pacemakers and electrical nerve stimulators help keep a heart beating. Some items are so commonplace we take them for granted, yet only 10 years ago, patients would be forced to stay home all day every day. Other products, such as wheelchairs, have evolved into more convenient and accommodating pieces of equipment.

Each item and every accessory cost money to build. Therefore, the health care facility or company should be reimbursed for giving, renting or leasing, or selling equipment. HCPCS Level II codes for durable medical equipment are used in the reimbursement process.

Durable Medical Equipment

Durable medical equipment (DME) includes such items as canes, wheelchairs, and ventilators. However, to be accurate, Medicare has four qualifiers to determine whether an item can be classified as DME. These qualifiers are:

1. The item can withstand repeated use.
2. The item is primarily used for medical purposes.
3. The item is used in the patient's home (rather than only in a health care facility).
4. The item would not be used if the individual were not ill or injured.

DMEPOS

Durable Medical Equipment, Prosthetic, and Orthotic Supplies.

Most often, **DMEPOS** dealers supply DME to the patient. Such companies submit their claims not to Medicare or the state's Medicare fiscal intermediary (FI) but to their assigned durable medical equipment regional carrier (DMERC), which is contracted by Centers for Medicare and Medicaid Services (CMS), formerly HCFA.

HCPCS E Code Subheadings

The DME section, codes E0100- E9999, is divided into subheadings. It is not the only section in the HCPCS Level II book having codes related to DME services and supplies; however, it is the section dedicated to them. Take a minute to look through its subheadings, and you should gain a clearer understanding of the items and services included here.

- Canes
- Crutches
- Walkers
- Attachments (i.e., accessories for walkers)
- Commodes (i.e., portable toilets)
- Decubitus Care Equipment (i.e., care for **decubitus ulcers** and related issues)
- Heat/Cold Application
- Bath and Toilet Aids
- Hospital Beds and Accessories

Decubitus ulcer

Bedsore, or wound created by lying in the same position, on the same irritant without relief.

- Oxygen and Related Respiratory Equipment
- Intermittent Positive-Pressure Breathing (IPPB) Machines
- Humidifiers/Compressors/Nebulizers for use with Oxygen IPPB Equipment
- Suction Pump/Room Vaporizers
- Monitoring Equipment (i.e., home blood glucose monitor)
- Pacemaker Monitor
- Patient Lifts (i.e., to lift a patient out of, or into, a bed, a bathtub, or other circumstance)
- Pneumatic Compressor and Appliances
- Safety Equipment
- Restraints
- **Transcutaneous** and/or Neuromuscular **Electrical Nerve Stimulators—TENS**
- Infusion Supplies
- Traction–All Types
- Traction–Cervical
- Traction–Overdoor
- Traction–Extremity
- Traction–Pelvic
- Trapeze Equipment, Fracture Frame, and Other Orthopedic Devices
- Rollabout Chair
- Wheelchairs–Fully reclining
- Wheelchair–Semireclining
- Wheelchair–Standard
- Wheelchair–Amputee
- Wheelchair–Power
- Wheelchair–Special Size
- Wheelchair–Lightweight
- Wheelchair–Heavy-duty
- Whirlpool–Equipment
- Repairs and Replacement Supplies
- Additional Oxygen Related Equipment
- Artificial Kidney Machines and Accessories
- Jaw Motion Rehabilitation System and Accessories
- Other Orthopedic Devices

Transcutaneous electrical nerve stimulators (TENS)

The use of electricity to agitate the skin to relieve pain

LET'S CODE IT! SCENARIO

Isadore McPherson, an 82-year-old male, had a stroke, and is coming to live with Grace, his granddaughter. In order to properly accommodate his needs, Chuck Michaels, a representative of Peterson's Medical Equipment, has come to Grace's home to deliver and set up a hospital bed. The bed has a variable height function to make caring for Isadore easier, and it has detachable side rails. The mattress is a firm one and is supplied with the bed.

Let's Code It!

You are the coding specialist working for Peterson's Medical Equipment and must send a claim to Medicare for the bed. The bed is described as a *hospital bed, variable height,* with detachable *side rails,* and a *mattress.* Let's go to the alphabetic index in the HCPCS Level II book.

Find the term *bed,* and you see *hospital* indented below. Beneath this, indented, are more descriptors, such as full electric, manual, or safety enclosure frame. We do not have any of those terms in our notes, so let's go to the suggested codes shown next to Bed, hospital, E0250–E0270.

E0250   Hospital bed, fixed height, with any type side rails, with mattress

E0251   Hospital bed, fixed height, with any type side rails, without mattress

Neither code is accurate because they describe beds with a *fixed* height, not *variable* height, as our notes describe. Let's keep reading.

E0255   Hospital bed, variable height, hi-lo, with any type side rails, with mattress

The code description matches our notes. Great job!

LET'S CODE IT! SCENARIO

Dean Bernard, a 12-year-old male, was born with spina bifida. His power wheelchair's motor has malfunctioned, and Wayne Dolan, a repair technician for Haverty's Medical Supplies and Repairs, has come to Dean's house to install a replacement motor.

Let's Code It!

You are the coding specialist working for Haverty's Medical Supplies and Repairs, and must send a claim to Dean's insurance carrier for the *replacement motor* for the *power wheelchair.* You have checked, and know that the third-party payer accepts HCPCS Level II codes.

Let's go to the alphabetic listing and find *wheelchair.* As you go down the list indented beneath the key term, you find *power.* Keep reading, and indented below *power,* you see *motor.* Hmm. This looks perfect. Let's check out Wheelchair, power, motor, E2368.

E2368   Power wheelchair component, motor, replacement only

Cool. It couldn't be a better description if you had written it yourself!

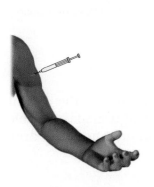
Intramuscular

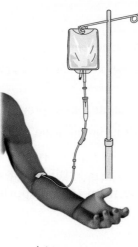
Intravenous

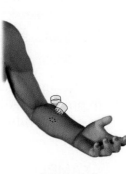
Intradermal

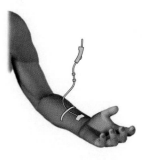
Intra-arterial

CODING PHARMACEUTICAL SERVICES

In Chap. 11, "Medicine Coding," you learned about coding for the administration of pharmaceuticals (drugs). Those codes are used for reporting the services—the labor—of the health care professional who gives the patient the drug. You may remember that the different methods of administering drugs include:

IA	Intra-arterial administration
IV	Intravenous administration (e.g., gravity infusion, injections, and timed pushes)
IM	Intramuscular administration
IT	Intrathecal
SC	Subcutaneous administration
INH	Inhaled solutions
VAR	Various routes for drugs that are commonly administered into joints, cavities, tissues, or topical applications, as well as other parenteral administrations
ORAL	Administered orally
OTH	Other routes of administration, such as suppositories or catheter injections

EXAMPLE

From the CPT book:

90782 Therapeutic, prophylactic or diagnostic injection (specify material injected); subcutaneous or intramuscular

90783   intra-arterial

90784   intravenous

The codes in HCPCS Level II enable you to report, and gain reimbursement for, the actual drug or medication, as well as the syringe or IV bag used. The codes cover the pharmaceutical materials only—*not* the administration of the drug.

J0760   Injection, colchicine, per 1 mg

J7613   Albuterol, inhalation solution, administered through DME, unit dose, 1 mg

S0012   Butorphanol tartrate, nasal spray, 25 mg

S5001   Prescription drug, brand name

In some cases, you may find DME has been supplied to the patient to provide medication, or drugs. When the equipment is made available to an individual, it may need to be reported separately from the drug itself.

S5560   Insulin delivery device, reusable pen; 1.5 ml size

J1817   Insulin for administration through DME (i.e., insulin pump) per 50 units

Note that S5560 only covers the DME, whereas J1817 only covers the medication.

Generic Names and Brand Names

As you look through the HCPCS Level II book, you will notice that the drugs are listed by their chemical, or generic, name. When the notes describe a medication or a drug by its brand name, or trade name, you may have to look for the drug in one of the following resources:

1. *Alphabetic index of the HCPCS Level II book.* Some—but not all—drugs are shown in the alphabetic index by both the generic name and a brand, or trade, name.

2. *Appendix 1, Table of Drugs, of the HCPCS Level II book.*

3. *Physicians' Desk Reference (PDR).*

The PDR has the correct generic name for any drug, along with other important data, such as indications (when the patient should be given this drug), contraindications (when a patient should *not* be given this drug), and possible side effects. Once you have the generic name for the drug supplied to the patient, you will be able to look it up in the HCPCS Level II book.

Proventil (brand name) is listed in the table of drugs but not in the alphabetic index.

Albuterol (generic name) is listed in both the alphabetic index and the table of drugs.

Appendix 1—Table of Drugs

In addition to the regular alphabetic index, you also have the table of drugs, located in Appendix 1 in the back of the book. The table lists many drugs, by their generic and/or brand names, alphabetically.

CODING TIP »»

The table of drugs is no different from the primary alphabetic index. You should never code from the table. Always confirm the code by its complete description in the alphanumeric listing.

Drug Name	Unit	Route	Code
Aldomet	250 mg	IV	J0210
Cipro	200 mg	IV	J0744

In the first column of the table, the name of the drug is listed in alphabetical order, from A to Z.

The second column identifies the most often used unit of measurement or dose for that particular drug.

The third column indicates the method of administration (the route), such as intravenous or inhalation.

The last column has the suggested code. You should still double-check the code's complete description in the alphanumeric listings contained in the body of the book.

You might find the table easier to use than the alphabetic index. Choose whichever helps you find the best, most appropriate code for the actual services delivered.

LET'S CODE IT! SCENARIO

Russell Bromwell, a 23-year-old male, was brought to the emergency department with severe abdominal cramps, vomiting, and nausea. Test results and examination led Dr. Camponetta to the diagnosis of an intra-abdominal infection caused by exposure to Escherichia coli. He prescribed ampicillin sodium and sulbactam sodium IV injection 1.5 g q6h. Code for the first 12 hours.

Let's Code It!

Dr. Camponetta prescribed *ampicillin sodium and sulbactam sodium,* to be *injected* intravenously (IV). Let's go the HCPCS Level II book's alphabetic index and look up the name of the drug: ampicillin sodium. You will see

Ampicillin sodium, J0290

    sodium/sulbactam sodium, J0295

It appears that you may only need one code for both drugs. Let's go to the alphanumeric listing to check the complete description for J0295.

J0295   Injection, ampicillin sodium/sulbactam sodium, per 1.5 g

That matches Dr. Camponetta's orders (and the nurses' notes indicate that Russell actually did receive the medication). Next, we must look at the quantity, or measurement, included in the code description and compare it to the dosage that Russell received. Russell was given a dosage of *1.5 grams* (g) and that matches the code description. Excellent! However, the case gives you the instruction to code for the first 12 hours of Russell's treatment. He was given the medication *every 6 hours* (q6h). Therefore, your claim form for Russell's first 12 hours of pharmaceutical, therapeutic treatment will show J0295×2. Great job!

Notations

In notations below many of the code descriptions, you will see the mention of an additional name, usually the brand name, which is also represented by that code.

The notations will help you confirm that a code for a generic drug is the correct code for a brand name drug shown on the patient's chart.

Quantity Specifications

Many codes also include the measurement of a typical dose in the code's description.

You may recognize the check mark in the box symbol ☑ next to almost every code in this section. You learned in Chap. 13 that the symbol means the code description includes a quantity or amount. In our example, the amount is 2 g (two grams). Therefore, if the procedure notes state that 4 grams of cyclophosphamide was given to the patient, the correct way to report this would be written J9092, J9092 (or J9092×2).

Measurement Equivalents

As you can see, many code descriptors for medications and pharmaceuticals include dosage measurements. Of course, if the notes you are coding from are written in a different type of measurement, you have to do the math. To make it easier, Table 14-1 has conversion rates.

J Codes

The J codes (J0000–J9999) in the HCPCS Level II book are used for reporting drugs administered by a health care professional and *cannot,* under usual circumstances, be self-administered.

Part 2 HCPCS Level II

Table 14-1 Conversions and Equivalents	
Measure	**Equivalent**
1 L (liter)	1,000 mL (milliliter)
1 L	1,000 cc (cubic centimeter)
1 mL (milliliter)	1 cc
1 oz (fluid ounce)	8 dr (fluid drams)
1 oz	30 cc
1 g (gram)	1,000 mg
1 g	15 gr (grain)
1 mg (milligram)	1,000 mcg (microgram)
1 kg (kilogram)	1,000 g
1 kg	2.2 lb (pounds)
1 in. (inch)	2.54 cm (centimeters)
1 T (tablespoon)	3 teaspoons

CODING AMBULANCE AND OTHER TRANSPORTATION SERVICES

If a severely ill or injured individual must be moved, whether from home or an accident scene to a health care facility or from one health care facility to another, transportation arrangements are made. The patient may need to be lying down or receiving continuous intravenous. The health care professional may have to monitor the patient's vital signs and other issues constantly. The room for additional personnel, the ability to keep special equipment secure and functional, and the configuration of the seating so everyone involved can be kept safe during the ride are all concerns that demand more than your average vehicle.

HCPCS Level II codes A0000–A0999 report the following transportation services:

- Ground ambulances
- Air ambulances (often a helicopter but not exclusively)
- Nonemergency transportation, such as a special van, a taxi cab, a car, or even a bus
- Additional or secondary related costs and fees

Coding Components

The codes in the transportation section are determined by several components.

1. What type of vehicle was used to transport the patient?
   a. Ground (ambulance, taxi, bus, minibus, van, etc.)
   b. Air–fixed wing (such as an airplane)
   c. Air–rotary wing (such as a helicopter)

«« CODING TIP

In order for transportation charges to be reimbursable from the third-party payer, the claim form must include diagnosis code(s) to identify the medical necessity of the special equipment.

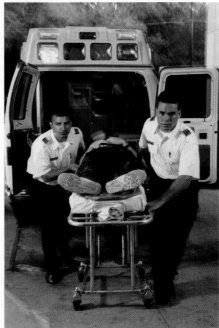

Advanced life support (ALS)

Life-sustaining, emergency care is provided, such as airway management, defibrillation, and/ or the administration of drugs.

Basic life support (BLS)

The provision of emergency CPR, stabilization of the patient, first aid, control of bleeding, and/or the treatment of shock.

Specialty care transport (SCT)

Continuous care provided by one or more health professionals in an appropriate specialty area, such as respiratory care, cardiovascular care, or a paramedic with additional training.

2. What type of services did the patient need?
    a. Emergency
    b. Nonemergency
    c. **Advanced life support (ALS)**
    d. **Basic life support (BLS)**
    e. **Specialty care transport (SCT)**
3. Did the ambulance have to wait? (See Table 14-2 on page 357, "Waiting Times.")
4. How many miles did the ambulance have to travel from origin to destination?
5. Were extra personnel required?

Answering the above questions will direct you to the best, most appropriate code or codes needed to properly report transportation services for a patient.

EXAMPLE

Hilda Camacho, an 87-year-old female, was taken by ambulance to the emergency room at Barton Hospital after experiencing a seizure and falling into a coma. The EMTs provided advanced life support (ALS) services during the transport. Use code A0427 to report these services.

LET'S CODE IT! SCENARIO

Abby Lennox, an EMT, was called in as an extra ambulance attendant for the ALS ground transportation of Ruby Premin, a 15-year-old autistic female.

Let's Code It!

Abby was called in as an *extra ambulance attendant.* When you look in the alphabetic index of the HCPCS book, you notice that this does not match any of the listings under *Ambulance* or *Attendant.* So let's turn to the range shown next to the term *Ambulance* in the index, A0021–A0999.

Although reading down the listing will take time, sometimes it is the best way to find the code you need. Fortunately, you won't have to read too far to reach:

A0424 Extra ambulance attendant, ground (ALS or BLS) or air (fixed or rotary winged); (requires medical review)

Transportation Codes in Other Sections

A few transportation codes in the HCPCS Level II book are in sections other than the A codes. This, of course, is an excellent example of why you should use the alphabetic index to find the best code in the alphanumeric listing—because there may be a better, more appropriate code in a section you might not otherwise examine. In all cases of temporary codes, you must confirm the acceptance of the temporary code by the third-party payer to whom you are billing.

The S series (S0000–S9999) are temporary codes and not accepted by Medicare, according to the HCPCS Level II book. Medicaid programs and some private insurers, such as Blue Cross and Blue Shield Association, do accept S codes. You must check with the organization or association in your state to confirm the acceptance of S codes. The S codes that relate to transportation are:

S0215 Non-emergency transportation; mileage, per mile

S9992 Transportation costs to and from trial location and local transportation costs (e.g., fares for taxicab or bus) for clinical trial participant and one caregiver/companion

The T codes (T1000–T9999) are used by Medicaid state agencies to report services, procedures, and other items for which there are no permanent national codes. You must communicate with the third-party payer to whom you are sending the claim to ensure that it accepts T codes. Transportation services that may be reported using T codes are:

T2001 Non-emergency transportation; patient attendant/escort

T2002 Non-emergency transportation; per diem

T2003 Non-emergency transportation; encounter/trip

T2004 Non-emergency transport; commercial carrier, multi-pass

T2005 Non-emergency transportation; stretcher van

T2007 Transportation waiting time, air ambulance and non-emergency vehicle, one-half (1/2) hour increments

T2049 Non-emergency transportation; stretcher van, mileage; per mile

EXAMPLE

Chad Nevins, a 91-year-old male, was being transferred to a nursing home closer to his daughter's home. Due to his health problems, he had to be transported on a stretcher. Code T2005 accurately reports that service.

LET'S CODE IT! SCENARIO

Ronald Stockman, an 81-year-old male, had a stroke three weeks ago. He has now recovered sufficiently to be discharged from the hospital. However, he is not completely well. Ronald is being transferred to a short-term rehabilitation facility to help him regain use of his legs and right arm. Terrell Peterson, from Link-Up Ambulance Services, drove the wheelchair van to take Ronald from Barton Hospital to Sunstate Nursing and Rehabilitation Center, a 12-mile ride.

CPT © 2007 American Medical Association. All Rights Reserved.

Terrell, the driver, will submit the documentation to you. He noted that he drove a *wheelchair van* to transport Ronald from the hospital to the nursing facility. The notes also indicate that Ronald is being discharged from the hospital and there is no indication that this is an emergency. In addition, the wheelchair van does not contain emergency equipment, so we know that this is a *nonemergency* trip. Let's go to the alphabetic index and turn to *wheelchair.* Go down the list to the indented term Van, non-emergency . . . A0130, S0209. Turn to the alphanumeric listing to check out the complete description of the first code.

A0130   Non-emergency transportation: wheelchair van

This matches Terrell's documentation, doesn't it? Yes. In addition, it is the only code shown for that portion of the service. However, you might also look in the alphabetic listing under Transportation, non-emergency, A0080–A0210, Q3020, T2001–T2005, T2049. Once you review the complete descriptions of the suggested codes, you will see rather quickly that A0130 is the most specific and accurate.

Now, you must include a code for the mileage traveled by the van. Under *Wheelchair, van, non-emergency* you get the suggestion for code S0209, and while under *Transportation, non-emergency, mileage,* you see S0215. Let's examine both codes.

S0209   Wheelchair van, mileage, per mile

S0215   Non-emergency transportation; mileage, per mile

You also might notice:

A0380   BLS mileage (per mile)

A0390   ALS mileage (per mile)

A0425   Ground mileage, per statute mile

Five different codes appear applicable to report the mileage component of the service. Look at S0209 versus S0215 versus A0380, A0390, and A0425. You can see that the descriptions of A0380 and A0390 are not truthful at all in comparison to our notes, and would be considered upcoding! S0209 is more accurate and more specific in its description of the type of vehicle involved in the transportation. Therefore, as long as the insurance carrier accepts S codes, the claim form should show:

A0130 Non-emergency transportation: wheelchair van

S0209 Wheelchair van, mileage, per mile;

Number of miles: twelve

Great job!

CODING TIP »»»

When you send a claim to Medicare for transportation services, you will most probably use CMS form #1491. The origin of service modifier goes in Box 12, and the destination of service modifier goes in Box 13. Appendix A of this text has a copy of the form.

Ambulance Origin/Destination

When reporting transportation services to insurance carriers, you have to identify the *origin of service* and the *destination of service.*

The most common modifiers for the origin and the destination of service are one-letter codes that categorize locations. Box 14-1 has a list of the modifiers.

BOX 14-1 Transportation Location Modifiers

D   Diagnostic or therapeutic site other than "P" or "H"

E   Residential domiciliary custodial facility (i.e., nursing home, but *not* a skilled nursing facility)

G   Hospital-based dialysis facility (hospital or hospital-related)

H   Hospital

I   Site of transfer (e.g., airport or helicopter pad) between types of ambulance

J   Nonhospital-based dialysis facility

N   Skilled nursing facility (SNF)

P   Physician's office (e.g., HMO, nonhospital facility, clinic, etc.)

R   Residence

S   Scene of accident or acute event

X   Intermediate stop at physician's office en route to the hospital (e.g., HMO nonhospital facility, clinic, etc. *Note:* Modifier X may only be used to identify a destination.)

Transportation Waiting Time

The HCPCS Level II book has a table of waiting times in the A code section, so that you can easily report time lapsed.

Waiting time is measured in units of 30 minutes or less but is not reported until the transportation vehicle has been waiting for 31 minutes or more. Table 14-2 shows you the waiting time data. The number of units indicated in the table tells you how many times to report either of the following codes:

A0420 Ambulance waiting time (ALS or BLS), one-half (1/2) hour increments

T2007 Transportation waiting time, air ambulance and non-emergency vehicle, one-half (1/2) hour increments

Ambulance Billing Indicators

An *ambulance billing indicator* is a two-character alphanumeric modifier consisting of one number and one letter. The modifiers can be used to supply important information regarding the patient's condition, reason for the transport, and the level of services provided during the transportation. Box 14-2 has a list of billing indicators.

Table 14-2	Waiting Times
Units	**Time, in Hours**
1	1/2 to 1
2	1 to 1 1/2
3	1 1/2 to 2
4	2 to 2 1/2
5	2 1/2 to 3
6	3 to 3 1/2
7	3 1/2 to 4
8	4 to 4 1/2
9	4 1/2 to 5
10	5 to 5 1/2

YOU CODE IT! CASE STUDY

Vernon Salisbury, a 31-year-old male, drove his car into an electrical pole. After the ambulance arrived at the scene, the EMTs waited 75 minutes for the electric company to turn off the power. Then the EMTs got Vernon out of the car and into the ambulance, and they drove him to the hospital. Code the waiting time.

BOX 14-2 Ambulance Billing Indicators

1A	Bedridden	2B	Possible cerebral vascular accident (CVA)
2A	Accidental injury home/nursing home	3B	Black out passed out
3A	Accidental injury car	4B	Laceration of head
4A	Patient in shock	5B	Dead on arrival (DOA) at hospital
5A	Oxygen used and/or heart monitor used	6B	Died en route to hospital
6A	Transported by stretcher	7B	Unresponsive or coma
7A	Fracture to hip, leg, knee, and/or trunk (same day as ambulance trip)	8B	Quadriplegia
		9B	Stroke (same day ambulance service)
8A	Hospital lacks facility (patient admitted to second hospital)	1C	Paralysis
		2C	Mentally retarded
9A	Rectal bleeding		
1B	Myocardial infarction		

You Code It!

Go through the steps of coding, and determine the codes that should be reported for this ambulance's waiting time.

Step 1: Read the case completely.

Step 2: Abstract the notes: Which key words can you identify relating to the procedures performed?

_____

Step 3: Query the provider, if necessary.

Step 4: Diagnosis: MVA.

Step 5: Code the Waiting time:

_____

Step 6: Link the procedure codes to at least one diagnosis code.

Step 7: Back code to double-check your choices.

Answer

Did you find the correct code to be:

A0420x2 Ambulance waiting time (ALS or BLS), one-half (1/2) hour increments; one to one and one-half hour total

CHAPTER SUMMARY

Learning the techniques and guidelines for accurately reporting HCPCS Level II codes is mandatory for coders submitting claims for patients covered by Medicare, as well as many other third-party payers. In addition, understanding the complexities of Level II codes opens many opportunities for employment, from skilled nursing facilities to durable medical equipment suppliers.

1. An example of a medical supply reported by HCPCS Level II codes is

   a. Bandages for use in the office.

   b. Paper liner for examination tables.

   c. Paper for the office ECG machine.

   d. Vascular catheter.

2. Incontinence supplies, reported with HCPCS Level II codes, are used

   a. In the hospital.

   b. In the physician's office.

   c. By the patient for personal, at home use.

   d. None of the above.

3. DME stands for

   a. Durable medical equipment.

   b. Diagnostic medical equipment.

   c. Diagnostic medical evaluators.

   d. Durable modern escalators.

4. Medicare uses all except one of the following qualifiers to determine an item as DME.

   a. The item can withstand repeated use.

   b. The item is used in the patient's home.

   c. The item has been paid for by the patient.

   d. The item is primarily used for medical purposes.

5. An example of DME is a(n)

   a. Plaster cast.

   b. Ostomy pouch.

   c. Albuterol inhaler.

   d. Pacemaker monitor.

6. A method of administering drugs where the medication is inserted into the patient's muscle is abbreviated

   a. IA

   b. IV

   c. IM

   d. IT

7. HCPCS Level II codes identifies certain pharmaceuticals by brand name and/or generic name in

   a. The alphabetic index.

   b. Notations beneath code descriptions.

   c. Appendix 3.

   d. The table of drugs.

8. The J codes report drugs administered by

   a. The patient himself or herself.

   b. A family member.

   c. A health care professional.

   d. All of the above.

9. Coding transportation services includes specifics about all except

   a. The type of vehicle used.

   b. The type of insurance that covers the service.

   c. The type of service provided.

   d. Whether extra personnel were required.

10. The codes used for reporting transportation of a patient may only be used

    a. In cases of extreme emergency.

    b. When the patient is taken more than 10 miles.

    c. When the patient cannot afford a taxi.

    d. Whenever medically necessary.

Find the best, most appropriate code from the HCPCS Level II book.

1. Maria Feshan, a 43-year-old female, was diagnosed with diabetes and must test her blood sugar (glucose) regularly. Grunion Medical Supplies sent her a bottle of 50 blood glucose reagent strips for use with her home glucose monitor.

   _____

2. Craig Owens, a 9-year-old male, was diagnosed with acute asthma. Johannsen Health Care delivered 3000 ml of distilled water for use with his nebulizer.

   _____

3. Samantha Woods, a 5-year-old female, was diagnosed with an immature bladder. Until her bladder grows and becomes more functional, she is using a youth-sized incontinence brief. Her mother ordered two briefs.

   _____

4. Dean Mulvanney, a 50-year-old male, suffers from chronic renal failure, and Dr. Fahud has him on hemodialysis. Today, Dean receives new arterial blood tubing.

   _____

5. Ned Houston was born today with indications of spina bifida. Dr. Kensington, his pediatrician, wants to transfer him to Barton Medical Center because it has the only Level III neonatal unit in the area. The ambulance that transports Ned is equipped with a special isolette to keep Ned safe.

   _____

6. Gina Loffelin, a 77-year-old female, had a heart attack at home. During the ambulance ride to the hospital, Raul Fresca, the EMT, administered oxygen along with other advanced life support services.

   _____

7. Jared Morrison, an 81-year-old male, was discharged from the hospital with a stress fracture of his left hip. A stretcher van was provided to take him from the hospital to the Barton Rehabilitation Center across town.

   _____

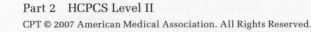

8. Paula Warren, a 23-year-old female, fell on the ski slopes. After her broken leg was stabilized by the ski patrol, she was airlifted by helicopter to the nearest hospital in Barton City.

_____

9. After a wonderful trip to South America and tours of the wilderness there, Gerard Stewart, a 41-year-old male, had signs of acute malaria. Dr. Sequoia gives him a 200 mg injection IM of chloroquine hydrochloride.

_____

10. Francine Cadwaller, a 47-year-old female, was in a great deal of pain and nothing seemed to help. Dr. Tershwell gave her an injection SC of 50 mg of codeine phosphate.

_____

11. Ryan Sparks, a 57-year-old male, was diagnosed with convulsive status epilepticus. Dr. Longwell orders Cerebyx; initial dose of 100 mg.

_____

12. Karyn Monmouth, an 83-year-old female, has been diagnosed with heparin-induced thrombocytopenia (HIT). Dr. Taman gave her a 25 mg injection of lepirudin.

_____

13. Roseanne Carter of Master's Medical brought a seat attachment for Joseph Starke's walker.

_____

14. Suzanne Headley's heel is irritated from the special brace ordered by her physician to assist the healing of her fractured ankle. She receives one heel protector from Jackson Medical Supplies.

_____

15. Larry Rodriquez has frequent bouts of respiratory distress, and his physician prescribed a portable negative pressure ventilator. Jason Braun delivered the equipment and taught Larry how to use it.

_____

YOU CODE IT! Simulation
Chapter 14. Coding Medical Supplies

On the following pages, you will see notes documenting services provided for patients of our textbook's health care facility, Cipher, Victors, & Associates. Carefully read through the notes, and find the best code or codes from the HCPCS Level II book for each of the cases.

CIPHER, VICTORS, & ASSOCIATES
A Complete Health Care Facility
234 MAIN STREET • ANYTOWN, FL 32711 • 407-555-1234

PATIENT: WEBBER, ROSE ANNE
ACCOUNT/EHR #:   WEBBRO001
Date: 10/21/08
Representative: Elizabeth Alexander

Attending Physician: James I. Cipher, MD

The Pt is a 27-year-old female who recently returned from working in Africa. She was diagnosed with variola, and has been on a gastric feeding tube to increase her fluids, electrolytes, and calories because the pharyngeal lesions make swallowing difficult.

    Nasogastric tubing without a stylet was supplied for this patient.

    DX: Variola

P: Service number given to caregiver

Elizabeth Alexander

EA/mg   D: 10/21/08 09:50:16   T: 10/22/08 12:55:01

Find the best, most appropriate HCPCS Level II code(s) for the tubing.

Part 2   HCPCS Level II

PATIENT: POWELL, FARRAH
ACCOUNT/EHR #:   POWEFA001
Date: 9/18/08
Representative Technician: LuAnn Hallmark

Attending Physician: James I. Cipher, MD

The Pt is a 69-year-old female diagnosed with adult kyphosis caused by poor posture. Dr. Cipher prescribed bed rest on a firm mattress with pelvic traction attached to the footboard.

At 5:00 p.m. on this date, I delivered a bed board and the traction frame to Ms. Powell's home. I placed the bed board underneath the existing mattress in order to create a firm surface upon which the patient could sleep. I then attached the traction frame to the footboard of the existing bed. I spent 45 minutes instructing the patient, her family, and caretaker on the proper use of the equipment, how to properly get into and out of the traction, and the expected sensations.

DX: Adult kyphosis

P: Follow-up in two weeks to see if patient has any questions or concerns.

_____

LuAnn Hallmark

LH/mg   D: 9/18/08 09:50:16   T: 9/20/08 12:55:01

Find the best, most appropriate code(s) for the DME delivered.

_____

_____

_____

CIPHER, VICTORS, & ASSOCIATES
A Complete Health Care Facility
234 MAIN STREET • ANYTOWN, FL 32711 • 407-555-1234

PATIENT: YAMIN, ANTON
MRN: YAMIAN001
Date: 12 November 2008

Attending Physician: Jacqueline Bennett, MD

Pt is a 61-year-old male with metastatic testicular tumors. He comes in today for the administration of cisplatin solution, IV, 20 mg. It is the first of five treatments he will receive this week.
   IV infusion given over 7 hours.
   Patient reports mild nausea. Refuses any pharmaceutical treatment for that side effect of this treatment.
   Patient discharged at 4:15 p.m.

Jacqueline Bennett, MD

JB//mg   D: 11/12/08 09:50:16   T: 11/15/08 12:55:01

Find the best, most appropriate code(s) for the pharmaceutical.

_____

_____

_____

CIPHER, VICTORS, & ASSOCIATES
A Complete Health Care Facility
234 MAIN STREET • ANYTOWN, FL 32711 • 407-555-1234

PATIENT: STRAUSS, EMILY
MRN: STRAEM001
Date: 4 October 2008

Attending Physician: Jacqueline Bennett, MD

Pt is a 21-year-old female in labor. Upon examination, her cervix is dilated and the presentation of the fetus has occurred. She is in the third stage of labor and her uterine contractions are not strong enough to complete delivery.

    10:12 a.m. IV is started with 1 mU/min of oxytocin.

    10:27 a.m. increase to 2 mU/min

    Contractions increase to proper level and delivery is completed at 10:59 a.m. Baby girl Strauss is handed over to the pediatrics team.

    Patient is taken to the recovery room in stable condition.

Jacqueline Bennett, MD

JB//mg   D: 10/04/08 09:50:16   T: 10/05/08 12:55:01

Find the best, most appropriate code(s) for the pharmaceutical.

_____

_____

_____

CIPHER, VICTORS, & ASSOCIATES
A Complete Health Care Facility
234 MAIN STREET • ANYTOWN, FL 32711 • 407-555-1234

PATIENT: DELGATO, DESIREE
ACCOUNT/EHR #:   DELGDE001
Date: 9/27/08

Attending Physician: James I. Cipher, MD
EMT/Attendant: Lance H. Reynoso, EMT

Pt is a 73-year-old female, who appears to have suffered a myocardial infarction in her nursing home's day room. Pt complained of numbness and tingling in the left arm and sharp pains in her chest. EKG shows abnormal activity. Pulse and respiration are abnormal.

    While preparing the patient for transport, she goes into arrest. Defibrillator restored heartbeat. Advance life support services were administered, and patient was transported immediately to Barton Hospital.

    Routine disposable supplies were used.

    Total Mileage: 4.5

___

Lance H. Reynoso, EMT

LHR/mg   D: 9/27/08 09:50:16   T: 9/27/08 12:55:01

Find the best, most appropriate transportation code(s).

___

___

___

HCPCS Level II Modifiers

Class A finding

Class B finding

Class C finding

Clinical Laboratory Improvement Amendment (CLIA)

Early and periodic screening, diagnostic, and treatment (EPSDT)

End-stage renal disease (ESRD)

Locum tenens physician

Liters per minute (LPM)

Parenteral enteral nutrition (PEN)

Urea reduction ratio (URR)

LEARNING OUTCOMES

- Apply the guidelines to correctly use HCPCS Level II modifiers.
- Determine when to appropriately use HCPCS Level II modifiers.
- Distinguish between the various functions of HCPCS Level II modifiers.
- Append multiple modifiers in the proper sequence.
- Utilize HCPCS Level II modifiers for statistical analysis of services.
- Differentiate between CPT modifiers and HCPCS modifiers.

EMPLOYMENT OPPORTUNITIES

Hospitals

Physicians' offices

Clinics

Ambulatory care centers

Assisted living facilities

Nursing homes

Skilled nursing facilities

Short-term facilities

Long-term care facilities

Pharmacies

Medical supply companies

Ambulance companies

Taxi companies

Public transportation services

Air ambulance services

Nonprofit organizations

Chapter 3 of this textbook introduced you to CPT modifiers. This chapter introduces you to HCPCS Level II modifiers. The modifiers can be used with both CPT (HCPCS Level I) codes and HCPCS Level II codes. However, you can only append them when submitting data to a third-party payer or organization that accepts Level II codes.

HCPCS Level II modifiers are two-character codes that are appended to the main code, as necessary, to provide additional information about a particular health care encounter. The modifiers have either two letters (alpha) or one letter and one number (alphanumeric). You will find the complete, and very long, list of the modifiers in Appendix 2 of the HCPCS Level II book.

EXAMPLE

Q3	Live kidney donor surgery and related services
ST	Related to trauma or injury

LEVEL II MODIFIER GUIDELINES

Just as with CPT modifiers, HCPCS modifiers are used to add detail or information to the description of the code. It is your responsibility to read the code's description carefully to make certain the information is not already there. As a coding specialist, you must determine whether or not a modifier is required.

EXAMPLE

96154 Health and behavior intervention, each 15 minutes, face-to-face; family (with the patient present)

When you carefully read this code's description, you can see that appending the modifier that follows would be duplicating information.

HR Family/couple with client present

In other cases, adding a modifier can provide important additional information to help care for the patient more effectively, now and in the future. Modifiers can be used to help avoid what might appear to the insurance carrier as a duplicate billing.

EXAMPLE

28008 Fasciotomy, foot and/or toe

Adding the following modifier would include very important information to the claim, especially if the patient had a preexisting condition involving a different toe.

T7 Right foot, third digit

YOU CODE IT! CASE STUDY

On January 5, a respiratory suction pump was provided to Annabelle Anderson who was diagnosed with Emphysema. On January 6, another suction pump was delivered to Annabelle. The first unit had to be replaced because of a defective piece.

CPT © 2007 American Medical Association. All Rights Reserved.

Go through the steps of coding, and determine the codes that should be reported for this service for Annabelle Anderson.

Step 1: Read the case completely.

Step 2: Abstract the notes: Which key words can you identify relating to the procedures performed?

_____

Step 3: Query the provider, if necessary.

Step 4: Diagnosis: Emphysema.

Step 5: Code the provision of the original pump and the replacement pump.

_____

Step 6: Link the procedure codes to at least one diagnosis code.

Step 7: Back code to double-check your choices.

Answer

Did you find the correct codes to be:

January 5: E0600 Respiratory suction pump, home model, portable or stationary, electric

January 6: E0600-RP Respiratory suction pump, home model, portable or stationary, electric; replacement and repair

Without the RP modifier to add the information that this code was to replace or repair the first pump, the insurance carrier would be certain to believe that the January 6 claim was a case of double billing.

When you need more than one modifier with a procedure or service code, you must place the modifiers in order of specificity, with the most important, most precise modifier closest to the main code.

YOU CODE IT! CASE STUDY

Dr. Curtis drained an abscess on Barry McClintock's left great toe and another on his second toe. Both were simple procedures.

You Code It!

Go through the steps of coding, and determine the codes that should be reported for this encounter between Dr. Curtis and Barry McClintock.

Step 1: Read the case completely.

Step 2: Abstract the notes: Which key words can you identify relating to the procedures performed?

_____

Step 3: Query the provider, if necessary.

Step 4: Diagnosis: Abscess, great toe; abscess, second toe.

Step 5: Code the procedure(s).

Step 6: Link the procedure codes to at least one diagnosis code.

Step 7: Back code to double-check your choices.

Answer

Did you find the correct code to be:

10060-TA Incision and drainage of abscess, simple or single; left foot, great toe

10060-T1-59 Incision and drainage of abscess, simple or single; left foot, second digit; separate procedure

Without the modifiers *TA* for left foot, great toe; *T1* for left foot, second digit; and *59* for distinct procedural service, the claim form could not clearly communicate that Dr. Curtis did work on two different toes.

THE MODIFIERS

The modifiers are listed in alphabetical order in Appendix 2. They are not grouped with regard to what each modifier represents anywhere in the HCPCS Level II book. In this chapter, we have reorganized and grouped the modifiers by content to help you better understand when to use each one.

Providers

The modifiers shown below specifically identify the qualifications of the health care professional who provided the service reported by the code to which this modifier is being attached.

You will note that some of the modifier descriptions also include a location as a part of its meaning.

EXAMPLE

| GF | Non-physician services in a critical access hospital |
| AQ | Physician providing a service in an unlisted health professional shortage area (HPSA) |

Other modifiers identify the special training that the provider may have.

EXAMPLE

| SD | Services provided by registered nurse with specialized, highly technical home infusion training |

AE   Registered dietician

AF   Specialty physician

AG   Primary physician

AH   Clinical psychologist

AK   Nonparticipating physician

AM   Physician, team member service

AR   Physician provider services in a physician scarcity area

AS   Physician assistant, nurse practitioner, or clinical nurse specialist services for assistant at surgery

GC   Service performed in part by a resident under the direction of a teaching physician

GE   Service performed by a resident without the presence of a teaching physician under the primary care exception

GF   Nonphysician services in a critical access hospital (e.g., nurse practitioner, certified registered nurse anesthetist, certified registered nurse, clinical nurse specialist, physician assistant)

GJ   "Opt out" physician or practitioner emergency or urgent service

GV   Attending physician not employed or paid under arrangement by the patient's hospice provider

HL   Intern

HM   Less than bachelor degree level

HN   Bachelors degree level

HO   Masters degree level

HP   Doctoral level

HT   Multidisciplinary team

Q4   Service for ordering/referring physician that qualifies as a service exemption

Q5   Service furnished by a substitute physician under a reciprocal billing arrangement

Q6   Service furnished by a **locum tenens physician**

SA   Nurse practitioner rendering service in collaboration with a physician

SB   Nurse midwife

SD   Services provided by registered nurse with specialized, highly technical home infusion training

SW   Services provided by a certified diabetic educator

TD   Registered nurse (RN)

TE   Licensed practical nurse (LPN) or LVN

Locum tenens physician

A physician that fills in, temporarily, for another physician.

Wound Care

Typically, a dressing change is required for a wound many times throughout the healing process. In addition, it is not unusual that a patient might have more than one wound that needs care at the same time. Therefore, to make the coding process easier and more efficient, one modifier can explain the extent of such care so that listing the same code multiple times is not necessary. The following list contains the modifiers for multiple wounds:

A1   Dressing for one wound

A2   Dressing for two wounds

A3   Dressing for three wounds

A4   Dressing for four wounds

A5   Dressing for five wounds

A6   Dressing for six wounds

A7   Dressing for seven wounds

A8   Dressing for eight wounds

A9   Dressing for nine or more wounds

LET'S CODE IT! SCENARIO

Victor Hirsch, a 29-year-old male, is a firefighter and sustained partial-thickness burns the entire length of his right arm when something exploded. He comes in to see Dr. Malvern to have the dressings changed on four wounds.

Let's Code It!

Victor came in to have his *dressings changed* on *four* burn wounds. First, we must find the CPT code for the procedure; second, we can address the modifier. Let's go to the alphabetic index and look up *dressings.* You find:

Dressings

Burns   16020–16030

Change

   Anesthesia   15852

You know that Dr. Malvern is changing Victor's dressings; however, there is nothing in the notes that states anesthesia was involved. In addition, Victor's wounds are burns, so let's turn to the numeric listing and carefully read the descriptions for the codes shown next to *burns.* Do you agree that the best code is:

16025 Dressings and/or debridement of partial-thickness burns, initial or subsequent; medium (e.g., whole face or whole extremity, or 5% to 10% total body surface area)

The notes indicate that Dr. Malvern changed the dressings for *four wounds.* So rather than just list this same code four times, we can use a modifier to communicate this fact: 16025-A4 tells the whole story clearly.

Good work!

Anesthesia Services

You should remember anesthesia modifiers from Chap. 3, "Introduction to Modifiers," and Chap. 6, "Anesthesia Coding," of this textbook. The following modifiers, used only with anesthesia codes, are actually HCPCS Level II modifiers:

«« CODING TIP

Chapter 6, "Anesthesia Coding," reviews the use of anesthesia modifiers thoroughly.

AA   Anesthesia services that are performed personally by anesthesiologist

AD   Medical supervision by a physician: more than four concurrent anesthesia procedures

G8   Monitored anesthesia care (MAC) for deep complex, complicated, or markedly invasive surgical procedure

G9   Monitored anesthesia care for patient who has history of severe cardiopulmonary condition

QK   Medical direction of two, three, or four concurrent anesthesia procedures involving qualified individuals

QS   Monitored anesthesia care (MAC) service

QX   CRNA (certified registered nurse anesthetist) service: with medical direction by a physician

QY   Medical direction of one certified registered nurse anesthetist (CRNA) by an anesthesiologist

QZ   CRNA service: without medical direction by a physician

Ophthalmology/Optometry

Sometimes, when ophthalmic or optometric services are provided, more detail is necessary to ensure proper reimbursement. Following are the HCPCS Level II modifiers used with these services:

AP   Determination of refractive state was not performed in the course of diagnostic ophthalmological examination

LS   FDA-monitored intraocular lens implant

PL   Progressive addition lenses

VP   Aphakic patient

ESRD/Dialysis

Dialysis, and other services for a patient with renal conditions, including those with **end-state renal disease (ESRD),** may involve extenuating circumstances requiring further explanation. The dialysis modifiers shown below provide that information.

End stage renal disease (ESRD)

Chronic, irreversible kidney disease requiring regular treatments.

CB   Service ordered by a renal dialysis facility (RDF) physician, as part of the beneficiary's benefit, is not part of the composite rate, and is separately reimbursable

CD   Automated Multi-Channel Chemistry (AMCC) test has been ordered by an ESRD facility or MCP physician that is part of the composite rate and is not separately billable

CE   AMCC test has been ordered by an ESRD facility or MCP physician that is a composite rate test but is beyond the normal

Urea reduction ratio (URR)

A formula to determine the effectiveness of hemodialysis treatment

frequency covered under the rate and is separately reimbursable based on medical necessity

CF   AMCC test has been ordered by an ESRD facility or MCP physician that is not part of the composite rate and is separately billable

EM   Emergency reserve supply (for ESRD benefit only)

G1   Most recent **URR** reading of less than 60

G2   Most recent URR reading of 60 to 64.9

G3   Most recent URR reading of 65 to 69.9

G4   Most recent URR reading of 70 to 74.9

G5   Most recent URR reading of 75 or greater

G6   ESRD patient for whom less than six dialysis sessions have been provided in a month

LET'S CODE IT! SCENARIO

Naomi Bridges, a 41-year-old female, was diagnosed with ESRD. Dr. Nashman prescribed her treatments to begin on May 29 at the Hammerlin Dialysis Center (HDC). Code for the services provided at HDC for the month of May.

Let's Code It!

As you remember from Chap. 11, *Medicine Coding*, ESRD services are billed on a monthly basis. However, Naomi only received three days of services during the month of May (May 29, May 30, and May 31) from Hammerlin Dialysis Center. In the alphabetic index, you find no listings for ESRD or end-stage renal disease. You need to turn to the following:

Dialysis

End-stage renal disease   90918–90925

After reading the complete code descriptions in the suggested range, you find the best procedure code to be:

90925 End-stage renal disease (ESRD) related services (less than full month), per day; for patients twenty years of age and over

This means you will have to list the code three times, because the code description says per day. The modifier that will complete this report is G6 because she has had fewer than six sessions in one month: 90925-G6; 90925-G6; 90925-G6 or 90925-G6 x3. Good job!

Pharmaceuticals

Pharmaceuticals, the industry term for drugs, are items that must be monitored very carefully: the purchase, the storage, and the dispensing. The modifiers shown below provide important information that must be tracked.

Modifier *RD* indicates that a particular pharmaceutical was given to the patient, but not administered. In other words, the provider may have given the patient the drugs in a bottle or other container, but did not inject or use any other means to deliver the drug into the patient's biological system.

Modifier *SV* might be used by a mail-order pharmaceutical service to show that the medications were delivered to the patient's house, but have nothing to do with how, when, or if the patient uses those drugs.

EXAMPLE

RD	Drug provided to beneficiary, but not administered incident to
SV	Pharmaceuticals delivered to patient's home but not utilized

Pharmaceutical Modifiers

JW   Drug amount discarded/not administered to any patient

KD   Drug or biological infused through DME

KO   Single drug unit dose formulation

KP   First drug of a multiple drug unit dose formulation

KQ   Second or subsequent drug of a multiple drug unit dose formulation

QE   Prescribed amount of oxygen is less than 1 **LPM**

QF   Prescribed amount of oxygen exceeds 4 LPM and portable oxygen is prescribed

QG   Prescribed amount of oxygen is greater than 4 LPM

QH   Oxygen conserving device is being used with an oxygen delivery system

RD   Drug provided to beneficiary, but not administered incident to

SL   State supplied vaccine

SV   Pharmaceuticals delivered to patient's home but not utilized

Liters per minute (LPM)

The measurement of how many liters of a drug or chemical is provided to the patient in 60 seconds.

Items/Services

The modifiers shown below cover a variety of circumstances relating to the provision of an item or a service.

AU   Item furnished in conjunction with a urological, ostomy, or tracheostomy supply

AV   Item furnished in conjunction with a prosthetic device, prosthetic or orthotic

AW   Item furnished in conjunction with a surgical dressing

AX   Item furnished in conjunction with dialysis services

BA   Item furnished in conjunction with **parenteral enteral nutrition (PEN)** services

BO   Orally administered nutrition, not by feeding tube

EY   No physician or other licensed health care provider order for this item or service

Parenteral enteral nutrition (PEN)

Nourishment delivered using a combination of means other than the gastrointestinal tract (e.g., IV) in addition to via the gastrointestinal tract.

GK Actual item/service ordered by physician, item associated with GA or GZ modifier

GL Medically unnecessary upgrade provided instead of standard item, no charge, no advance beneficiary notice (ABN)

GY Item or service statutorily excluded or does not meet the definition of any Medicare benefit

GZ Item or service expected to be denied as not reasonable and necessary

KS Glucose monitor supply for diabetic beneficiary not treated with insulin

KZ New coverage not implemented by managed care

QV Item or service provided as routine care in a Medicare qualifying clinical trial

QW **CLIA** waived test

SC Medically necessary service or supply

SF Second opinion ordered by a professional review organization (PRO)

SM Second surgical opinion

SN Third surgical opinion

SQ Item ordered by home health

Purchase/Rental Items

Often, when durable medical equipment (DME) is supplied, the patient has a choice to rent the equipment or purchase it outright. This will depend upon the patient's personal situation. Following is a list the modifiers relating to the services and provision of DME:

BP The beneficiary has been informed of the purchase and rental options and has elected to purchase the item

BR The beneficiary has been informed of the purchase and rental options and has elected to rent the item

BU The beneficiary has been informed of the purchase and rental options and after 30 days has not informed the supplier of his/her decision

KH DMEPOS item, initial claim, purchase or first month rental

KI DMEPOS item, second or third month rental

KJ DMEPOS item, parenteral enteral nutrition (PEN) pump or capped rental, months four to fifteen

KR Rental item, billing for partial month

LL Lease/rental (use when DME rental payments are to be applied against the purchase price)

MS Six-month maintenance and servicing fee for reasonable and necessary parts and labor not covered under any manufacturer or supplier warranty

NR New when rented (use when DME was new at the time of rental and then, purchased later)

RR Rental DME

Nickolas Sawyer, a 67-year-old male, fell and broke his hip last winter. Even though it healed, Nickolas experienced difficulty in walking long distances. Dr. Estevez prescribed a power wheelchair for him. Nickolas decided to purchase a lightweight, portable, motorized/power wheelchair from Wentworth Medical Supply Systems.

You Code It!

Go through the steps of coding, and determine the codes that should be reported for the supply of Nickolas Sawyer's new equipment.

Step 1: Read the case completely.

Step 2: Abstract the notes: Which key words can you identify relating to the procedures performed?

_____

Step 3: Query the provider, if necessary.

Step 4: Diagnosis: Osteoarthrosis, pelvic region and thigh.

Step 5: Code the provision of the wheelchair:

_____

Step 6: Link the procedure codes to at least one diagnosis code.

Step 7: Back code to double-check your choices.

Answer

Did you find the correct code to be:

K0012-KH Lightweight portable motorized/power wheelchair; DMEPOS item, initial claim, purchase or first month rental

Deceased Patient

Should a patient expire (i.e., die) while services are in the process of being rendered, certainly the situation changes and there must be some indication of the death. The following modifiers are used in such circumstances:

CA   Procedure payable only in the inpatient setting when performed emergently on an outpatient who expires prior to admission

QL   Patient pronounced dead after ambulance called

Claims and Documentation

The following modifiers directly provide additional information relating to the claims and documentation involved in certain health care encounters:

CC   Procedure code change (used to indicate that a procedure code previously submitted was changed either for an administrative reason or because an incorrect code was filed)

GA   Waiver of liability statement on file

GB   Claim being resubmitted for payment because it is no longer covered under a global payment

KB   Beneficiary requested upgrade for ABN, more than 4 modifiers identified on claim

KX   Specific required documentation on file

QP   Documentation is on file showing that the laboratory test(s) was ordered individually or ordered as a CPT-recognized panel other than automated profile codes 80002–80019, G0058, G0059, and G0060

Anatomical Sites

In Chap. 3, some of the HCPCS Level II modifiers were reviewed that identify a very specific anatomical site upon which a procedure was performed. The following list contains all these modifiers:

E1   Upper left, eyelid

E2   Lower left, eyelid

E3   Upper right, eyelid

E4   Lower right, eyelid

FA   Left hand, thumb

F1   Left hand, second digit

F2   Left hand, third digit

F3   Left hand, fourth digit

F4   Left hand, fifth digit

F5   Right hand, thumb

F6   Right hand, second digit

F7   Right hand, third digit

F8   Right hand, fourth digit

F9   Right hand, fifth digit

LC   Left circumflex coronary artery

LD   Left anterior descending coronary artery

LT   Left side (i.e., procedures performed on the left side of the body)

RC   Right coronary artery

RT   Right side (i.e., procedures performed on the right side of the body)

TA   Left foot, great toe

T1   Left foot, second digit

T2   Left foot, third digit

T3   Left foot, fourth digit

T4   Left foot, fifth digit

T5   Right foot, great toe

T6   Right foot, second digit

T7   Right foot, third digit

T8   Right foot, fourth digit

T9   Right foot, fifth digit

Gregory Kendall, a 51-year-old male, had a mass on his left upper eyelid. Dr. Denning performed a biopsy on the eyelid. The pathology report determined it was a benign neoplasm.

Let's Code It!

Go through the steps of coding, and determine the codes that should be reported for this encounter between Dr. Denning and Gregory Kendall.

Step 1: Read the case completely.

Step 2: Abstract the notes: Which key words can you identify relating to the procedures performed?

_____

Step 3: Query the provider, if necessary.

Step 4: Diagnosis: Neoplasm, benign, eyelid.

Step 5: Code the procedure(s).

_____

Step 6: Link the procedure codes to at least one diagnosis code.

Step 7: Back code to double-check your choices.

Answer

Did you find the correct code to be:

67810-E1 Biopsy of eyelid; upper left, eyelid

Family Services

Services provided under Medicaid's **early and periodic screening, diagnostic, and treatment (EPSDT)** program must be identified with the EP modifier. In addition, other family services may benefit from further explanation by the use of one of the modifiers found in the following list:

EP   Service provided as part of Medicaid early periodic screening diagnosis and treatment (EPSDT) program

FP   Service provided as part of family planning program

G7   Pregnancy resulted from rape or incest or pregnancy certified by physician as life threatening

TL   Early intervention/individualized family service plan (IFSP)

TM   Individualized education plan (IEP)

TR   School-based individualized education program (IEP) services provided outside the public school district responsible for the student

Early and periodic screening, diagnostic, and treatment (EPSDT)

Medicaid preventive health program for children under 21.

CPT © 2007 American Medical Association. All Rights Reserved.

Treatments/Screenings

The modifiers shown in the following list are directly related to the provision of mammography and infusion therapeutic services:

GG Performance and payment of a screening mammogram and diagnostic mammogram on the same patient, same day

GH Diagnostic mammogram converted from screening mammogram on same day

SH Second concurrently administered infusion therapy

SJ Third, or more, concurrently administered infusion therapy

Transportation

The following list has the modifiers that provide additional details with relation to transportation services provided to patients:

GM Multiple patients on one ambulance trip

LR Laboratory round trip

QM Ambulance service provided under arrangement by a provider of services

QN Ambulance service furnished directly by a provider of services

TK Extra patient or passenger, non-ambulance

TP Medical transport, unloaded vehicle

TQ Basic life support transport, by a volunteer ambulance provider

Funded Programs

When a service or treatment is provided under the terms or conditions of a formalized program or plan, the services must be identified so that statistical tracking can be accomplished accurately and that reimbursement is not received from two sources. The modifiers in the following list enable that tracking:

GN Services delivered under an outpatient speech language pathology plan of care

GO Services delivered under an outpatient occupational therapy plan of care

GP Services delivered under an outpatient physical therapy plan of care

H9 Court-ordered

HA Child/adolescent program

HB Adult program, nongeriatric

HC Adult program, geriatric

HD Pregnant/parenting women's program

HF Substance abuse program

HG Opioid addiction treatment program

Part 2   HCPCS Level II

HH	Integrated mental health/substance abuse program
HI	Integrated mental health and mental retardation/ developmental disabilities program
HJ	Employee assistance program
HK	Specialized mental health programs for high-risk populations
HU	Funded by child welfare agency
HV	Funded by state addictions agency
HW	Funded by state mental health agency
HX	Funded by county/local agency
HY	Funded by juvenile justice agency
HZ	Funded by criminal justice agency
SE	State and/or federally funded programs/services

Individual/Group

Most often, but not always, modifiers for individuals or groups are going to be used in conjunction with psychiatric and psychotherapeutic codes to clarify how many patients were involved in the session. The modifiers in the following list relate to the number, and sometimes the type, of patient(s) being helped at one time:

HQ	Group setting
HR	Family/couple with client present
HS	Family/couple without client present
TJ	Program group, child and/or adolescent
TT	Individualized service provided to more than one patient in same setting
UN	Two patients served
UP	Three patients served
UQ	Four patients served
UR	Five patients served
US	Six or more patients served

Prosthetics

When services are provided relating to the supply or adjustment of a prosthetic device, you might have to include additional information by using one of the following modifiers:

| K0 | Lower extremity prosthesis functional level 0—does not have the ability or potential to ambulate or transfer safely with or without assistance and prosthesis does not enhance their quality of life or mobility |
| K1 | Lower extremity prosthesis functional level 1—has the ability or potential to use a prosthesis for transfers or ambulation on level surfaces at fixed cadence. Typical of the limited and unlimited household ambulatory |

K2 Lower extremity prosthesis functional level 2—has the ability or potential for ambulation with the ability to traverse low-level environmental barriers such as curbs, stairs, or uneven surfaces. Typical of the limited community ambulator

K3 Lower extremity prosthesis functional level 3—has the ability or potential for ambulation with variable cadence. Typical of the community ambulatory who has the ability to transverse most environmental barriers and may have vocational, therapeutic, or exercise activity that demands prosthetic utilization beyond simple locomotion

K4 Lower extremity prosthesis functional level 4—has the ability or potential for prosthetic ambulation that exceeds the basic ambulation skills, exhibiting high impact, stress, or energy levels, typical of the prosthetic demands of the child, active adult, or athlete

KM Replacement of facial prosthesis including new impression/moulage

KN Replacement of facial prosthesis using previous master model

LET'S CODE IT! SCENARIO

Rafael Longbranch, a 23-year-old male, returned home after being in a rehabilitation center for three months. He had a BKA after he was hurt in a rescue mission after a major hurricane. Carol Ann Burkett fitted him for an initial, below knee PTB type socket prosthesis because he has the ability to walk and even maneuver with such low obstacles as sidewalk curbs and stairs.

Let's Code It!

Carol Ann Burkett ordered and supplied Rafael with an *initial, below knee PTB type socket prosthesis.* In the HCPCS Level II alphabetic index, you find:

Prosthesis

Fitting, L5400–L5460, L6380–L6388

The notes did say that Carol Ann fitted him, so this should provide a good lead. When you get to this section, beginning with L5400, you find a code whose description matches the notes very well:

L5500 Initial, below knee PTB type socket, non-alignable system, pylon, no cover, SACH foot, plaster socket, direct formed.

NOTE: SACH stands for solid ankle, cushioned heel.

You also have to support the service with a modifier to explain Rafael's abilities:

K2 Lower extremity prosthesis functional level 2—has the ability or potential for ambulation with the ability to traverse low-level environmental barriers such as curbs, stairs, or uneven surfaces. Typical of the limited community ambulator

Durable Medical Equipment

When the services relate to the provision or adjustments to a piece of durable medical equipment (DME), a modifier from the following list may be needed to clarify a certain condition or circumstance:

KA   Add on option/accessory for wheelchair

KC   Replacement of special power wheelchair interface

KF   Item designated by FDA as Class III device

NU   New equipment

QA   FDA investigational device exemption

RP   Replacement and repair of DME, orthotic, and/or prosthetic device

TW   Backup equipment

UE   Used durable medical equipment (DME)

Location

The modifiers shown below describe situations when you will need to clarify the location at which services were provided.

SG   Ambulatory surgical center (ASC) facility service

SU   Procedure performed in physician's office (i.e., to denote use of facility and equipment)

TN   Rural/outside providers' customary service area

Podiatric Care

There are times when particular services are recategorized, determined by certain signs and/or symptoms that the patient may be exhibiting. The following list identifies modifiers used to indicate some of these circumstances when a podiatrist provides treatment to a patient:

Q7   One **class A finding**

Q8   Two **class B findings**

Q9   One class B and two **class C findings**

Recording

The following modifiers indicate the use of recording equipment as a part of the service, treatment, or procedure provided to the patient:

QC   Single-channel monitoring

QD   Recording and storage in solid-state memory by a digital recorder

QT   Recording and storage on tape by an analog tape recorder

Other Services

The following modifiers do not seem to fit into any of the other categories we have established. Review all the modifiers in the list, and see if you can come up with examples of how and when they would be used.

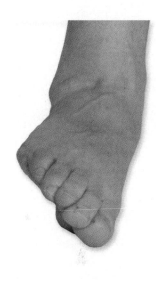

Class A finding

Nontraumatic amputation of a foot or an integral skeletal portion.

Class B finding

Absence of a posterior tibial pulse; absence or decrease of hair growth; thickening of the nail, discoloration of the skin, and/or thinning of the skin texture; and/or absence of a posterior pedal pulse.

Class C finding

Edema; burning sensation; temperature change (cold feet); abnormal spontaneous sensations in the feet; and/or limping.

AT   Acute treatment (to be used only with 98940, 98941, 98942)

EJ   Subsequent claims for a defined course of therapy

ET   Emergency services

GQ   Via asynchronous telecommunications system

GT   Via interactive audio and video telecommunication systems

GW   Service not related to the hospice patient's terminal condition

QJ   Services/items provided to a prisoner or patient in state or local custody, however, the state or local government, as applicable

Q2   HCFA/ORD demonstration project procedure/service

Q3   Live kidney donor surgery and related services

SK   Member of high-risk population (to be used only with immunization codes)

ST   Related to trauma or injury

SY   Persons who are in close contact with member of high-risk population [use with immunization codes only]

TC   Technical component

TG   Complex/high-tech level of care

TH   Obstetrical treatment/services, prenatal or postpartum

TS   Follow-up service

UF   Services provided in the morning

UG   Services provided in the afternoon

UH   Services provided in the evening

UJ   Services provided at night

UK   Services provided on behalf of the client to someone other than the client (collateral relationship)

Medicaid Services

Each state administers its own version of the federal Medicaid program and determines its own specific descriptions of the different levels of care. To maintain consistency, HCPCS Level II has the following modifiers that can be used nationwide—even though the description of each modifier will change, as defined by each state.

U1   Medicaid level of care 1, as defined by each state

U2   Medicaid level of care 2, as defined by each state

U3   Medicaid level of care 3, as defined by each state

U4   Medicaid level of care 4, as defined by each state

U5   Medicaid level of care 5, as defined by each state

U6   Medicaid level of care 6, as defined by each state

U7   Medicaid level of care 7, as defined by each state

U8   Medicaid level of care 8, as defined by each state

U9   Medicaid level of care 9, as defined by each state

UA   Medicaid level of care 10, as defined by each state

UB   Medicaid level of care 11, as defined by each state

UC   Medicaid level of care 12, as defined by each state

UD   Medicaid level of care 13, as defined by each state

Special Rates

The two modifiers shown below are used to indicate that a service or procedure was provided to a patient during an unusual time frame, that is, not during regular working hours.

TU   Special payment rate, overtime

TV   Special payment rates, holidays/weekends

LET'S CODE IT! SCENARIO

Betsy Conchran, a 43-year-old female, came into the hospital for a screening mammogram with computer-aided detection, due to a lump that Dr. Erlich found in her left breast during her annual checkup. Betsy has a prior history of breast cancer. Later that day, after the films were analyzed, Dr. Erlich made the decision to perform a simple, complete mastectomy. Betsy agreed, and she was immediately taken to the OR for the surgery.

Let's Code It!

Betsy came in for a *screening mammogram with computer-aided detection* on her *left breast*. Let's go to the alphabetic index of the CPT book, and find the best, most appropriate code or codes:

> 77057 Screening mammography, bilateral (two view film study of each breast)

> 77052 Computer-aided detection (computer algorithm analysis of digital image data for lesion detection) with further physician review for interpretation, with or without digitization of film radiographic images; screening mammography (List separately in addition to code for primary procedure.)

There are two points you must address with regard to the above codes. First, Betsy only had one breast examined, but code 77057 describes a bilateral exam. Therefore, you must use a modifier to identify what was actually done.

> 77057-52 Screening mammography, bilateral (two view film study of each breast), reduced services

The addition of modifier 52 explains that the services were only for one side (unilateral), not two sides (bilateral).

Second, once the results of the mammogram became the basis for a decision to have surgery, the screening mammogram became a diagnostic mammogram. Betsy's insurance carrier accepts HCPCS Level II codes and modifiers, so you must adapt the definition of the mammogram from screening to diagnostic by appending a modifier 77057-52-GH. The GH modifier means that a diagnostic mammogram was converted from a screening mammogram on the same day.

This is also why you use 77052 for the computer-aided detection.

Dr. Erlich then performed a "simple, complete mastectomy" on Betsy's *left breast.* The alphabetic index directs you to 19303. The numeric listing shows the complete description:

19303 Mastectomy, simple, complete

You know that Betsy's insurer accepts HCPCS Level II codes and modifiers, so you need to complete the description of the procedure Dr. Erlich performed.

19303-LT Mastectomy, simple, complete, left side

Great job!

CHAPTER SUMMARY

The general concept of using modifiers is the same for both HCPCS Level II and CPT modifiers, as you learned here and in Chap. 3 of this text. The two-character HCPCS Level II codes help identify specific situations or conditions that may be out of the ordinary and enable your facility to receive additional compensation. At the very least, you know that modifiers help offer additional information that may avoid a delay in payment from the insurance carrier or third-party payer.

1. HCPCS Level II modifiers can be appended to

   a. Level II codes only.

   b. CPT codes only.

   c. Category III codes only.

   d. (a) and (b).

2. HCPCS Level II modifiers can identify

   a. An anatomical part.

   b. A replacement part.

   c. A professional's qualifications.

   d. All of the above.

3. LPM stands for

   a. Local procedure modality.

   b. Liters per minute.

   c. Licensed practical medicine.

   d. Local patient median.

4. When both a CPT modifier and a HCPCS Level II modifier are needed, place them in the following order:

   a. CPT and then HCPCS Level II.

   b. HCPCS Level II and then CPT.

   c. They cannot be reported together.

   d. The most important modifier should be placed closest to the code.

5. An example of a DME is

   a. Aspirin.

   b. The administration of a vaccination.

   c. A wheelchair.

   d. Removal of a cyst.

6. CLIA stands for

   a. Clinical Laboratory Internal Assessment.

   b. Clinical Laboratory Improvement Amendment.

   c. Catastrophic Laboratory Inventory Allotment.

   d. Clinical Lateral Improvement Amendment.

7. Early and periodic screening, diagnostic, and treatment is a program of

   a. Medicare.

   b. Medicaid.

   c. Blue Cross Blue Shield.

   d. American Medical Association.

8. A prosthetic is

   a. A treatment plan.

   b. A type of diagnostic exam.

   c. An artificial body part.

   d. A specially trained health care professional.

9. A podiatric Class C finding includes all except

   a. Edema.

   b. Bleeding.

   c. Burning sensation.

   d. Temperature change.

10. Medicaid provides modifiers at _____ levels for use by each state.

   a. ten

   b. five

   c. thirteen

   d. twelve

YOU CODE IT! Practice
Chapter 15. HCPCS Level II Modifiers

Identify the HCPCS Level II modifier that would be used in each scenario.

1. Dr. Mathers performed a blepharotomy on Georgie Anne McAfee, draining the abscess on her upper left eyelid.

   _____

2. Wilma Certifano, a nurse midwife, helped Cloris Dana deliver her first baby, a girl.

   _____

3. Jasper Jons, a 71-year-old male diagnosed with terminal bone cancer, has been in the hospice facility for three weeks, and is showing signs of an ear infection. Dr. Lieber was called in to attend Jasper's ear problem.

   _____

4. Frank Ferguson, an EMT, answered a call, with his partner, to Barton Nursing Home. There was a small fire in the laundry room, and two patients were overcome by smoke enough to require hospitalization. Frank transported both patients at the same time in his ambulance and made one trip to the hospital.

   _____

5. Allen Ashcroft, a licensed psychotherapist, began the first of a series of court-ordered therapy sessions with Neil Scranton.

   _____

6. Dr. Horvath was called in to provide monitored anesthesia care for a procedure that will be performed on Sophia Applot. Sophia has a history of acute cardiopulmonary problems.

   _____

7. Juan Gonzalez, a registered nurse, works at the Barton Nursing Facility. He changed the dressing on three wounds that Miriam Warner had on her leg.

   _____

8. Elaine Everidge is the coding specialist for Barton Dialysis Center. She is preparing the claim for services provided to Grace Boxer, a patient with ESRD, who moved to the area just last week. Barton Dialysis provided four dialysis treatments for Grace during the month.

   _____

9. Linda Meyers, one of the coding specialists at Barton Hospital, discovered that a claim was submitted with an incorrect code. She has corrected the procedure code and is resubmitting the claim.

_____

10. Nadine Stuart works at Barton Medical Equipment Inc. She meets with Arthur Lynch who was recently prescribed an electric wheelchair by Dr. Bryan. Nadine explains the options of purchasing and renting the chair, and Arthur decides to purchase the wheelchair.

_____

11. Dr. Quimby excised a lesion from Gary McDonald's right thumb.

_____

12. Glenda Javlin gave Blanche Hansel, a 77-year-old female, a flu shot.

_____

13. Dr. Helen Messina saw Virginia Cromwell and provided service defined as level 3 by Medicaid in her state.

_____

14. Ashley Polk is a certified diabetic educator. She met with Amos Brahma to provide services.

_____

15. The PRO ordered Dr. Filippelli to provide a second opinion on the surgical options for Marcel Daquan.

_____

YOU CODE IT! Simulation
Chapter 15. HCPCS Level II Modifiers

On the following pages, you will see notes documenting encounters with patients at our textbook's health care facility, Cipher, Victors, & Associates. Carefully read through the notes and find the best code or codes from the CPT and/or HCPCS Level II books for each of the cases. Include all necessary modifiers.

Note: All insurance carriers and third-party payers for these patients accept HCPCS Level II codes and modifiers.

CIPHER, VICTORS, & ASSOCIATES
A Complete Health Care Facility
234 MAIN STREET • ANYTOWN, FL 32711 • 407-555-1234

PATIENT: LEE, CHARLENE
ACCOUNT/EHR #:   LEECHA001
Date: 11/23/08

Attending Physician: James I. Cipher, MD

S: New Pt is a 67-year-old female who works at a car dealership and spends a lot of time on her feet. She has been suffering from a cyst on the fourth toe of her left foot that is filled with fluid. She presents today to have the cyst drained.

O: Pt lies back on the examination table, and her left foot is elevated and draped in a sterile fashion. A topical antiseptic is applied, and I incised the cyst located below the fascia and drained it. The tendon sheath is not involved. The incision area is bandaged. The patient tolerated the procedure well.

A: Cyst of bursa

P: Follow-up in two weeks.

_____

James I. Cipher, MD

JIC/mg   D: 11/23/08 09:50:16   T: 11/25/08 12:55:01

Find the best, most appropriate code(s) and modifiers.

_____

_____

_____

CIPHER, VICTORS, & ASSOCIATES
A Complete Health Care Facility
234 MAIN STREET • ANYTOWN, FL 32711 • 407-555-1234

PATIENT: GENTRY, BRIAN
ACCOUNT/EHR #:   GENTBR001
Date: 11/10/08

Attending Physician: James I. Cipher, MD

S: Pt is a 36-year-old male who has not been seen in the office in just over a year. He recently began working for a landscaping company and presents today with a rash covering both hands and arms up to the elbow. Pt states that the rash itches and is uncomfortable. Scabs have formed over spots where he has scratched and bled. Patient has no history of allergies or other dermatological reactions. However, he also states that he has not previously worked with pesticides, particularly the new brand being used at his job.

O: HEENT is unremarkable with the exception of some redness in the back of the throat. Upper extremities show pustular eruptions anteriorly and posteriorly. Herve Sanchez, a nurse practitioner, in collaboration with me, gave the patient an injection subcutaneously of Benadryl, 40 mg.

A: Exanthem

P: 1. Rx Benadryl ointment prn
     2. Follow-up in two weeks.

_____

James I. Cipher, MD

JIC/mg   D: 11/10/08 09:50:16   T: 11/12/08 12:55:01

Find the best, most appropriate code(s) and modifiers.

_____

_____

_____

CIPHER, VICTORS, & ASSOCIATES
A Complete Health Care Facility
234 MAIN STREET • ANYTOWN, FL 32711 • 407-555-1234

PATIENT: BRINKLEY, ALISSA
ACCOUNT/EHR #:   BRINAL001
Date: 11/21/08

Attending Physician: Rodney Southern, MD
Referring Physician: Valerie R. Victors, MD

S: Pt is a 41-year-old female who was injured in a car accident. She presents today, at the recommendation of Dr. Victors, for a fitting for a prosthetic spectacle.

O: HEENT is unremarkable. Monofocal measurements are taken, and data for the creation of an appropriate prosthesis are recorded.

A: Aphakia, left eye

P: Return in two weeks for final fitting.

_____

Rodney Southern, MD

RS/mg   D: 11/21/08 09:50:16   T: 11/23/08 12:55:01

Find the best, most appropriate code(s) and modifiers.

_____

_____

_____

Part 2   HCPCS Level II
CPT © 2007 American Medical Association. All Rights Reserved.

PATIENT: DAHL, WILLIAM
ACCOUNT/EHR #:   DAHLWI001
Date: 12/10/08

Attending Physician: Kristen Tremaine, MD
Referring Physician: James I. Cipher, MD

Upon orders from Dr. Cipher, I transported a portable x-ray machine to the
Barton Nursing Facility to take chest x-rays of three patients with suspicion of tuberculosis.

Patients served:
    Joselyn Gano, a 73-year-old female
    Barbara Ann Forrester, an 83-year-old female
    Martin Bloomington, a 79-year-old male

All three patients show nodular lesions and patchy infiltrates in the upper lobes.

_____

Kristen Tremaine, MD

KT/mg   D: 12/10/08 09:50:16   T: 12/12/08 12:55:01

Find the best, most appropriate code(s) and modifiers.

_____

_____

_____

CIPHER, VICTORS, & ASSOCIATES
A Complete Health Care Facility
234 MAIN STREET • ANYTOWN, FL 32711 • 407-555-1234

PATIENT: TRUMBLE, HORACE
ACCOUNT/EHR #:   TRUMHO001
Date: 9/7/08

Locum Tenens Physician: Roxan J. Platt, MD
Attending Physician: James I. Cipher, MD

S: Pt is a 17-year-old male who has been a patient of Dr. Cipher for many years. He presents today with a sore throat. I explained to the patient that I am just filling in for Dr. Cipher while he is on vacation.

O: HEENT is relatively unremarkable with the exception of white spots in the back of the throat. Patient still has his tonsils. His throat is swabbed for a culture (immunoassay with direct optical observation to detect Streptococcus group B).

A: Streptococcal sore throat

P: 1. Rx Antibiotic
     2. Follow-up in 10 days.

_____

Roxan J. Platt, MD

RJP/mg   D: 9/7/08 09:50:16   T: 9/9/08 12:55:01

Find the best, most appropriate code(s) and modifiers.

_____

_____

_____

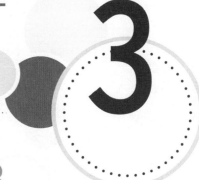

PART THREE

ICD-9-CM VOLUME 3

CHAPTER 16 ICD-9-CM Volume 3 Procedure Codes

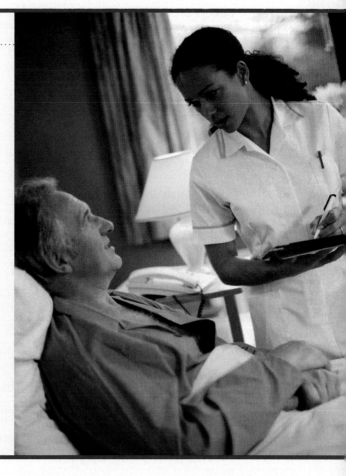

16

ICD-9-CM Volume 3 Procedure Codes

LEARNING OUTCOMES

- Identify the circumstances when Volume 3 codes are used.
- Interpret the notations shown in Volume 3.
- Apply the correct terminology used in Volume 3.
- Identify the necessary documentation specifics required to code accurately.
- Distinguish between CPT and Volume 3 codes.
- Determine the most accurate code to report services rendered.

Hospital

A facility that provides diagnostic, therapeutic (both surgical and nonsurgical), and rehabilitation services by, or under, the supervision of physicians to patients admitted for a variety of medical conditions; also known as acute care facility.

Inpatient

An individual admitted for an overnight or longer stay in a hospital.

Reimbursement

Payment for services provided.

CODING TIP »»

ICD-9-CM Volume 3 codes do not use modifiers.

Hospitals use a different set of codes to report services and procedures provided to their patients, called **inpatients** (for *in* the hospital). The codes come from the third section of the ICD-9-CM book called *ICD-9-CM Volume 3*. Different from CPT codes that you learned about in Part 1 of this textbook, the hospital's codes are used to ensure **reimbursement** to the facility for the use of its resources, including:

- On-staff personnel such as registered nurses, nurses' aides, and orderlies
- Equipment and supplies, such as x-ray machines, linens, and sterilization units
- Overhead, such as electricity, telephones, and taxes

You might notice that physicians are not listed as a hospital's resource. That is because physicians are not typically employed by the hospital. They are given privileges to attend to patients inside the facility and to use the resources within that facility for the benefit of their patients. So a coder employed at the physician's office uses CPT codes to report physician services, and a coder employed at the hospital uses ICD-9-CM Volume 3 codes to report what the facility provided.

ICD-9-CM Volume 3 does not include codes for evaluation and management or for anesthesiologist's services because they are provided by a health care professional who is not employed by the facility—a physician.

CPT codes may be used, in conjunction with Volume 3 codes, if necessary to report the encounter properly.

EXAMPLE

Dr. Cantor performed a lamellar keratoplasty with autograft on Victor Kerper at Barton Hospital. Victor's insurance carrier will actually receive three different claim forms for this one procedure.

Dr. Cantor's coder will report 65710 Keratoplasty (corneal transplant); lamellar from the CPT book to be reimbursed for his professional services in performing the surgery.

Barton Hospital's coder will report 11.61 Lamellar keratoplasty with autograft from the ICD-9-CM Volume 3 to be reimbursed for the use of the operating room, the nurses, the instruments and equipment, and the supplies.

The anesthesiologist's coder will report 00144 Anesthesia for procedures on eye; corneal transplant (plus the appropriate physical status modifier).

DIFFERENT PROCEDURE CODES

You can distinguish between CPT, HCPCS Level II, and ICD-9-CM Volume 3 codes by examining the structure of the code.

CPT codes have five numbers with no dot.

12345   CPT (HCPCS Level I) codes are used to report outpatient procedures and physician's services.

HCPCS Level II codes begin with a letter followed by four numbers.

A1234   HCPCS Level II codes are used to report durable medical equipment (DME), transportation, medications, etc.

ICD-9-CM Volume 3 codes have two numbers, which are sometimes followed by a dot and one or two numbers after that dot.

12.34   ICD-9-CM Volume 3 are used to report inpatient procedures and services.

However, even though they look different, the coding process is still the same. You will abstract the physician's notes to identify key words relating to the procedures and services provided to the patient during a specific visit, query the doctor for clarifications and additional information, and go through the appropriate book to find the best, most accurate code. Let's review the elements used in ICD-9-CM Volume 3.

NOTATIONS

Just as with coding from CPT and HCPCS Level II, ICD-9-CM Volume 3 helps you—via abbreviations, punctuation, and notations—find the most accurate code.

Abbreviations and Punctuation

NOS (Not Otherwise Specified)

Just like the code description "unspecified," *not otherwise specified (NOS)* identifies a code to use if the physician's notes have not provided additional or sufficient detail to enable you to choose a more specific code.

EXAMPLE

Excision, disc, intervertebral [NOS] 80.50

NEC (Not Elsewhere Classifiable)

Similar to "other specified," *not elsewhere classifiable (NEC)* explains that although the health care provider actually gave you more specifics, the coding book does not offer any other code that shares that same definition.

EXAMPLE

Amputation, leg NEC 84.10

[ ] (Brackets)

Brackets are used in the tabular (numeric) listing to add alternative phrases, terminology, synonyms, and/or acronyms intended to be included in the particular code's description. It is similar to an "includes" note (see the section "Instructional Notes" below).

EXAMPLE

57.33 Closed [transurethral] biopsy of bladder

[ ] (Slanted Brackets)

Found in the alphabetic index, *italic brackets* direct the coder to report a second code as well as the first code. The additional code provides further details.

EXAMPLE

Ileal, bladder, closed 57.87 [*45.51*]

( ) (Parentheses)

The tabular (numeric) listing and the alphabetic index both use *parentheses* to provide the coder with additional terms or modifiers that are used to further describe the code's meaning. Such terms are **optional.**

EXAMPLE

Division, vein (with ligation) 38.80

: (Colon)

When a *colon* is used within a code's description, it is followed by a list of terms that may be used to further modify or elaborate on the code's meaning. The colon saves space by indicating that each of the following words can be used with the previous description.

EXAMPLE

07 Operations on other endocrine glands

INCLUDES operations on:

adrenal glands   pituitary glands

pineal gland   thymus

} (Brace)

A *brace* indicates that a word or phrase shown to the right of the brace is to be appended to each of the terms to the left of the brace.

EXAMPLE

01.51 Excision of lesion or tissue of cerebral meninges

Decortication

Resection   } of (cerebral) meninges

Stripping of subdural membrane

Therefore, in this example, the terms included with the brace will be read: Decortication of (cerebral) meninges; Resection of (cerebral) meninges; and Stripping of subdural membrane of (cerebral) meninges.

Instructional Notes

INCLUDES

The *includes* note provides a listing of alternate terms, phrases, and other descriptors that might be used by the physician in his or her notes and that are also incorporated in the meaning of the code.

EXAMPLE

82.6 Reconstruction of thumb

INCLUDES digital transfer to act as thumb

The opposite of the includes note, the *excludes* note tells you specific terms and phrases that are *not* described by the code. The book goes one step further and suggests the code you might use instead.

EXAMPLE

20.51 Excision of lesion of middle ear

EXCLUDES biopsy of middle ear (20.32)

Code Also

Code Also Any

Code Also Any Synchronous

Similar to the intent of the italic brackets in the alphabetic index, *code also, code also any,* and *code also any* **synchronous** direct you to include another code along with the use of this code, when applicable. Essentially, it is telling you that if additional components of the procedure have been performed, they are to be coded separately.

EXAMPLE

08.2 Excision or destruction of lesion or tissue of eyelid

Code also any synchronous reconstruction (08.61–08.74)

See; See Also

A *see* or *see also* note is the book's way of telling you to check out another term or phrase in the alphabetic index.

EXAMPLE

Function, study (*see also* Scan, radioisotope)

Omit Code

The *omit code* note tells you that the procedure is a component of another, more extensive procedure and *should not* be coded separately.

EXAMPLE

Costectomy, associated with thoracic operation—*omit code*

And

When *and* is used in a code's description, read it as "and/or." In other words, both terms do not have to be applicable as long as at least one term is appropriate.

EXAMPLE

38.5 Ligation and stripping of varicose veins

Synchronous

Simultaneous; occurring at the same time.

The "and" in the example means that 38.5x is a correct code if the physician performed (1) the ligation of the varicose veins; (2) the stripping of the varicose veins, or (3) both ligation and stripping.

Color Highlighting

The color notations in Volume 3 are used to identify **Medicare code edits (MCE)** and other possible reimbursement issues. Remember, though, that these notations pinpoint national approval, or coverage, concerns. While Medicare is a federal program, each state administers the plan and can make its own decisions with regard to coverage over and above the national standards. Therefore, the highlighting of a noncovered procedure in the book, for example, may not apply in your state. When working with codes, you are responsible for finding out from your state's **fiscal intermediary (FI),** or the state office of a private insurer, its coverage parameters with regard to your facility's procedures.

Note: Not all publishers of the ICD-9-CM Volume 3 use these same color schemes. Refer to the legend, located across the bottom of a page, to confirm the colors used in your edition.

Blue-Gray Highlighting

Blue-gray indicates a *non-OR procedure;* that is, a procedure that is not typically performed in the operating room. If for some reason, this procedure was performed in a surgical suite in the operating room, you have to attach a report to explain the circumstances that required the additional precaution.

EXAMPLE

00.10 Implantation of chemotherapeutic agent

Gray Highlighting

The highlight represents a *valid OR procedure,* which is approved to be performed in the operating room.

EXAMPLE

03.94 Removal of spinal neurostimulator lead(s)

Pink Highlighting

Pink identifies an **adjunct code.** An adjunct code is the same as a CPT add-on code. The code cannot be reported by itself, and must be reported along with the code for the main portion of the procedure. Technically, such codes are not considered procedure codes, in and of themselves, but serve to add more details about the primary procedure.

EXAMPLE

00.16 Pressurized treatment of venous bypass graft [conduit] with pharmaceutical substance

Medicare code edit (MCE)

A computerized system that identifies coding errors and/or concerns regarding medical necessity; part of the Correct Coding Initiative.

Fiscal intermediary

A company that administers the day-to-day operation of reviewing and reimbursement of claims for state Medicare programs.

Adjunct code

The equivalent of CPT's add-on code. This code may not be reported alone or as a first-listed code.

✓ 3ʳᵈ (The red box with a check mark and 3)

Unlike CPT codes, which are always five digits long, Volume 3 codes begin with just two digits. However, a third digit is sometimes required to include more specific information about the procedure. *It is not a suggestion.* When the book tells you—via a red box with a check mark and "3ʳᵈ"—that a third digit is required, you *must* include it; otherwise the code is **invalid.**

EXAMPLE

> ✓ 3ʳᵈ 19 Reconstructive operations on middle ear
>
> 19.0 Stapes mobilization

✓ 4ᵗʰ (The red box with a check mark and 4)

Exactly like the third-digit indicator, the red box with a check mark and "4ᵗʰ" simply means you need to provide even more specifics about the procedure by using the next level of coding. Again, it is not a suggestion; *it is a requirement!*

EXAMPLE

> ✓ 4ᵗʰ 48.9 Other operations on rectum and perirectal tissue
>
> 48.91 Incision of rectal stricture

NC (The red box with an NC)

The red box with an NC, shown to the right of a code, identifies a procedure that the national Medicare program considers a noncovered (NC) procedure. Referring to Medicare code edit 11, it warns you of the possibility that Medicare will not reimburse your facility for providing the service. Again, it is a national determination. Always check with your state administrator.

EXAMPLE

> 66.21 Bilateral endoscopic ligation and crushing of fallopian tubes NC

BI (The dark gray box with a BI)

The dark gray box with a BI, located to the right of a code, indicates that it is a **bilateral** (BI) edit. When the procedure (reported with this code) is performed on both of the bilateral joints of a patient's lower extremity, you have to report the code twice—once for each side. It refers directly to Medicare code edit 13.

EXAMPLE

> 81.54 Total knee replacement BI

LC (The blue-green box with an LC)

When you see the blue-green box with an LC, located to the right of a code, it tells you that it is a limited coverage (LC) procedure. Medicare

Part 3 ICD-9-CM Volume 3

code edit 17 limits reimbursement to only a portion of the costs connected with an extremely complicated and serious procedure.

EXAMPLE

33.51 Unilateral lung transplantation `LC`

THE ALPHABETIC INDEX

At the beginning of Volume 3, you will find its alphabetic index. Designed like the alphabetic index in CPT, the main terms for procedures and services are in bold at the left margin of the column. Then indented underneath those terms may be additional descriptions.

As you read through the alphabetic index, you may notice something different in Volume 3. While both CPT and Volume 3 use common surgical and procedural words, the books don't always choose the same term.

For example, the alphabetic index of CPT gives you listings under *x-ray* and sends you to code descriptions that begin with *radiologic examination*. However, Volume 3 has a limited number of listings under x-ray, and almost all tell you to look under the term *radiography*. Then the suggested codes under *radiography* all send you to code descriptions that begin with *x-ray*.

≪≪≪ **CODING TIP**

Be very careful when reading down a long list of indented terms. It is easy to misread.

Example

In Volume 3, find:

Radiography, clavicle 87.43

87.43 X-ray of ribs, sternum, and clavicle

In CPT, find:

X-ray, clavicle 73000

73000 Radiologic examination; clavicle, complete

The different way in which the two books use the same health care terms illustrates the importance of learning medical terminology and having a good medical dictionary by your side.

LET'S CODE IT! SCENARIO

Elias Morrison, a 57-year-old male, was admitted into Barton Hospital to have Dr. Yanni excise Elias's thymus.

Let's Code It!

Dr. Yanni *excised* Elias's *thymus.* This seems pretty straightforward, so let's go to the alphabetic index of Volume 3 to find the most accurate code to reimburse the hospital for the procedure.

Excision

Thymus (*see also* Thymectomy) 07.80

You learned in medical terminology class that the excision of the thymus is called a *thymectomy,* so this should be the same thing. However, it is always good to double-check, so let's go ahead and look this up as well.

Thymectomy 07.80
    Partial (open)(other) 07.81
        thoracoscopic 07.83
    Total (open)(other) 07.82
        thoracoscopic 07.84
        transcervical 07.99

The alphabetic index is telling you two things:

1. The excision of the thymus *is* a thymectomy. Good for you!

2. You need more information before you can choose the correct code because the book has five choices:

07.80 Thymectomy, not otherwise specified
07.81 Partial excision of thymus
07.82 Total excision of thymus
07.83 Thoracoscopic partial excision of thymus
07.84 Thoracoscopic total excision of thymus

You have to check further in the notes or query the physician to find out if the thymectomy performed on Elias was a total or a partial, and whether or not it was done with a thoracoscope. Code 07.80 is an NOS code for the procedure, and you want to avoid using that, if at all possible.

<table>
<tr><td>

CODING TIP »»

Never, never, never code from the alphabetic index. *Always* confirm the code in the tabular (numeric) listing before using a code to report a service.

</td></tr>
</table>

THE TABULAR LISTING

The tabular listing of Volume 3 shows all the codes available in numeric order, from 00 to 99.99. Once you find a suggested code in the alphabetic index, you must turn to the tabular (numeric) listing to confirm that the code is the best possible choice for reporting the service provided.

Third and Fourth Digits

You have learned a lot already about how to read the tabular section. You read about the required third- and fourth-digit codes to provide additional specificity. Signified by a symbol next to a two- or three-digit code, you *must* read carefully to find that complete code. Sometimes you have to read further down the column; other times you have to refer back up the column to a special last-digit box. Failure to include a required digit will result in the rejection of your claim due to using invalid codes.

EXAMPLE

✓ **3rd**   04 Operations on cranial and peripheral nerves

   ✓ **4th**   04.0 Incision, division, and excision of cranial and peripheral nerves

      04.01 Excision of acoustic neuroma

As you look at the codes shown in our example, the symbols tell you that codes 04 and 04.0 are both invalid. They do not exist and cannot be used to report a service. Here, the only valid code you see is 04.01 Excision of acoustic neuroma.

Tabular Descriptors

Earlier in this chapter, you learned about the differences in how Volume 3 uses terminology to describe codes. In the tabular listings, there are additional elements you have to know about the procedures performed that differ from CPT.

In the section "The Alphabetic Index," you learned that Volume 3 lists x-rays under the term *radiography*. The tabular listing uses different descriptors for codes as well.

Let's go back and look at the same department's services and review the differences between CPT and Volume 3 in the code descriptors.

CPT Codes

73600 Radiologic examination, ankle; *two views*

73610 Radiologic examination, ankle; complete, *minimum of three views*

Volume 3 Codes

88.28 *Skeletal x-ray* of ankle and foot

88.37 Other *soft tissue x-ray* of lower limb

In addition to the difference in terms (x-ray versus radiologic examination), there is also a difference in the information you will need to choose the correct code. Volume 3 requires that you know exactly the *type* of x-ray (e.g., skeletal versus soft tissue), whereas CPT requires that you know how many views were taken (e.g., two views or minimum of three views).

The bottom line is that when coding, you must match the descriptions in the coding book (whichever you are using) to the information you have from the physician. If the physician's notes and the supporting documentation, such as lab and radiology reports, do not provide the information and details you need to code accurately, you *must* query.

LET'S CODE IT! SCENARIO

Gail Samuelson, a 50-year-old female, was admitted into the hospital because of rectal bleeding and extreme diarrhea. She was brought down to the hospital's endoscopy department for a colonoscopy. Dr. Tapper performed the procedure and reported to Gail that her colon looked healthy and saw no concerns. Gail was taken back to her room to await the next part of her diagnostic testing.

Let's Code It!

To report Dr. Tapper's service of performing the colonoscopy, you use CPT code 45378. As the coder for the hospital, however, you must use a

Volume 3 code so that the facility can be reimbursed for its costs related to Gail's procedure.

Let's go to the alphabetic index of Volume 3 and look up *colonoscopy:*

Colonoscopy 45.23

>with biopsy 45.25

>>rectum 48.24

Remember, the indented portions of the column are additional descriptors or definitions that attach to the term immediately above at the margin. So the three lines are read:

Colonoscopy 45.23

Colonoscopy with biopsy 45.25

Colonoscopy with biopsy, rectum 48.24

Also, as with all the other coding sections, we *never code from the alphabetical index.* So let's turn to the section directly after this one to find the numeric listings for the ICD-9-CM procedure codes and locate 45. We see the code:

✓ 3rd 45 Incision, excision, and anastomosis of intestine

Code also any application or administration of an adhesion barrier substance (99.77)

Dr. Tapper's notes do not mention anything about an adhesion barrier substance, so the *code also* notation does not apply to this case.

Let's keep looking down the column to find a more accurate definition. *Note:* The red box next to the 45 is telling us we must have a third digit.

✓ 4th 45.2 Diagnostic procedures on large intestine

The red box instructs you to keep reading down the column to find the correct *four*-digit code.

45.21 Transabdominal endoscopy of large intestine

45.22 Endoscopy of large intestine through artificial stoma

45.23 Colonoscopy

The code 45.23 Colonoscopy matches the physician's notes, exactly!

YOU CODE IT! CASE STUDY

Harrison Ming, a 27-year-old male, was admitted into Barton Hospital so that Dr. Houghton can perform an arthroplasty of the carpometacarpal joint to repair the torn tendon in Harrison's right wrist.

Go through the steps of coding, and determine the code(s) that should be reported for Barton Hospital for the procedure Dr. Houghton performed on Harrison Ming.

Step 1: Read the case completely.

Step 2: Abstract the notes: Which key words can you identify relating to the procedures performed?

_____

Step 3: Query the provider, if necessary.

Step 4: Diagnosis: Torn tendon, wrist.

Step 5: Code the procedure(s).

_____

Step 6: Link the procedure codes to at least one diagnosis code.

Step 7: Back code to double-check your choices.

Answer

Did you find the correct code to be:

81.75 Arthroplasty of carpocarpal or carpometacarpal joint without implant

Good job!

CHAPTER SUMMARY

A professional coding specialist must know how to determine the best, most accurate code to obtain proper reimbursement. When coding for a hospital, ICD-9-CM Volume 3 codes are used to report inpatient services, procedures, and other treatments. The process is essentially the same as coding from CPT, with alternative terminology being used.

In the near future, ICD-10-PCS will replace ICD-9-CM Volume 3. Appendix B will walk you through the changes expected with ICD-10-PCS. You will find that the same coding process you have learned throughout this textbook will still get you to the most accurate code or codes.

1. ICD-9-CM Volume 3 codes are used only by

    a. Physician's offices.

    b. Laboratories.

    c. Hospitals.

    d. Imaging centers.

2. Volume 3 includes codes for all except

    a. Surgical procedures.

    b. Anesthesia.

    c. Radiology.

    d. Injections.

3. Dr. Gerard goes to see his patient who has been admitted into the hospital. You will code his visit from which book?

    a. ICD-9-CM Volume 3.

    b. HCPCS Level II.

    c. CPT.

    d. None of the above.

4. NOS has the same meaning as

    a. Not elsewhere classified.

    b. Other specified.

    c. Specified elsewhere.

    d. Unspecified.

5. Terms shown in (parentheses) in the tabular listing are

    a. Mandatory.

    b. Required.

    c. Optional.

    d. Eliminated.

6. An adjunct code in Volume 3 is the same as a CPT

    a. Add-on code.

    b. Mutually exclusive code.

    c. Modifier.

    d. Qualifying circumstances code.

7. A small box with the letters NC next to a code means

    a. Noncompliant.

    b. No copayment.

    c. Newly established procedure.

    d. Noncovered by Medicare.

8. You are required to code to the highest specificity. This means if a four-digit code is correct and available,

    a. Use is mandatory.

    b. Use is optional.

    c. Use with a modifier.

    d. Use with another code only.

9. Volume 3 codes report the use of all except

    a. On-staff personnel such as certified nurse assistants.

    b. Attending physicians.

    c. Equipment such as x-ray machines.

    d. Cost of doing business, such as utilities.

10. An example of a Volume 3 code is

    a. 537.89

    b. 65270

    c. 36.09

    d. L0100

YOU CODE IT! Practice
Chapter 16. ICD-9-CM Volume 3 Procedure Codes

Find the best Volume 3 procedure code(s) for these patients.

1. Alexander Frienze, 52-year-old male, is admitted into the hospital with a concussion. A skull x-ray and brain MRI are both performed.

   _____

2. Rose Neiman, a 39-year-old female, was admitted into the hospital with suspected appendicitis. An ultrasound of the abdomen was performed.

   _____

3. Rob Nalley, a 35-year-old male in Barton Hospital, is given aerosol inhalation of pentamidine.

   _____

4. Dorothy Dubois, a 73-year-old female, was admitted to the hospital for surgery. A routine ECG was taken in preparation for her surgery the following day.

   _____

5. Charlene Bahaman, a 45-year-old female, in the hospital since yesterday, has a laparoscopic cholecystectomy by laser.

   _____

6. Kenneth Caten, a 39-year-old male, goes to the hospital to have an operative esophageal endoscopy.

   _____

7. Helene Ruboni, a 58-year-old female, has a bunionectomy with a soft tissue correction.

   _____

8. Anton Fraison, an 8-year-old male, is admitted into the hospital for a suspected broken clavicle. An x-ray is taken. A plaster cast is applied.

   _____

9. Stacey Highland, a 5-year-old female, is in Barton Hospital and given a blood transfusion of packed cells.

   _____

10. After cutting his foot on the beach, Burt Dennis, a 19-year-old male, is admitted into the hospital for cellulitis and inflammation of the foot. He is given an administration of a tetanus antitoxin.

_____

11. Manuel Sedaka, a 19-year-old male, has had a bad cough for the last two months. Therefore, Dr. Fabiole admitted him into the hospital and performed a diagnostic fiber-optic bronchoscopy with hopes of determining the cause of the irritation.

_____

12. Renee Beecher, a 39-year-old female, is a professional runner and has won three marathons. Today, she is admitted to the hospital for a total arthroplasty of her right knee.

_____

13. Calvin Moriarity, a 25-year-old male, was taken to the OR from the emergency department so that Dr. Neilson could do an exploration of Calvin's wound. He was stabbed in the abdomen during a mugging.

_____

14. Dr. Zorman, a pediatrician, admitted his patient, Katy Cooper, a 4-year-old female, into the hospital to surgically repair her deviated septum. Dr. Zorman performed a septoplasty with a cartilage scoring.

_____

15. Denise Mosure, a 33-year-old female, was having a nosebleed and went to see Dr. Vickmann right away. She was admitted into the hospital, and Dr. Vickmann performed extensive cautery in the anterior portion of her right nasal passage to control the bleeding.

_____

YOU CODE IT! Simulation
Chapter 16. ICD-9-CM Volume 3 Procedure Codes

On the following pages, you will see physician notes documenting encounters with patients at our textbook's hospital, Barton Hospital. Carefully read through the notes and find the best code or codes from Volume 3 for each of these cases.

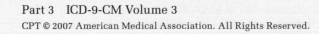

BARTON HOSPITAL
239 MAIN STREET • ANYTOWN, FL 32711 • 407-555-1243

PATIENT: BRUTUS, JOHN
ACCOUNT/EHR #:   BRUTJO001
Date: 09/20/08

Attending Physician: Julio Yearlin, MD

Pt is a 27-year-old male who was involved in a fistfight at a local bar the previous evening. He is admitted to the hospital today complaining of an ache in the area of his left eye as well as severe pain around his right ear.
    After examination, the patient is taken to the operating room for a repair of the left eye rupture.
    Dx: Ruptured eyeball, left

___

Julio Yearlin, MD

JY/mg   D: 09/20/08 09:50:16   T: 09/22/08 12:55:01

Find the best, most appropriate ICD-9-CM Volume 3 code(s).

___

___

___

BARTON HOSPITAL
239 MAIN STREET • ANYTOWN, FL 32711 • 407-555-1243

PATIENT:	BACHELDER, JEFFREY
MRN:	BACHJE001
Admission Date:	13 October 2008
Discharge Date:	15 October 2008
Date:	13 October 2008
Preoperative DX:	Malignant neoplasm, scrotum, CA in situ
Postoperative DX:	same
Procedure:	Resection of scrotum, needle biopsy of testis
Surgeon:	Daniel Macintosh, MD
Assistant:	None
Anesthesia:	General

Indications: The patient is a 59-year-old male with a recent diagnosis of malignancy of the scrotum.

Procedure: The patient was placed on the table in supine position. General anesthesia was administered by Dr. Cattan. He was placed in proper position. A needle biopsy was taken of the testis, and then a surgical resection of the scrotum was performed.

10/15/08 11:47:39

Find the best, most appropriate ICD-9-CM Volume 3 code(s).

_____

_____

_____

PATIENT: BAKER, DORITTA
MRN: BAKEDO001
Date: 19 September 2008

Procedure Performed: Endocervical specimen,

                                     Intraepithelial lesion of the cervix, cytopathology smear

Pathologist: Caryn Simonson, MD

Referring Physician: Rodney L. Cohen, MD

Indications: Lesion of cervix

Impressions: Uncertain behavior neoplasm
Cytopathology, cervical, collected in preservative fluid, automated thin layer preparation; manual screening and rescreening

Caryn Simonson, MD

CS/mg   D: 9/19/08 09:50:16   T: 9/23/08 12:55:01

Find the best, most appropriate ICD-9-CM Volume 3 code(s).

_____

_____

_____

BARTON HOSPITAL
239 MAIN STREET • ANYTOWN, FL 32711 • 407-555-1243

PATIENT:	KLOTSKY, STACY
MRN:	KLOTST001
Date:	5 October 2008
Procedure Performed:	Bladder, biopsy gross and microscopic examination
Pathologist:	Caryn Simonson, MD
Referring Physician:	Leonard Dupont, MD
Indications:	R/o bladder tumor
Impressions:	Chronic cystits with squamous cell metaplasia Surgical pathology, gross and microscopic examination, urinary bladder, biopsy

Caryn Simonson, MD

CS/mg   D: 10/5/08 09:50:16   T: 10/7/08 12:55:01

Find the best, most appropriate ICD-9-CM Volume 3 code(s).

_____

_____

_____

BARTON HOSPITAL
239 MAIN STREET • ANYTOWN, FL 32711 • 407-555-1243

PATIENT: SOUSA, NORMAN
ACCOUNT/EHR #:   SOUSNO001
Date: 11/05/08

DX: Cervical sprain C1-C7; lumbar strain L4-L5; multiple subluxation of cervical spine

Attending Physician: Terrence Fontaine, MD

This 23-year-old male was admitted after being involved in a 2-car MVA two weeks ago. He saw his family physician, Dr. Ashley Proctor, after experiencing constant neck pain radiating into the shoulders. Pain medication and rest (no movement) provided temporary relief. Dr. Proctor suggested admission for further evaluation.

In addition to neck pain, Pt states pain radiating across the lower back area beginning approximately 2 hours after the MVA. He states it hurts to move, bend, walk. Pt denies similar pain in back or neck before.

BP 122/85 P60 After review of patient history questionnaire, PE indicates general appearance is age appropriate with average build and a protective gait. Normal lymph nodes: cervical; axillae; groin. Upper and lower extremities appear normal with the exception of muscle strength in both arms and left leg. Toe walk exam rates 3 of 5. Limited-to-no ROM with pain C1–C7 and L4–L5. Pt exhibits spinal tenderness: cervical; dorsal; lumbar. Evidence of edema: cervical and lumbar regions. Muscle spasms evident: scalenes, traps, lat, and paraspinal.

Patient sent to Radiology for x-rays: cervical and lumbar. Radiologic results show multiple subluxations of the cervical vertebrae with pain on movement. Dens and spinous process are intact. No breaks or fractures. Lumbar spine is intact with no breaks or fractures.

Terrence Fontaine, MD

TF/mg   D: 11/05/08 09:50:16   T: 11/07/08 12:55:01

Find the best, most appropriate ICD-9-CM Volume 3 code(s).

_____

_____

_____

PRACTICUM

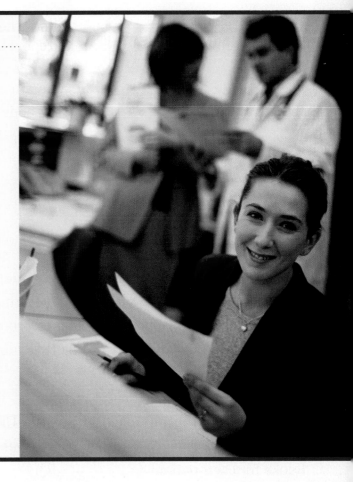

17 Procedure Coding Practicum

LEARNING OUTCOMES

- Interpret the physician's notes carefully.
- Correctly abstract physician's notes and operative reports.
- Identify any missing or unclear documentation and query the doctor.
- Determine the best, most accurate code or codes for each case to report the procedures provided.
- Connect each procedure code to at least one diagnosis, as stated in the notes, to support medical necessity.
- Back code to confirm that the codes correctly, and completely, report the encounter

The following pages include selections from actual physicians' notes and operative reports that document services and treatments performed for patients at various health care facilities. The names, ages, and dates have been changed to protect patient confidentiality, and the facility name has been changed, as well.

Abstract the reports, and determine the best, most appropriate codes from the CPT, ICD-9-CM Volume 3, and HCPCS Level II books for each patient.

In the real world, you would only code one portion of a patient's chart, because you would be working for only one of the facilities or pro-

fessionals. However, to benefit the most from this chapter, you should code for the person who wrote and signed the notes:

- Attending physician
- Surgeon
- Anesthesiologist
- Radiologist
- Pathologist
- Physical therapist
- Hospital

By coding for everyone, you will practice all types of coding, and be prepared to work for any type of facility.

The names of the facilities, health care professionals, and patients have all been changed to protect the privacy and confidentiality of all concerned in all case scenarios and physician notes contained in this textbook.

Any similarities to actual persons or places are purely coincidental. The cases are to be used for educational purposes only.

《《《 **CODING TIP**

In this practicum, HCPCS level II codes and modifiers are accepted by insurance carriers.

CIPHER, VICTORS, & ASSOCIATES
A Complete Health Care Facility
234 MAIN STREET • ANYTOWN, FL 32711 • 407-555-1234

PATIENT:	HUMPHREY, DONALD
MRN:	HUMPDO01
Date:	23 August 2008
Procedure Performed:	Neurosurgical evaluation
Physician:	Patrick B. Reynoso, MD

This is the first visit for this 79-year-old right-handed male who comes for evaluation of possible normal pressure hydrocephalus. The patient's family has been noting that the patient has symptoms consistent with normal pressure hydrocephalus and apparently was made aware of this in recent publications. The patient has had mental deterioration. He has a history of urinary urgency and has been seen by Dr. Jackson for this. Problems with his gait, which he describes as "vertigo in the legs" and he "minces his steps." His primary care physician is Dr. Thomas.

The patient has allergies to pollen and hay fever. His medications include Plavix, aspirin, Lipitor, Avodart, Uroxatral, Hyzaar, calcium 600 + vitamin D, and multivitamins.

Pertinent Medical History:
The patient does not smoke cigarettes or drink alcohol.

Social History:
He is married and is a retired dentist.

Family History:
His mother died at the age of 96 of "dementia" and possible stroke. His father died at the age of 96 of an unknown cause.

Review of Systems:
The patient has had several transient ischemic attacks in January, April, and July. He is status post cataract surgery. He is status post a syncopal episode in January. He has a history of hypertension, asthma, bronchitis, and a history of bilateral inguinal hernia repairs 45 years ago. In January, he had a urinary tract infection and also had a cardiac evaluation, which was negative. Otherwise, his review of systems is negative for cardiac, pulmonary, gastrointestinal, genitourinary, or musculoskeletal disease.

Physical Examination:
This is a well-developed, well-nourished elderly white male in no acute distress that appears to be awake, alert, and oriented. His blood pressure is 170/70. His pulse is 70. His respiration is 16. His head is atraumatic, normocephalic. He is status post cataracts. He has dentures. His neck is subtle without jugular venous distention or bruits. His lungs are clear to auscultation. His heart is regular rhythm. His abdomen is soft. His extremities are without clubbing, cyanosis, or edema. Examination of his spine does not demonstrate any direct cervical spine tenderness. The patient has kyphoscoliosis of the thoracolumbar spine. Neurological examination of cranial nerves II–XII demonstrate a decrease in upward gaze and a decrease in hearing. He wears hearing aides. Otherwise, they appear to be grossly unremarkable. Motor function is 5/5 = in all major motor groups. Sensory examination appears to be grossly intact in all extremities. Deep tendon reflexes are 0= for the biceps, triceps, and brachioradialis. In the lower extremities, the patellars, suprapatellars, and hamstrings are 0=. The right Achilles is 2+, the left is absent. The toes are downgoing bilaterally. The patient's cerebellar testing is intact for finger to nose function. On regular gait testing, the patient has a magnetic/shuffling gait. Station testing does not demonstrate any drift or Romberg's sign.

(Continued)

Review:
There are no x-rays available for review.

Impression:
The patient has possible normal pressure hydrocephalus verses ischemic cerebrovascular disease.

Recommendations:
The patient will have an MRI scan, MR angiogram of the brain and MR angiogram of the carotid and vertebral arteries and then return to see me in the office.

Patrick B. Reynoso, MD

PBR/mg   D: 8/23/08 09:50:16   T: 8/25/08 12:55:01

Find the best, most appropriate code(s).

CIPHER, VICTORS, & ASSOCIATES
A Complete Health Care Facility
234 MAIN STREET • ANYTOWN, FL 32711 • 407-555-1234

PATIENT: HUMPHREY, DONALD
MRN: HUMPDO01
Date: 25 August 2008

Procedure Performed: MRI, brain, no contrast
                              MR angiogram, brain, no contrast
                              MR angiogram, neck, no contrast

Radiologist: Michelle H. McNair, MD

Clinical Information: Evaluate for VP shunt
                              No prior studies available for a comparison

Technical Information:
The examination was performed without the use of intravenous contrast material.

Interpretation:
Evaluation of the posterior fossa demonstrates hydrocephalus versus low pressure communicating hydrocephalus.

Michelle H. McNair, MD

MHM/mg   D: 8/25/08 09:50:16   T: 8/27/08 12:55:01

Find the best, most appropriate code(s).

_____

_____

_____

Part 4   Practicum

CIPHER, VICTORS, & ASSOCIATES
A Complete Health Care Facility
234 MAIN STREET • ANYTOWN, FL 32711 • 407-555-1234

PATIENT: HUMPHREY, DONALD
MRN: HUMPDO01
Date: 15 September 2008

Procedure Performed: Test Evaluation

Physician: Patrick B. Reynoso, MD

The patient was last seen on August 23. The MRI scan of the brain demonstrates that the patient has hydrocephalus with transependymal edema.

Impression:
The patient has either normal pressure hydrocephalus or a low pressure communicating hydrocephalus.

Recommendations:
In either case, he requires a ventricular shunt placement. I have explained to the patient and his family the shunt procedure, its indications, risks, benefits, and alternatives in detail including the risk of bleeding, infection, and injury to the brain tissue with hemorrhages, stroke, paralysis, blindness, coma, or even death. All of their questions have been answered. No guarantees have been given. I have advised that the patient will need to have medical clearance from his primary care physician, Dr. Roger Thomas, 407-555-9899. Once we have the medical clearance, we can schedule him for surgery. Chest x-ray is taken to confirm patient is OK for surgery.

Patrick B. Reynoso, MD

PBR/mg   D: 9/15/08 09:50:16   T: 9/20/08 12:55:01

Find the best, most appropriate code(s).

_____

_____

_____

PATIENT: HUMPHREY, DONALD
MRN: HUMPDO01
Admission Date: 17 September 2008
Discharge Date: 19 September 2008

Operative Report:
Preoperative Diagnosis: Normal pressure hydrocephalus
Postoperative Diagnosis: Normal pressure hydrocephalus
Operation: Right parieto-occipital ventriculoperitoneal shunt placement with cerebro-
                                spinal fluid manometry and Hakim valve programming.

Surgeon: Patrick B. Reynoso, MD

Assistant:
Anesthesia: General endotracheal
Anesthesiologist: Carter H. Beauman, MD
Estimated Blood Loss: Less than 10 cc.
Complications:

Procedure:
This 79-year-old gentleman had progressive urinary, gait, and memory problems with MRI study demonstrating significant ventriculomegaly consistent with normal pressure hydrocephalus. Because of the patient's deterioration, he was offered the option of ventriculoperitoneal shunt placement to try to stop the downward deterioration of his mental faculties.

Following the obtaining of informed consent, the patient was taken to the operating table for the procedure.

The patient was placed supine on the operating table, inducted under general anesthesia and intubated. His right parieto-occipital scalp was shaved, and then the scalp, neck, chest, and abdomen on the right side were washed with alcohol and prepped with DuraPrep solution and then draped with sterile drapes with additional Ioban dressing. The skin incision was marked out with a skin marker for the right parieto-occipital scalp, centered on a point approximately 3 cm lateral to and 8-to-9 cm rostral to the inion, and in the right upper quadrant of the abdomen at the midcostal line. These incisions were then infiltrated with 1/2% lidocaine with 1:200,000 epinephrine solution. The skin incision was then made in the scalp with a #10 blade, and hemostasis was obtained with Bovie cauterization. A pneumatic perforator was used to drill a hole in the cranium, and then the margins of the bur hole were waxed with bone wax for hemostasis. Blunt dissection of the occipital scalp was used to create a subcutaneous cul-de-sac for placement of the value system, and following this, a subcutaneous passer was used to create a track for passing the distal Bactocill peritoneal catheter between the two incisions. The abdominal incision was also opened with a #10 blade to facilitate passage.

Once the distal catheter was in place, the dura was cauterized using the Bovie cautery bayonet technique, and then a ventricular catheter was passed into the ventricles without difficulty. The cerebrospinal fluid pressure was measured to be approximately 9 cm of water and cerebrospinal fluid was also sent for routine culture and Gram stain. Once the cerebrospinal fluid pressure had been measured, the Hakim valve was programmed to

(Continued)

a pressure resistance of 60 mm of water. The valve was then connected to the ventriculostomy catheter, which was 10 cm in length. It was a Bactocill catheter that was used for this also. The connection was made with a 2-0 silk ligature. The valve was also connected to the distal peritoneal catheter with a 2-0 silk ligature. The valve was then pulled underneath the scalp and anchored to the pericranium with 3-0 Prolene anchoring sutures to prevent migration of the valve. There was good spontaneous flow of cerebrospinal fluid from the distal portion of the peritoneal catheter. Excess length of the peritoneal cavity was removed, and then several slits were made in the sides of the peritoneal catheter to provide additional egress points for cerebrospinal fluid as needed.

   Once this was done, the abdominal incision was opened further with a Bovie cautery and cutting current. The anterior abdominal fascia was divided with a Bovie cautery, and then blunt dissection with a hemostat was used to split the fibers of the rectus abdominus muscles. The posterior abdominal fascia was then identified and lifted up with hemostats and then divided with Metzenbaum scissors. The peritoneum was then identified, lifted up with hemostats, and again divided with Metzenbaum scissors. Following this, the peritoneal cavity was easily visualized. A hemostat and then a peritoneal trocar were able to be passed into the peritoneal cavity without difficulty. Following this, the distal portion of the ventriculoperitoneal shunt was passed into the peritoneal cavity without difficulty, after once again ascertaining that there was spontaneous flow of spinal fluid. Once the catheter was in the peritoneal cavity, #0 Vicryl sutures were used to reapproximate the posterior abdominal fascia, and then the anterior abdominal fascia. The Scarpa's fascia was then closed with #0 Vicryl interrupted sutures with inverted knots. Gelfoam soaked in Thrombin was placed overlying the point of insertion of the ventriculostomy catheter, and then the galea was closed with #0 Vicryl interrupted sutures with inverted knots. The areas were irrigated with bacitracin irrigation solution during the closure process, and then the skin incisions were closed with 3-0 nylon simple running sutures with good skin approximation. The skin incisions were then washed again with bacitracin irrigation solution, and then dressed with triple antibiotic ointment and coverlet dressings. The patient was awakened from general anesthesia, extubated, and taken to the recovery room for further observation. Estimated blood loss from the entire procedure was less than 10 cc. The patient appeared to have tolerated the procedure well.

Patrick B. Reynoso, MD

PBR/mg   D: 9/17/08 12:50:14   T: 9/21/08 11:02:01

Find the best, most appropriate code(s).

_____

_____

_____

PATIENT: HUMPHREY, DONALD
MRN: HUMPDO01
Admission Date: 17 September 2008
Discharge Date: 19 September 2008

Operative Report:
Preoperative Diagnosis: Normal pressure hydrocephalus
Postoperative Diagnosis: Normal pressure hydrocephalus
Operation: Right parieto-occipital ventriculoperitoneal shunt placement with cerebro-spinal fluid manometry and Hakim valve programming.

Surgeon: Patrick B. Reynoso, MD

Assistant:
Anesthesia: General endotracheal
Anesthesiologist: Carter H. Beauman, MD

Procedure:
This 79-year-old gentleman had progressive urinary, gait, and memory problems with MRI study demonstrating significant ventriculomegaly consistent with normal pressure hydrocephalus. Because of the patient's deterioration, he was offered the option of ventriculoperitoneal shunt placement to try to stop the downward deterioration of his mental faculties.

    Following the obtaining of informed consent, the patient was taken to the operating table for the procedure.

    The patient was placed supine on the operating table, inducted under general anesthesia and intubated. His right parieto-occipital scalp was shaved, and then the scalp, neck, chest, and abdomen on the right side were washed with alcohol and prepped with DuraPrep solution and then draped with sterile drapes with additional Ioban dressing.

    Vital signs maintained at appropriate level.

    The patient was awakened from general anesthesia, extubated, and taken to the recovery room for further observation. Estimated blood loss from the entire procedure was less than 10 cc. The patient appeared to have tolerated the procedure well.

Carter H. Beauman, MD

CHB/mg   D: 9/17/08 12:50:14   T: 9/21/08 11:02:01

Find the best, most appropriate code(s).

_____

_____

_____

PATIENT: HUMPHREY, DONALD
MRN: HUMPDO01
Date: 19 September 2008

Procedure Performed: Subsequent Inpatient Visit

Physician: Patrick B. Reynoso, MD

The patient was admitted for surgery on September 17, 2008, and underwent a right parieto-occipital ventricular peritoneal shunt placement with a Hakim valve, which was programmed to 60 mm after CSF manometry demonstrated higher pressures. The procedure was uneventful. Postoperatively, the patient was awake, alert, and conversant. His postoperative CT scan demonstrated excellent position of the ventriculostomy catheter and the ventricles without the evidence of hemorrhage. The patient was noted to have a marked improvement in his gait according to his family within 12 hours of surgery. He had no headaches, and he was felt to be sufficiently stable. He is able to be discharged home for outpatient follow-up. His condition at discharge was stable/improved.

Recommendations:
Patient to be seen in the office in one week for removal of external sutures.

Patrick B. Reynoso, MD

PBR/mg   D: 9/19/08 09:50:16   T: 9/20/08 12:55:01

Find the best, most appropriate code(s).

CIPHER, VICTORS, & ASSOCIATES
A Complete Health Care Facility
234 MAIN STREET • ANYTOWN, FL 32711 • 407-555-1234

PATIENT: HUMPHREY, DONALD
MRN: HUMPDO01
Date: 18 September 2008

Procedure Performed: CT Brain w/o Contrast
Radiologist: Michelle H. McNair, MD
Clinical Information: Evaluate for VP shunt, postsurgical
                                No prior studies available for a comparison

Technical Information:
Contiguous 3 mm thick axial images were obtained through the skull base and posterior fossa structures followed by 7 mm thick axial images through the remainder of the brain. The examination was performed without the use of intravenous contrast material.

Interpretation:
Evaluation of the posterior fossa demonstrates bilateral vertebral artery calcification. No abnormal intra or extra-axial collections are noted. There is no evidence of midline shift.

    Analysis of the region of the sella turcica demonstrates calcification, likely atherosclerotic involving the cavernous carotid arteries bilaterally seen on series 2 image 7.

    Supratentorially, the lateral ventricles are prominent in size. A ventriculostomy catheter is seen coursing from the region of the post central sulcus with its distal tip terminating within the frontal horn of the right lateral ventricle abutting the septum pellucidum. Hypodensity is seen within the periventricular white matter particularly abutting the frontal horns of the lateral ventricles bilaterally. There is a mild degree of cerebral volume loss. No abnormal intra or extra-axial collections are noted.

    Evaluation of the visualized skull and paranasal sinuses demonstrates a right parietal burr hole defect for placement of the patient's ventriculostomy catheter. A subcutaneous ventriculostomy valve is seen on series 2 image 23.

Recommendations:
1. There is mild prominence of the lateral ventricles bilaterally without evidence of dilation of the cerebral aqueduct or fourth ventricle.

Michelle H. McNair, MD

MHM/mg   D: 9/18/08 09:50:16   T: 9/20/08 12:55:01

Find the best, most appropriate code(s).

_____

_____

_____

Part 4   Practicum

CIPHER, VICTORS, & ASSOCIATES
A Complete Health Care Facility
234 MAIN STREET • ANYTOWN, FL 32711 • 407-555-1234

PATIENT: VANCE, NICOLE
MRN: VANCNI01
Admission Date: 1 September 2008
Discharge Date: 3 September 2008

Procedure Performed: Newborn Evaluation

Attending Physician: Pravdah H. Jeppard, MD

The patient is a female, gestational age 39 weeks, 4 days, born vaginally in this facility, 9/1/08, 02:35.

Impression:
Neonate was of a single birth, BWT 2,857 grams without significant OR procedures with a normal newborn diagnosis. 19″ long. Head circumference: 32 cm. Amniotic fluid: clear. Cord: 3 vessels. Evidence of a benign tumor of blood vessels; due to malformed angioblastic tissues (vascular hamartomas) at right groin. Appears pale, poor skin turgor, mucousy, and transitional stool.
    Apgar Score: 1 min = 9; 5 min = 9. Heart rate: >100; Respiratory Effort: Good, Muscle tone: Active, Response to catheter in nostril: Cough, Color: Body pink, extremities blue

Maternal History:
30 yo, G1, blood type O+, spontaneous labor, 16 h, 24 min, Epidural anesthesia, HIV tested during pregnancy: neg

Administrations:
Hepatitis B, Peds Vaccine (Recomb) 5 mcg/0.5 ml, given: 9/2/08
Newborn hearing screening: passed.

Recommendations:
Follow-up in office 2 days

_____

Pravdah H. Jeppard, MD

PHJ/mg   D: 9/01/08 09:50:16   T: 9/05/08 12:55:01

Find the best, most appropriate code(s).

_____

_____

_____

CIPHER, VICTORS, & ASSOCIATES
A Complete Health Care Facility
234 MAIN STREET • ANYTOWN, FL 32711 • 407-555-1234

PATIENT: VANCE, NICOLE
MRN: VANCNI01
Procedure Date: 1 September 2008

Procedure Performed: Newborn routine pathological evaluation

Laboratory Technician: Constance L. Hall

Attending Physician: Pravdah H. Jeppard, MD

GENERAL CHEMISTRY:
    BILI TOTAL   7.1   (0.0–10.0)   M
    BILIRUBIN DIRECT 0.6   (0.0–0.6)   M

SEROLOGY/IMMUNOLOGY STUDIES:
    SYPHILIS   RPR   NON-REAC   (NON-REAC)

BLOOD BANK:
    ANTIBODY SCREENING AND TESTING   DIRECT ANTIGLOB   NEG

CORD BLOOD EVALUATION:
    DIRECT ANTIGLOB   NEGATIVE

Constance L. Hall

CLH/mg   D: 9/01/08 09:50:16   T: 9/05/08 12:55:01

Find the best, most appropriate code(s).

_____

_____

_____

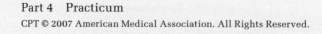

Part 4   Practicum

CIPHER, VICTORS, & ASSOCIATES
A Complete Health Care Facility
234 MAIN STREET • ANYTOWN, FL 32711 • 407-555-1234

PATIENT: KLAUSING, CLARENCE
MRN: KLAUCL01
Admission Date: 15 October 2008

Attending Physician: Tracy R. Stover, MD
Location: Emergency Department visit

History of Present Illness:
The patient is a 37-year-old white male with underlying acquired immunodeficiency syndrome, whom we initially evaluated in the Emergency Room this past Friday with complaints of right-sided back pain radiating to the anterior abdominal wall. On examination, blisters were noted compatible with the diagnosis of herpes zoster. The patient was started on oral Zovirax at a dose of 800 mg five times a day, plus Percocet for pain.

Over the weekend, the patient began complaining of nausea, vomiting, and inability to continue taking the medications, accompanied by constipation. The patient called in today with these complaints, and we asked the patient to come into the hospital for admission for intravenous therapy and management of this problem.

Past Medical History:
He has been human immunodeficiency virus positive for 3-1/2 years. The patient is originally from Chicago and has been 1-1/2 years here. Currently, he is not being followed by any physician for his underlying problem. He cannot recall his last CD4 count.

Prior medical problems include a history of oral candidiasis, but he denies any sexually transmitted diseases, PCP or other opportunistic infections. At age four, he had trauma to the left eye, causing his eye to be completely opacified. He has been previously treated with AZT and D4T.

Allergies:
He has no known drug allergies.

Social History:
He is divorced. He is currently living with a friend of many years. He has two children with his first marriage, ages 10 and 8. He smokes one pack of cigarettes per day for the last 15 years. He denies any alcohol use. He has a prior history of intravenous drug use—cocaine—but according to him, he has been clean for the last 3-1/2 years. He has no pets. He has been disabled secondary to his eye trauma.

Family History:
The family history is essentially noncontributory.

Physical Exam:
Appearance: The patient is alert and oriented times three, complaining of pain.
Head: Normocephalic.
Eyes: The right eye pupil is reactive. The left eye is completely opacified secondary to prior trauma.
Ears: Unremarkable.
Nose: Unremarkable.
Mouth/Tongue/Pharynx: The patient has complete upper dentures. No oral lesions detected, i.e., candidiasis or oral hairy leukoplakia.
Lungs: Clear to auscultation.
Cardiovascular: The heart is rhythmic, with no murmurs or gallops.
Abdomen: His abdomen is flat, soft, nontender, with no palpable organomegaly.
Genitalia: The examination is normal. He is circumcised. The testicles are bilaterally descended, with no lesions detected.

(Continued)

Extremities: Both lower extremities—good peripheral pulses and no edema.

Skin: He has numerous blisters and bullae on the right side of his body, approximately at the level of T10-T12, midline upper back going down to the anterior portion of the abdomen at the same level. Blisters with surrounding erythema. He has no other lesions.

Neurological: Nonfocalized.

Diagnoses:
1. Herpes zoster involving T10–T12 dermatome.
2. Nausea/vomiting secondary to oral medications.
3. History of being positive with the human immunodeficiency virus.

Plan/Recommendations:
1. Admit to the hospital for initiation of intravenous Acyclovir plus analgesics for pain management.
2. Domeboro compresses have also been ordered.

Tracy R. Stover, MD

TRS/mg   D: 10/15/08 09:50:16   T: 10/20/08 12:55:01

Find the best, most appropriate code(s).

Part 4   Practicum

CIPHER, VICTORS, & ASSOCIATES
A Complete Health Care Facility
234 MAIN STREET • ANYTOWN, FL 32711 • 407-555-1234

PATIENT: KLAUSING, CLARENCE
MRN: KLAUCL01
Admission Date: 16 October 2008

Procedures/Testing: Pathology and Lab

Laboratory Technician: Patrick Jensen
Attending Physician: Tracy R. Stover, MD

Hematology:

WBC	4.2L	5.1	4.8-10.8 K/UL
RBC	5.12	5.15	4.7-6.1 M/UL
HGB	15.5	15.3	14-18 G/DL
HCT	44.9	43.8	42-52 %
PLT	200,000/mm^3	200,000/mm^3	150,000–400,000/mm^3

Immuno/Serol:

RPR	NR	NR=NON-REACTIVE
CMV IGM	PEND	NEG
TOXOPLASMOS IGM	PEND	NEG

Patrick Jensen

PJ/mg   D: 10/16/08 09:50:16   T: 10/16/08 12:55:01

Find the best, most appropriate code(s).

_____

_____

_____

PATIENT: REILLY, BARBARA
MRN: REILBA01
Admission Date: 02 October 2008

Attending Physician: Charles L. Beckman, MD

History of Present Illness:
This is the first Barton Hospital admission for this 63-year-old female, with a known history of hypertension, depression, hypothyroidism, and kidney stones. The patient developed symptoms of frequency with dysuria for several days associated with mild flank discomfort. She has been taking cranberry juice, hoping for resolution of symptoms. The severe right flank pain occurred yesterday, associated with several bouts of vomiting. The patient presented to the emergency room, and at that time her evaluation included an IVP, which showed an obstructing calculus at the right ureterovesicular junction and with a urinalysis that was positive. The patient was admitted for IV fluid, pain control, and urological evaluation.

Past Medical History:
Includes hypertension, hypothyroidism, depression, and history of kidney stones—last bout several years ago. She has no history of myocardial infarction.

Social History:
The patient is a truck driver. She is a heavy smoker with a 45-pack year history. She drinks daily.

Review of Systems:
Negative for fever or chills. There is no hematuria, but there is dysuria and flank pain, as described in HPI. She has no chest pain, no exertional shortness of breath, no melena, no hematemesis, no headaches, or blurred vision.

Physical Exam:
General: She is currently quite comfortable in bed. She is in no pain.
Vital Signs: Blood pressure 120/80, she is afebrile, respirations 18 and not labored.
HEENT: Normocephalic, Atraumatic. Pupils equal, round and reactive to light. Conjunctive not injected.
Neck: Supple, no JVD, no carotid bruits
Lungs: Clear
Cardiac: Normal S1, S2, without S3, S4, murmurs, gallops or rubs
Abdomen: Soft, normoactive bowel sounds. Negative hepatosplenomegaly.
Extremities: Without cyanosis, clubbing, or edema
GU: Unremarkable
Lab Results: IVP report, as stated above. Her urinalysis is positive for white cells and red cells. Her electrolytes today showed a sodium of 136, potassium 3.6, chloride 97, bicarb 30, glucose 106, BUN 18, creatinine 1.5, calcium 8.5. White count 9.5

Diagnoses:
1. Renal calculus with obstruction

(Continued)

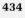

Assessment:

1. This is a 63-year-old, who is presenting with a bout of renal calculus with obstruction, associated with a urinary tract infection. She has not passed a stone, as evidenced by repeat KUB, and she is tentatively scheduled for retrograde studies with laser lithotripsy in the AM by the urologist. In the interim, will continue with parenteral antibiotic coverage, IV fluid, and antibiotics.
2. Hypothyroidism. Will resume Synthroid replacement.
3. History of hypertension, currently controlled. Continue with antihypertensive therapy.
4. Perform an EKG and chest x-ray, 2 views, to complete pre-op evaluation
5. NPO pending surgery
6. Control patient's blood pressure with IV Aldomet until postoperatively.

Charles L. Beckman, MD

CLB/mg   D: 10/02/08 09:50:16   T: 10/05/08 12:55:01

Find the best, most appropriate code(s).

CIPHER, VICTORS, & ASSOCIATES
A Complete Health Care Facility
234 MAIN STREET • ANYTOWN, FL 32711 • 407-555-1234

PATIENT: REILLY, BARBARA
MRN: REILBA01
Date: 03 October 2008

Attending Physician: Charles L. Beckman, MD

Reason for Exam: Stent Placement
Radiologist: Neal R. Williams, MD

Examination:
Abdomen Single View
Two films are submitted. Supine view of the abdomen including pelvis demonstrates contrast material within the urinary bladder, which is smooth in contour with no filling defects seen.
    Film #1: A nonspecific bowel gas pattern and faint calcification over the right hemipelvis.
    Film #2: A double pigtail ureteral stent has been placed. The proximal pigtail ureteral stent appears to be somewhat low in position and is likely in the proximal ureter. The stones have apparently been removed.

Impression:
Contrast material has cleared the kidneys such that status of the right renal collecting structures again cannot be ascertained. Suggest a right renal sonogram in further evaluation of suspected right-sided hydronephrosis. A right retrograde pyelogram could also be obtained to determine the site of suspected ureteral obstruction.

Neal R. Williams, MD

NRW/mg   D: 10/03/08 09:50:16   T: 10/04/08 12:55:01

Find the best, most appropriate code(s).

_____

_____

_____

Part 4   Practicum

CIPHER, VICTORS, & ASSOCIATES
A Complete Health Care Facility
234 MAIN STREET • ANYTOWN, FL 32711 • 407-555-1234

PATIENT: REILLY, BARBARA
MRN: REILBA01
Date: 03 October 2008

Attending Physician: Charles L. Beckman, MD

Reason for Exam: MD order—pre-op clearance
Radiologist: Neal R. Williams, MD

Examination:
1. Chest two views
   Chest—PA and lateral views.
   Clinical history states evaluation, kidney stone with obstruction.
   Slightly elongated thoracic aorta. Prominent left ventricle. No pulmonary vascular congestion. No acute inflammatory infiltrates in the lungs.
   There are orthopedic screws transfixing the acromioclavicular joint, probably related with old shoulder fracture.
2. ECG, 12 leads
   Unremarkable.

_____

Neal R. Williams, MD

NRW/mg D: 10/03/08 09:50:16 T: 10/04/08 12:55:01

Find the best, most appropriate code(s).

_____

_____

_____

CIPHER, VICTORS, & ASSOCIATES
A Complete Health Care Facility
234 MAIN STREET • ANYTOWN, FL 32711 • 407-555-1234

PATIENT: REILLY, BARBARA
MRN: REILBA01
Date: 03 October 2008

Attending Physician: Charles L. Beckman, MD

Reason for Exam: Groin pain
Radiologist: Neal R. Williams, MD

Examination:
IVP with Tomo
Intravenous pyelogram

There are several calcifications of the pelvis. There is one which is somewhat triangular shaped and measures approximately 8 mm in length and approximately 5 mm in diameter in the region of the right side of the pelvis in the proximal course of the right ureter.

There is prompt function on the left side and prompt filling of a normal appearing collecting system with dumping into the urinary bladder.

The right kidney has not begun functioning, even on the 30-minute delayed film. I suspect that this is because the calcification described above represents an obstructing distal right ureterovesical junction calculus.

We plan to obtain additional radiographs, and addendum reports will be issued.

Neal R. Williams, MD

NRW/mg   D: 10/03/08 09:50:16   T: 10/04/08 12:55:01

Find the best, most appropriate code(s).

_____

_____

_____

Part 4   Practicum

CIPHER, VICTORS, & ASSOCIATES
A Complete Health Care Facility
234 MAIN STREET • ANYTOWN, FL 32711 • 407-555-1234

PATIENT: REILLY, BARBARA
MRN: REILBA01
Date: 03 October 2008

Attending Physician: Charles L. Beckman, MD

Preoperative Diagnosis: Right ureteral calculus
Postoperative Diagnosis: Same
Operative Procedure: Cystoscopy, right retrograde pyelogram, ureteroscopy, Holmium laser
lithotripsy, and double-J stent placement

Surgeon: Sarah Lyndale, MD

Assistant:
Anesthesiologist: Lorenzo Garrett, MD
Anesthesia: General

Description of Operation:
The patient was prepped and draped in the usual manner after induction of general anesthesia. Examination of the anterior urethra using a 21 French cystourethroscope revealed no anterior lesions or strictures. Examination of the bladder revealed normal bladder mucosa, however, bulging of the intramural ureter was prominent on the right side. After the bladder was examined, using the 30° and 70° lens of the cystoscope, a #8 French cone-tipped catheter was inserted in the right ureteral orifice. Under fluoroscopic control, the contrast material was instilled. Stone was noted to be impacted in the distal intramural ureter with proximal hydronephrosis. Next, a 0.35 glide wire followed by a guide wire introducer and a second glide wire were introduced under fluoroscopic and x-ray control. The balloon dilators were used, 4 cm in size, to dilate the intramural ureter. The mini-ureteroscope was then inserted under direct vision and the stone was identified in the distal ureter and impacted in the wall. Using the Holmium dye laser, lithotripsy at 3–4 watts range for 414 seconds at 2,070 hertz with a total joules of 489.2. The stone fragmented and most of the stone material washed out and could not be easily retrieved. The stone appeared to be uric acid in nature. At this point, although no stone fragments could actually be basketed, a 7x26 double-J ureteral stent was placed under fluoroscopic and x-ray control and noted to be in the proximal upper ureter, which was quite tortuous because of previous hydronephrosis, and in the bladder. The string was brought out externally. The bladder was then emptied. A #15 French Foley catheter was passed. The patient was brought to the recovery room in fair condition.

Sarah Lyndale, MD

SL/mg   D: 10/03/08 09:50:16   T: 10/04/08 12:55:01

Find the best, most appropriate code(s).

_____

_____

_____

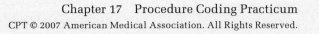

CIPHER, VICTORS, & ASSOCIATES
A Complete Health Care Facility
234 MAIN STREET • ANYTOWN, FL 32711 • 407-555-1234

PATIENT: REILLY, BARBARA
MRN: REILBA01
Date: 03 October 2008

Attending Physician: Charles L. Beckman, MD

Scheduled Medications: MD order

MEDICATIONS:
 Levofloxacin, 250 mg, IV
 Ciprofloxacin 500 mg IV (Cipro)
 Compazine, 10 mg, IM
 Meperidine HCL 75 mg, IM
 Hydroxyzine HCL 100 mg IM

_____

David C. Samuels, RN

DCS/mg D: 10/03/08 09:50:16 T: 10/04/08 12:55:01

Find the best, most appropriate code(s).

_____

_____

_____

CIPHER, VICTORS, & ASSOCIATES
A Complete Health Care Facility
234 MAIN STREET • ANYTOWN, FL 32711 • 407-555-1234

PATIENT: FLEMINGTON, EUGENE
MRN: FLEMEU01
Date: 11 November 2008

Attending Physician: Pravdah H. Jeppard, MD

Transportation: Acute care—MD order
Receiving Facility: Harrison Medical Center
Sending Facility: Barton Hospital
Diagnosis: Hyponatremia, hypopotassemia, fever, anemia
Transportation Protocol: Pediatric ALS, nonemergency
Patient Age: 17 months
Mileage: 12

Joleen L. Abernathy, EMT

JLA/mg   D: 11/11/08 09:50:16   T: 11/11/08 12:55:01

Find the best, most appropriate code(s).

PATIENT: FLEMINGTON, EUGENE

MRN: FLEMEU01

Date: 11 November 2008

Attending Physician: Pravdah H. Jeppard, MD

History of Present Illness:
The patient is a 17-month-old male brought in by ambulance. Pt has fever over 101°, nonproductive cough, and vomiting for the past 6 days. He was seen by his primary care physician, Dr. Golden, and started on antibiotics for otitis media. Also, Dr. Golden notes that the child's abdomen has been getting distended.

Patient is developmental on track for age, with no signs of impairment. Since illness began, patient is noted to be lethargic. Decreased appetite 6 days, when started to get sick.

Allergies:
NKA

Physical Examination:
Patient is alert and crying. Abdomen distended. Tympanic membrane diffused. Bowel sounds are hypoactive; last BM 6 days ago.

Pupils are equal and reactive. Breath sounds are clear, breathing regular.

Skin is warm, heart rhythm is regular, peripheral pulses normal, edema none.

HR 174, R 36, T 100.4°

Diagnosis:
Hyponatremia, hypopotassemia, fever, anemia

Testing/Procedures:
CBC, comprehensive metabolic panel, performed. Results pending.

Recommendations:
Admission to pediatric unit for observation

Pravdah H. Jeppard, MD

PHJ/mg   D: 11/11/08 09:50:16   T: 11/11/08 12:55:01

Find the best, most appropriate code(s).

_____

_____

_____

Part 4   Practicum

CIPHER, VICTORS, & ASSOCIATES
A Complete Health Care Facility
234 MAIN STREET • ANYTOWN, FL 32711 • 407-555-1234

PATIENT: FLEMINGTON, EUGENE
MRN: FLEMEU01
Date: 12 November 2008

Radiologist: Pedro L. Pacheco, MD

Attending Physician: Pravdah H. Jeppard, MD

Examination: Chest and abdomen
Clinical History: Fever

Chest:
AP supine and lateral films demonstrate no evidence of alveolar infiltrate or consolidation or pleural effusion. The mediastinal structures are not enlarged. There is very mild increase in central bronchovascular markings. There is no evidence of focal destructive bone lesion.

Impression:
No infiltrate.

Abdomen:
Supine and erect films demonstrate mild to moderate dilatation of loops of small bowel with short air/fluid levels on the erect film. The large bowel is within normal limits in size but is visualized to the level of the splenic flexure. There is no air visualized in the remainder of the colon. The findings are not specific but consistent with ileus. Further clinical correlation is advised. There is no evidence of focal destructive bone lesion. There is no suspicious calcification in the upper abdomen.

Impressions:
Abdominal bowel pattern, not specific, consistent with ileus.

Pedro L. Pacheco, MD

PLP/mg   D: 11/12/08 09:50:16   T: 11/12/08 12:55:01

Find the best, most appropriate code(s).

CIPHER, VICTORS, & ASSOCIATES
A Complete Health Care Facility
234 MAIN STREET • ANYTOWN, FL 32711 • 407-555-1234

PATIENT: FLEMINGTON, EUGENE
MRN: FLEMEU01
Date: 12 November 2008

Attending Physician: Pravdah H. Jeppard, MD

Patient Services:
    IV fluid replacement for dehydration, intravenous
    Continuous pulse oximetry
    Therapeutic warm water enema for intussusception

Renee K. McDonald, RN

RKM/mg   D: 11/12/08 09:50:16   T: 11/12/08 12:55:01

Find the best, most appropriate code(s).

_____

_____

_____

CIPHER, VICTORS, & ASSOCIATES
A Complete Health Care Facility
234 MAIN STREET • ANYTOWN, FL 32711 • 407-555-1234

Patient Name: GERRERRA, RAUL
MRN: GERRRA01
Date: 27 October 2008

Physical Therapist: Kevin Bryant

Attending Physician: Harvey Bradshaw, MD

DX: Postsurgical Carpal Tunnel Release LT
Type of Therapy: Occupational Therapy (Hand) B. I. W. x 3 week

Visit # 1/6
Reported Pain Level: 5/10
Patient Reports: "I am still having pain in my hand and fingers."

1. Ultrasound for 6 minutes, 3 mgHz, 0.4 u/cm2 100% to scar at LT CT area
2. Massage: Retrograde, 3 minutes to LT hand
3. Manual therapy: soft tissue mobilization, 5 minutes to scar at LT wrist
4. AROM and Stretching
5. Therapeutic Exercise: 12 minutes tendon glides, joint blocking, digit extension, median nerve glides and desensitization with cold towels (tolerated up until #6)

Pain Level: 4–5/10 Pt. still with heavy scar tissue adhesions in CT area. Pt still having pain in fingertips and numbness, reportedly up arm and into his neck.

Kevin Bryant

KB/mg   D: 10/27/08 09:50:16   T: 10/29/08 12:55:01

Find the best, most appropriate code(s).

_____

_____

_____

CIPHER, VICTORS, & ASSOCIATES
A Complete Health Care Facility
234 MAIN STREET • ANYTOWN, FL 32711 • 407-555-1234

Patient Name: GERRERRA, RAUL
Account #:   GERRERA01
Date: 3 November 2008

Physical Therapist: Kevin Bryant

Attending Physician: Harvey Bradshaw, MD

DX: Postsurgical Carpal Tunnel Release LT
Type of Therapy: Occupational Therapy (Hand) B. I. W. x 3 weeks

Visit # 3/6
Reported Pain Level: 5/10
Patient Reports: "The scar still feels very hard, and when I rest my palm on something, it is very uncomfortable."

1. Cold pack
2. Fluidotherapy: 15 minutes LT hand
3. Massage: Retrograde, 4 minutes to LT hand and wrist
4. Manual therapy: soft tissue mobilization, scar tissue 8 minutes MFR to scar at LT wrist
5. AROM, AAROM, PROM, and Stretching: Gentle carpal stretches
6. Therapeutic Exercise: 10 minutes of wrist AROM, joint blocking, place + hold FDS glides, rubber band–finger extensions, desensitizing (rods and rice bucket).

Pain Level: 4/10. Pt demonstrated decreased scar tissue adhesions at wrist scar. Pt did not tolerate rubber band exercises well.

Kevin Bryant

KB/mg   D: 11/03/08 09:50:16   T: 11/05/08 12:55:01

Find the best, most appropriate code(s).

_____

_____

_____

Part 4   Practicum
CPT © 2007 American Medical Association. All Rights Reserved.

Patient Name: PHELPS, MAXINE
Account #:   PHELMA01
Date: 13 December 2008

Attending Physician: Yamira E. Newadha, MD
Location: Office

History of Present Illness: This is a 51-year-old female who a month ago noted a lump in her right breast (8 o'clock position of the right breast just outside the areola). This prompted bilateral screening mammography. The mammo demonstrated a linear area of increased density and architectural distortion at the 12 o'clock position in the right periareolar region.

This was suspicious mammographically, and a biopsy of this was recommended. The patient had follow-up ultrasound as well. The ultrasound demonstrated a lobulated cyst of 3 mm at the 8 o'clock position corresponding to the patient's area of palpable abnormality. No other lesions were noted.

Due to the mammogram, the patient has an incidental finding of an area of increased density at the 12 o'clock position and requires biopsy. This is not appreciable on examination and requires needle localization and excisional biopsy for which she is here today.

The patient has no family history of breast cancer. Age of menarche 13. She was pregnant three times with one child, first child born at age 20.

Past Medical History: No coronary disease, hypertension, or diabetes
Past Surgical History: None
Medications: None
Allergies: None
Social History: The patient does not smoke, does not drink. No history of drug use.

Physical Examination:
Breasts: The patient examined in erect and supine. Both breast are symmetric. There is no skin dimpling. There is no nipple inversion. There is no mass appreciated in either breast with careful attention paid to the right breast overlying the 8 o'clock region as well as the 12 o'clock region. Again, no mass was appreciated. She has no axillary, cervical, supraclavicular, or infraclavicular adenopathy notes.
Lungs: Clear
Heart: Regular rhythm
Impression: Right breast mass

This is a 51-year-old who has an incidental finding of an area of increased density at the 12 o'clock position of the right breast. This cannot be appreciated on physical examination. She will require needle loc/excisional biopsy. The indication, alternatives, and complications of the procedure have been discussed with this patient. She understands and wishes to proceed.

Yamira E. Newadha, MD

YEM/mg   D: 12/13/08 12:55:01   T: 12/18/08 09:50:16

Find the best, most appropriate code(s).

CIPHER, VICTORS, & ASSOCIATES
A Complete Health Care Facility
234 MAIN STREET • ANYTOWN, FL 32711 • 407-555-1234

Patient Name: PHELPS, MAXINE
Account #:   PHELMA01
Date: 14 December 2008

Radiologist: Harry O. Leu, MD

Attending Physician: Yamira E. Newadha, MD

Examination of: Right Breast Needle localization

Clinical History:
Ridge-like area of increased density in upper right periareolar region; for preoperative localization.
A signed informed consent was obtained from the patient prior to the procedure, after an explanation of the relative benefits, risks, and potential side effects.

     After sterile preparation, a 3 mm Homer Mammalok needle/wire combination was advanced percutaneously via a superior approach, and its tips localized at the site of a ridge-like density in the upper periareolar region, utilization an alphanumeric grid. The wire was advanced through the needle and secured in place. Repeat views confirmed the localization of needle and wire tips to be at the site of the ridge-like density.

     The patient tolerated the procedure well, without immediate complications and left the mammography suite with needle and wire secured in place.

Impression:
Percutaneous needle/wire localization of ridge-like right upper periareolar density.

Harry O. Leu, MD

HOL/mg   D: 12/14/08 12:55:01   T: 12/18/08 09:50:16

Find the best, most appropriate code(s).

_____

_____

_____

CIPHER, VICTORS, & ASSOCIATES
A Complete Health Care Facility
234 MAIN STREET • ANYTOWN, FL 32711 • 407-555-1234

Patient Name:	PHELPS, MAXINE
Account #:	PHELMA01
Date:	15 December 2008
Preoperative Diagnosis:	Right Breast Mass
Postoperative Diagnosis:	Same (pending pathology)
Operation:	Excision of right breast mass, intermediate wound closure—4 cm
Surgeon:	Roweena L. Macomba, MD
Assistant:	None
Anesthesiologist:	Terence Abnernathy, MD
Anesthesia:	MAC/1% lidocaine diluted 50% with bicarbonate (10 cc)

History:
This is a 51-year-old female admitted to the minor surgery suite for excision of a 3 cm palpable nodule in the superficial aspect of the right breast in the 12 o'clock axis near the periphery. The indications, alternatives and possible complications were reviewed, and consent was obtained.

Procedure:
With the patient in the supine position, the area in question was prepped and draped in the usual sterile fashion using Betadine. After adequate IV sedation, 1% lidocaine without epinephrine was used to infiltrate the soft tissues at that level to create a field block.

An elliptical incision was made about the lesion itself, considering its intimate association with the overlying skin. The 4 cm incision was deepened into the subcutaneous space. The mass was excised in its entirety with a rim of normal appearing breast, fat, and surrounding skin. Adequate hemostasis was secured within the depths of the wound. The wound was closed in layers. The deeper breast tissue was approximated using interrupted 3-0 chromic sutures. The subcuticular layer was approximated using interrupted 4-0 Biosyn sutures. The skin edges were closed using 4-0 Vicryl in the subcuticular space in a continuous fashion. Mastisol and Steri-Strips were applied. A dressing was applied. The procedure was terminated. Needle, sponge and instrument counts were correct. Estimated blood loss was minimal.

Disposition:
The patient tolerated the procedure and was discharged from the minor operating department in satisfactory condition.

Roweena L. Macomba, MD

RLM/mg   D: 12/15/08 12:55:01   T: 12/18/08 09:50:16

Find the best, most appropriate code(s).

_____

_____

_____

CIPHER, VICTORS, & ASSOCIATES
A Complete Health Care Facility
234 MAIN STREET • ANYTOWN, FL 32711 • 407-555-1234

Patient Name: PHELPS, MAXINE
Account #:   PHELMA01
Date: 15 December 2008

Preoperative Diagnosis: Right Breast Mass
Postoperative Diagnosis: Same (pending pathology)
Operation: Excision of right breast mass, intermediate wound closure—4 cm

Surgeon: Roweena L. Macomba, MD

Assistant: None
Anesthesiologist: Terence Abnernathy, MD
Anesthesia: MAC/1% lidocaine diluted 50% with bicarbonate (10 cc)

History:
This is a 51-year-old female admitted to the minor surgery suite for excision of a 3 cm palpable nodule in the superficial aspect of the right breast in the 12 o'clock axis near the periphery. The indications, alternatives and possible complications were reviewed, and consent was obtained.

Procedure:
With the patient in the supine position, the area in question was prepped and draped in the usual sterile fashion using Betadine. After adequate IV sedation, 1% lidocaine without epinephrine was used to infiltrate the soft tissues at that level to create a field block.

    Vital signs were maintained at an acceptable level.

    The patient tolerated the procedure and was discharged from the minor operating department in satisfactory condition.

Terence Abnernathy, MD

TA/mg   D: 12/15/08 12:55:01   T: 12/18/08 09:50:16

Find the best, most appropriate code(s).

Part 4   Practicum

CIPHER, VICTORS, & ASSOCIATES
A Complete Health Care Facility
234 MAIN STREET • ANYTOWN, FL 32711 • 407-555-1234

Patient Name: BATCHELDER, LINDA
Account #:   BATCLI01
Date: 24 November 2008

Consulting Physician: Robert R. Forester, MD
Attending Physician: Giselle R. Usher, MD
Reason for Consultation: Retroperitoneal abscess

History of Present Illness: The patient is well known to me from her earlier hospitalization. This is a s 73-year-old white female with a past history of metastatic follicular carcinoma of the thyroid who had been recently treated for superior vena cava syndrome and obstruction with anticoagulation. At that time, she developed a febrile illness, at which time infectious diseases department was consulted.

It turned out that an infectious disease workup was negative, and it was felt that she had an underlying autoimmune type basis to her fever and was put on prednisone. On the prednisone, her fever resolved and all the other symptoms resolved, and she had been doing quite well.

In the interim, it was determined that she did have metastatic thyroid carcinoma disease and so, she was admitted on 11/24/08 for radioactive iodine therapy. However, during the physical examination at the clinic yesterday, Dr. Harrel discovered an abdominal mass. The patient had, totally, no symptoms from this mass. She denied any history of trauma; denied fevers, chills, sweats, or other systemic symptoms. She had been doing quite well actually since going home on low-dose maintenance prednisone therapy.

A CT was done that showed a retroperitoneal mass, and a CT-guided biopsy was done this morning that revealed rank pus. She subsequently underwent drainage of 500 cc of grossly purulent material, described as pea-green soup. We are now asked to consult to help with the antibiotic management. The fluid did not apparently appear to be foul smelling but did look green and thick.

The patient, again, continues to deny any fevers, chills, sweats, or systemic symptoms. At the time the subsequent drainage was done today, two drainage catheters were placed into the abscess. She experienced hypotension, nausea, and diaphoresis, which resolved with some fluid boluses. She is now in the intermediate care for further management because of the episode of hypotension and a concern of sepsis.

Again, on talking to the patient, she denies any history of trauma to the area. She denies any history of abdominal pain, fevers, chills, sweats, nausea, vomiting, diarrhea, or systemic symptoms. She has no past history of diverticulitis or diverticular disease. She has not had any diarrhea or abdominal pain.

The preliminary gram stain results shows a few white blood cells; no organisms. Cultures are pending.

Her white count at this time was 12,800, with a left shift but she is on oral prednisone. The sedimentation rate was 42. The PT was 12.4 and the PTT is 25. The chemistries are remarkable for a glucose of 115, albumin of 3.6, cholesterol of 235, and the liver function tests were normal.

Past Medical History: As stated, the past medical history is significant for follicular cell carcinoma of the thyroid, status post subtotal thyroidectomy, 10/08/08; status post right internal jugular repair from tumor invasion into the jugular; and biopsy of mediastinal metastatic disease. The patient also has a history of superior vena cava syndrome, status post her carcinoma. She is status post mastectomy for breast carcinoma in 07/05. She has post thoracotomy syndrome in 03/08, with fever and effusion, which resolved. She has a history of a small clot at the site of the venogram entry of the left leg. She had been on Coumadin and may possibly have had a retroperitoneal bleed. She also has a history of hypocalcemia secondary to her thyroidectomy and is on calcium maintenance.

Medications: Her medications at this time include Nolvadex 10 mg po bid; Os-Cal 1000 mg po tid; Rocaltrol 0.25 mcg po bid; and prednisone 10 mg po qam.

Allergies: She is allergic to penicillin and sulfa.

(Continued)

Review of Systems: As stated, the review of systems is essentially unremarkable. She denies fevers, chills, sweats, abdominal pain, nausea, vomiting, and diarrhea. The fevers had resolved on the prednisone.

Physical Exam: B/P: 100/60; P 90; T 98.4

Appearance: Alert, oriented, 73-year-old female lying in bed, in no acute distress
Head: Normocephalic, atraumatic
Eyes: Pupils are equal, round, and reactive to light and accommodation. Extraocular movements full.
Mouth/tongue/pharynx: Throat clear, no thrush or exudates.
Neck: Supple. No stiffness
Lungs: Few crackles at both bases. Scattered rhonchi bilaterally. Good air exchange.
Cardiovascular: Regular rhythm. Normal S1 and S2. No murmurs.
Abdomen: Soft. Some tenderness in the right middle quadrant, with two drainage catheters in place and no definite mass appreciated at this time.
Extremities: No joint effusions or deformities. Trace edema of the ankles.
Skin: Some scattered ecchymoses. No significant rashes or lesions noted.
Neurological: Grossly normal. No focal deficits.

Impression:
1. Retroperitoneal mass appears to be an abscess; may possibly have been secondary to a possible bleed that secondarily got infected. She has had no preceding systemic signs of infection or trauma to the area. Other etiologies would be some type of relationship to possible abdominal disease, but she has no history of diverticular disease and this would be less likely. The most likely organisms to consider, again, would be staphylococcus, streptococcus, anaerobes, and gut flora.
2. Penicillin allergic.
3. Metastatic thyroid follicular carcinoma; to receive radiation therapy.

Plan/Recommendations:
1. Will start her empirically on intravenous antibiotic therapy with clindamycin and Cipro, which should cover staphylococcus, streptococcus, anaerobes, and gram-negatives, until more culture results are known.
2. Monitor vital signs carefully and supportive care if she becomes hypotensive again.
3. Will check blood cultures as well as urine culture.
4. Would not give radioactive iodine at this time until we have cleared up her infection.

Thanks for this consultation. Will follow.

Robert R. Forester, MD

RRF/mg   D: 11/24/08   T: 11/27/08

CC: Giselle R. Usher, MD

Find the best, most appropriate code(s).

_____

_____

_____

CIPHER, VICTORS, & ASSOCIATES
A Complete Health Care Facility
234 MAIN STREET • ANYTOWN, FL 32711 • 407-555-1234

Patient Name: OSGOOD, BENITA
Account #:   OSGOBE01
Date: 15 September 2008

Attending Physician: Roland F. LaScala, MD

Interval History:
The patient is a 29-year-old female G1 P0 who presents at term with regular uterine contractions. The patient's antepartum course has been uncomplicated to date. Sonogram and amniocentesis were normal. GBS culture was negative.

Physical Examination:

HEENT:	unremarkable
Neck:	supple
Chest:	clear
Abd:	guarded, soft
Contractions:	Q3–4 minutes, 40–50 seconds duration
Membrane:	ruptured @ 2:45 with clear fluids
Vaginal discharge:	"Show"
Vaginal Exam:	3 cm dilated Eff: 80%, Sta: –2
Vital Signs:	T98.7, P82, R20, FHR 130s, Location LLQ
Fetal Status:	Reassuring
Assessment:	Term pregnancy, in spontaneous labor
Plan:	Admit, expectant management for delivery

Roland F. LaScala, MD

RFL/mg   D: 9/15/08   T: 9/20/08

Find the best, most appropriate code(s).

_____

_____

_____

CIPHER, VICTORS, & ASSOCIATES
A Complete Health Care Facility
234 MAIN STREET • ANYTOWN, FL 32711 • 407-555-1234

Patient Name: OSGOOD, BENITA
Account #:   OSGOBE01
Date: 15 September 2008

Attending Physician: Roland F. LaScala, MD

Admission to Labor and Delivery

Pathology and Laboratory:
CBC w/diff & PLT
Hold Clot
Urinalysis

Medications:
IV Ringer's Lactate, 1000 ml @ 125 ml/hr
Oxytocin 10 units in 500 ml, D5W (premixed) to run via infusion device
Fentanyl 200 mcg/100 ml + Ropivacaine (naropin) 0.2% 100 ml premixed bag

Roland F. LaScala, MD

RFL/mg   D: 9/15/08   T: 9/20/08

Find the best, most appropriate code(s).

_____

_____

_____

Patient Name: OSGOOD, BENITA
Account #:   OSGOBE01
Date: 15 September 2008

Attending Physician: Roland F. LaScala, MD

Anesthesia: Epidural
Type of Delivery: NSVD
Condition of Perineum: MLE
Episiotomy: Midline preformed
Vagina/Cervix: Intact
Delivered: Live, single born, female, weight 6 lb, 4 oz
Type of Stimulation: Mouth suction
Condition: Good
Birth Injury: None
Apgar Rating: 1 min = 9
                                          5 min = 9

Roland F. LaScala, MD

RFL/mg   D: 9/15/08   T: 9/20/08

Find the best, most appropriate code(s).

_____

_____

_____

CIPHER, VICTORS, & ASSOCIATES
A Complete Health Care Facility
234 MAIN STREET • ANYTOWN, FL 32711 • 407-555-1234

Patient Name: OSGOOD, BENITA
Account #:   OSGOBE01
Date: 15 September 2008

Anesthesiologist: Sabine Suwani, MD
Anesthesia: Epidural
Type of Delivery: NSVD
Condition of Perineum: MLE
Episiotomy: Midline preformed
Vagina/Cervix: Intact
Delivered: Live, single born, female, weight 6 lb, 4 oz
Type of Stimulation: Mouth suction
Condition: Good
Birth Injury: None
Apgar Rating: 1 min = 9
                        5 min = 9

Sabine Suwani, MD

SS/mg   D: 9/15/08   T: 9/20/08

Find the best, most appropriate code(s).

_____

_____

_____

CIPHER, VICTORS, & ASSOCIATES
A Complete Health Care Facility
234 MAIN STREET • ANYTOWN, FL 32711 • 407-555-1234

Patient Name:	COOKE, CARLEEN
Account #:	COOKCA01
Date:	5 January 2009
Indications:	Ulcerative enterocolitis
Procedure:	Colonoscopy
Attending Physician:	Dean Sing, MD
Instrument:	Olympus video colonoscope CF 100L
Anesthesia:	Versed 4 mg; Demerol 75 mg MAC < 30 min

History: This is a 71-year-old female admitted to the ambulatory surgical center for a colonoscopy. Due to her chronic enterocolitis, she is at high risk for a malignancy of the colon, and therefore, this screening is being done. She has been informed of the nature of the procedure, the risks and consequences, as well as told of alternative procedures. She consents to the procedure.

Procedure: The patient is placed in the left lateral decubitus position. The rectal exam reveals normal sphincter tone and no masses. A colonoscope is introduced into the rectum and advanced to the distal sigmoid colon. Due to a marked fixation and severe angulation of the rectosigmoid colon, the scope could not be advanced any further and the procedure was aborted.

On withdrawal, no masses or polyps are noted, and the mucosa is normal throughout. Retroflexion in the rectal vault is unremarkable.

Disposition: The patient tolerated the procedure and was discharged from the minor operating department in satisfactory condition.

Impressions: Normal colonoscopy, only to the distal sigmoid colon

Plan: Strong recommendation for a barium enema

Dean Sing, MD

DS/mg   D: 01/05/09 12:55:01   T: 01/08/09 09:50:16

Find the best, most appropriate code(s).

_____

_____

_____

PATIENT:	MAGOO, MARGARET
ACCOUNT/EHR #:	MAGOMA01
Date of Operation:	06/17/08
Preoperative Diagnosis:	Nuclear sclerosis 2+ with a 2+ posterior subcapsular cataract, right eye
Postoperative Diagnosis:	same
Operation:	Phacoemulsification of cataract with posterior chamber intraocular lens implantation, right eye
Surgeon:	Mark C. Marcus, MD
Assistant:	Ralph Malphini, MD
Anesthesia:	Local

Description of Operative Procedure:
Local anesthesia was obtained with retrobulbar and modified Van Lint injection using a 50-50 mixture of 4% lidocaine and 0.75% Marcaine with Wydase. A Honan balloon was placed for approximately 15 minutes. The patient was positioned, prepped, and draped in the usual sterile fashion. A wire lid speculum was inserted, and the operating microscope was brought into position. A temporal limbal corneal incision was made with a 2.75 mm keratome, and Viscoat was injected into the anterior chamber. Using a cystotome and Utrata forceps, a continuous tear capsulorrhexis was performed. A limbal paracentesis stab incision was made at 6 o'clock with a diamond blade. Hydrodissection and hydrodelineation of the lens was accomplished with balanced salt solution via cannular injection. Phacoemulsification of the lens proceeded as the lens was sectioned into quadrants with each quadrant removed. Residual lens cortex was removed with irrigation and aspiration. The posterior capsule was polished with an irrigating Graether collar button. Viscoat was injected into the capsular bag, and the cataract incision was opened with the keratome. Using lens-folding forceps, an Alcon, model MA60VM, 6.0 mm optic, 21.5 diopter posterior chamber intraocular lens was inserted into the capsular bag. A Sinskey hook was used to facilitate rotation and centration of the lens. Residual anterior chamber Viscoat was removed with irrigation and aspiration. Balanced salt solution was injected into the anterior chamber, and the wound was observed to be watertight. Subconjunctival Celestone and Cefazolin were injected. Topical Iopidine solution and Maxitrol ophthalmic ointment were instilled. Dressing included eye pad and Fox shield. The patient tolerated the procedure well without complications.

Mark C. Marcus, MD

MCM/mg   D: 06/17/08 09:50:16   T: 06/19/08 12:55:01

Find the best, most appropriate code(s).

_____

_____

_____

CIPHER, VICTORS, & ASSOCIATES
A Complete Health Care Facility
234 MAIN STREET • ANYTOWN, FL 32711 • 407-555-1234

PATIENT: DOE-SMITH, JANE
ACCOUNT/EHR #:   DOESJA01
Date of Operation: 11/9/2008

Preoperative Diagnosis: Hallux limites, right foot
Postoperative Diagnosis: Same
Operation: Shortening, osteotomy, first metatarsal, right foot, with screw fixation and cheilectomy, first metatarsal head, right foot.

Surgeon: Allen Roberston, DPM

Assistant: n/a
Anesthesia: IV sedation with local anesthesia

Description of Operative Procedure:
Following the customary sterile preparation and draping, the right limb was elevated approximately 5 minutes in order to facilitate circulatory drainage at which time the pneumatic cuff, which had previously been placed on her right ankle, was inflated to a pressure of 250 mmHg. The right limb was then placed in the operative position. The operative site was injected with 2% Xylocaine mixed with 0.5% Marcaine. Upon having achieved anesthesia, a curvilinear incision was created on the plantar medial aspect of the first metatarsophalangeal joint of the right foot. The incision was deepened with sharp dissection, traversing veins were cauterized. Capsule was identified on the medial and dorsomedial aspect. Capsule was longitudinally incised on the dorsomedial aspect and meticulously dissected on to expose the head of the first metatarsal into the operative site. At this point, it was noted that the cartilage of the first metatarsal head was healthy; however there was distinct irritation to the dorsal portion of the metatarsal head with an apparent flattening of the metatarsal head secondary to the hallux limites. Using a rongeur, the hypertrophic exuberant portion of the first metatarsal head was resected, and the remaining surface was rasped smooth in order to recreate a ball joint. Using an oscillating saw, an osteotomy was performed from medial to lateral in a V-shaped fashion with the apex centrally located and the dorsal arm longer than the plantar arm. A segment of bone was removed from the dorsal arm in order to shorten and plantar flex the metatarsal head. Upon having done so, two 2.0 mm screws were obliquely driven into the osteotomy site, following range of motion was noted that the osteotomy remained stable. At this point, the hallux had approximately 90 degrees of motion to the metatarsal shaft. The area was copiously irrigated with sterile saline. The capsular tissue was repaired using 4-0 Vicryl; subcutaneous tissue was repaired using 5-0 Vicryl. Operative site was injected with dexamethasone, Betadine-soaked Adaptic was applied to the incision site, sterile gauze, and Kling. The pneumatic cuff was deflated. Normal color, circulation was noted to return to all digits immediately. The patient tolerated the surgery well. Vital signs remained stable throughout the entire procedure. The patient returned to the recovery room in good condition.

Allen Robertson, DPM

AR/mg   D: 11/9/08 09:50:16   T: 11/12/08 12:55:01

Find the best, most appropriate code(s).

_____

_____

_____

CIPHER, VICTORS, & ASSOCIATES
A Complete Health Care Facility
234 MAIN STREET • ANYTOWN, FL 32711 • 407-555-1234

PATIENT: HUNTER, ASHLEY
MRN: HUNTAS01
Admission Date: 7 September 2008
Discharge Date: 8 September 2008
Date: 7 September 2008

Preoperative DX: Stenotic cervical os with hematometrium
Postoperative DX: same
Operation: Cervical dilatation with release of old blood. This was done under ultrasound guidance followed by endometrial curettage.

Surgeon: Rodney L. Cohen, MD

Assistant: None
Anesthesia: General by LMA
Complications: None
Findings: See body of dictation
Specimens: Endometrial curettings to pathology
Disposition: Stable to recovery room

Procedure: The patient was taken to the OR where she was placed in the supine position and administered general anesthesia per LMA. She was then placed in candy-cane stirrups and prepped and draped in the usual sterile fashion. A weighted speculum was placed in the vagina, and with the aid of a Deaver retractor, the anterior portion of the cervix was grasped with single-toothed tenaculum. There were no evident holes or dimples or scenes suggestive of where the external cervical os might be, as the cervix had completely agglutinated across the entire surface. Using lacrimal ducts and gentle tension, the area of suspicion was gently poked until a perforation gave way. This tract was followed with serial dilators until ultimately brown old blood was released ensuring that I was in the right place. This was done with the aid of abdominal ultrasound guidance for the risk of false tracking and missing the endocervical canal uterus was real. The uterus was emptied. The cervix was dilated up to approximate 8 mm. This allowed for free flow of the contained old blood. This was followed by sharp curette of all the uterine lining surfaces. This specimen was captured and sent to pathology. Lastly a small 7 size suction catheter was inserted to ensure the remainder of any old captured blood that may be sitting in the deep recesses of this severely retroverted uterus was obtained and this concluded the case. The instruments were removed. The patient was taken down from cane stirrups. The patient was awakened from anesthesia and taken to the recovery room in stable condition.

9/7/08 11:47:39

Find the best, most appropriate code(s).

_____

_____

_____

Part 4   Practicum

PATIENT: KLOTSKY, STACY
MRN: KLOTST01
Admission Date: 5 October 2008
Discharge Date: 5 October 2008
Date: 5 October 2008

Preoperative DX: Rule out bladder tumor
Postoperative DX: same
Procedure: Cystoscopy, biopsy, and fulguration of bladder

Surgeon: Leonard Dupont, MD

Assistant: None
Anesthesia: Spinal

Indications: The patient is a 73-year-old female with a history of grade II superficial transitional cell carcinoma of the bladder. Cystoscopy showed a suspicious erythematous area on the right trigone. She presented today for cystoscopy, biopsy, and fulguration. Findings—the urethra was normal, the bladder was 1+ trabeculated, the mid and right trigone areas were slightly erythematous and hypervascular. No papillary tumors were noted, no mucosal abnormalities were noted.

Procedure: The patient was placed on the table in supine position. Satisfactory spinal anesthesia was obtained. She was placed in dorsolithotomy position. She was prepped sterilely with Hibiclens and draped in the usual manner. A #22 French cystoscopy sheath was passed per urethra in atraumatic fashion. The bladder was resected with the 70-degree lens with findings as noted above. Cup biopsy forceps were placed, and three biopsies were taken of the suspicious areas of the trigone. These areas were fulgurated with the Bugby electrode; no active bleeding was seen. The scope was removed, the patient was returned to recovery having tolerated the procedure well. Estimated blood loss was minimal.

Pathology report: Chronic cystitis (cystica) with squamous cell metaplasia.

Leonard Dupont, MD

10/5/08 11:47:39

Find the best, most appropriate code(s).

_____

_____

_____

CIPHER, VICTORS, & ASSOCIATES
A Complete Health Care Facility
234 MAIN STREET • ANYTOWN, FL 32711 • 407-555-1234

PATIENT:	DENNISON, DANIEL
MRN:	DENNDA01
Date:	23 November 2008
Procedure Performed:	Vasectomy
Physician:	Sunil Kaladuwa, MD
Indications:	Elective sterilization
Procedure:	The patient was given Versed for anxiety, and local anesthesia was administered. Removal of a segment of the deferent duct was accomplished bilaterally. Patient tolerated the procedure well.
Impression:	Successful outcome
Plan:	Postoperative semen examination is scheduled for one week.

Sunil Kaladuwa, MD

SK/mg   D: 11/23/08 09:50:16   T: 11/25/08 12:55:01

Find the best, most appropriate code(s).

_____

_____

_____

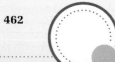

Part 4   Practicum

CIPHER, VICTORS, & ASSOCIATES
A Complete Health Care Facility
234 MAIN STREET • ANYTOWN, FL 32711 • 407-555-1234

PATIENT: KLACKSON, KEVIN
MRN: KLACKE01
Date: 15 September 2008

Diagnosis: Primary cardiomyopathy with chest pain
Procedure: Arterial catheterization

Physician: Frank Vincent, MD

Anesthesia: Local

Procedure: The patient was placed on the table in supine position. Local anesthesia was administered. Once we were assured that the patient had achieved no nervous stimuli, the incision was made and the catheter was introduced percutaneously. The incision was sutured with a simple repair. The patient tolerated the procedure well and was transferred to the recovery room.

_____

Frank Vincent, MD

FV/mg   D: 9/15/08 09:50:16   T: 9/15/08 12:55:01

Find the best, most appropriate code(s).

_____

_____

_____

CIPHER, VICTORS, & ASSOCIATES
A Complete Health Care Facility
234 MAIN STREET • ANYTOWN, FL 32711 • 407-555-1234

PATIENT: GIRALDI, MELODY
MRN: GIRAME01
Date: 02 October 2008

Diagnosis: Lumbar stenosis, Sciatica
Procedure: CMT; Traction, manual

Physician: Roxan K. Paschal, DC

Procedure: The patient was placed on the table.
    Chiropractic manipulative treatment: spinal, thoracic
    Chiropractic manipulative treatment: lower extremity, left
    Manual traction: cervical & lumbar regions x 30 minutes

Roxan K. Paschal, DC

RKP/mg   D: 10/02/08 09:50:16   T: 10/05/08 12:55:01

Find the best, most appropriate code(s).

_____

_____

_____

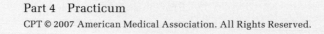

Forms

CMS-1500 CLAIM FORM

CMS-1500 is used for reporting the provision of outpatient and physician services.

1500

HEALTH INSURANCE CLAIM FORM

APPROVED BY NATIONAL UNIFORM CLAIM COMMITTEE 08/05

[ ][ ] PICA   PICA [ ][ ]

| 1. MEDICARE ☐ (Medicare #) | MEDICAID ☐ (Medicaid #) | TRICARE CHAMPUS ☐ (Sponsor's SSN) | CHAMPVA ☐ (Member ID#) | GROUP HEALTH PLAN ☐ (SSN or ID) | FECA BLK LUNG ☐ (SSN) | OTHER ☐ (ID) | 1a. INSURED'S I.D. NUMBER (For Program in Item 1) |

2. PATIENT 'S NAME (Last Name, First Name, Middle Initial)

3. PATIENT 'S BIRTH DATE MM DD YY   SEX   M ☐   F ☐

4. INSURED'S NAME (Last Name, First Name, Middle Initial)

5. PATIENT 'S ADDRESS (No., Street)

6. PATIENT RELATIONSHIP TO INSURED   Self ☐ Spouse ☐ Child ☐ Other ☐

7. INSURED'S ADDRESS (No., Street)

CITY   STATE

8. PATIENT STATUS   Single ☐ Married ☐ Other ☐

CITY   STATE

ZIP CODE   TELEPHONE (Include Area Code) ( )

Employed ☐ Full-Time Student ☐ Part-Time Student ☐

ZIP CODE   TELEPHONE (Include Area Code) ( )

9. OTHER INSURED 'S NAME (Last Name, First Name, Middle Initial)

10. IS PATIENT 'S CONDITION RELATED TO:

11. INSURED'S POLICY GROUP OR FECA NUMBER

a. OTHER INSURED'S POLICY OR GROUP NUMBER

a. EMPLOYMENT? (Current or Previous) ☐ YES ☐ NO

a. INSURED'S DATE OF BIRTH MM DD YY   SEX   M ☐   F ☐

b. OTHER INSURED'S DATE OF BIRTH MM DD YY   SEX   M ☐   F ☐

b. AUTO ACCIDENT?   PLACE (State) ☐ YES ☐ NO

b. EMPLOYER'S NAME OR SCHOOL NAME

c. EMPLOYER'S NAME OR SCHOOL NAME

c. OTHER ACCIDENT? ☐ YES ☐ NO

c. INSURANCE PLAN NAME OR PROGRAM NAME

d. INSURANCE PLAN NAME OR PROGRAM NAME

10d. RESERVED FOR LOCAL USE

d. IS THERE ANOTHER HEALTH BENEFIT PLAN? ☐ YES ☐ NO *If yes*, return to and complete item 9 a-d.

READ BACK OF FORM BEFORE COMPLETING & SIGNING THIS FORM.
12. PATIENT 'S OR AUTHORIZED PERSON'S SIGNATURE I authorize the release of any medical or other information necessary to process this claim. I also request payment of government benefits either to myself or to the party who accepts assignment below.

SIGNED _____ DATE _____

13. INSURED'S OR AUTHORIZED PERSON'S SIGNATURE I authorize payment of medical benefits to the undersigned physician or supplier for services described below.

SIGNED _____

14. DATE OF CURRENT: MM DD YY ◄ ILLNESS (First symptom) OR INJURY (Accident) OR PREGNANCY(LMP)

15. IF PATIENT HAS HAD SAME OR SIMILAR ILLNESS. GIVE FIRST DATE MM DD YY

16. DATES PATIENT UNABLE TO WORK IN CURRENT OCCUPATION MM DD YY   MM DD YY
FROM   TO

17. NAME OF REFERRING PROVIDER OR OTHER SOURCE

17a.
17b. NPI

18. HOSPITALIZATION DATES RELATED TO CURRENT SERVICES MM DD YY   MM DD YY
FROM   TO

19. RESERVED FOR LOCAL USE

20. OUTSIDE LAB? $ CHARGES   ☐ YES ☐ NO

21. DIAGNOSIS OR NATURE OF ILLNESS OR INJURY (Relate Items 1, 2, 3 or 4 to Item 24E by Line)

1. |___.___| 3. |___.___|

2. |___.___| 4. |___.___|

22. MEDICAID RESUBMISSION CODE   ORIGINAL REF. NO.

23. PRIOR AUTHORIZATION NUMBER

24. A. DATE(S) OF SERVICE						B. PLACE OF SERVICE	C. EMG	D. PROCEDURES, SERVICES, OR SUPPLIES (Explain Unusual Circumstances)		E. DIAGNOSIS POINTER	F. $ CHARGES	G. DAYS OR UNITS	H. EPSDT Family Plan	I. ID. QUAL.	J. RENDERING PROVIDER ID. #
From			To					CPT/HCPCS	MODIFIER						
MM	DD	YY	MM	DD	YY										
														NPI	
														NPI	
														NPI	
														NPI	
														NPI	
														NPI	

25. FEDERAL TAX I.D. NUMBER   ☐ SSN ☐ EIN

26. PATIENT 'S ACCOUNT NO.

27. ACCEPT ASSIGNMENT? (For govt. claims, see back) ☐ YES ☐ NO

28. TOTAL CHARGE $

29. AMOUNT PAID $

30. BALANCE DUE $

31. SIGNATURE OF PHYSICIAN OR SUPPLIER INCLUDING DEGREES OR CREDENTIALS (I certify that the statements on the reverse apply to this bill and are made a part thereof.)

SIGNED _____ DATE _____

32. SERVICE FACILITY LOCATION INFORMATION

a. NPI   b.

33. BILLING PROVIDER INFO & PH # ( )

a. NPI   b.

NUCC Instruction Manual available at: www.nucc.org

APPROVED OMB-0938-0999 FORM CMS-1500 (08/05)

CARRIER

PATIENT AND INSURED INFORMATION

PHYSICIAN OR SUPPLIER INFORMATION

UB-04 CLAIM FORM (CMS 1450)

UB-04 is the new form used for reporting the provision of inpatient services. This replaced the UB-92.

Appendix A   Forms

UB-92 CLAIM FORM

UB-92 is an older form used for inpatient services.

APPROVED OMB NO. 0938-0279

UB-92 HCFA-1450   OCR/ORIGINAL

I CERTIFY THE CERTIFICATIONS ON THE REVERSE APPLY TO THIS BILL AND ARE MADE A PART HEREOF.

CPT © 2007 American Medical Association. All Rights Reserved.

CM-1491 CLAIM FORM

CM-1491 is used for reporting the provision of ambulance services.

REQUEST FOR MEDICARE PAYMENT – AMBULANCE
MEDICAL INSURANCE BENEFITS - SOCIAL SECURITY ACT
(SEE INSTRUCTIONS ON BACK - TYPE OR PRINT INFORMATION)

FORM APPROVED
OMB NO 0938-0042

PART 1 – PATIENT TO FILL IN ITEMS 1 THROUGH 6 ONLY

No Part B Medicare Benefits may be paid unless a completed application form has been received as required by existing law and regulations (20 C.F.R. 405-251). NOTICE – Anyone who misrepresents or falsifies essential information requested by this form may upon conviction be subject to fine and imprisonment under Federal law.

COPY FROM YOUR OWN HEALTH INSURANCE CARD *(See Example on Back)*

1 Name of Patient (First Name, Middle Initial, Last Name)

2 Health Insurance Claim No.   ☐ Male   ☐ Female

3 Patient's complete mailing address *(including Apt. No.)* City, State, ZIP code   Telephone Number ( )

4 Was your illness or injury:	Yes	No
a. Connected with your employment?		
b. Result of an auto accident?		
c. Result of other type accident?		

5 If any of your medical expenses will be or could be paid by another insurance organization or government agency, show below

Name and address of organization or agency	Policy or Identification Number

Note: If you **Do Not** want information about this Medicare claim released to the above upon request, check (X) the following block ☐

6 I authorize any holder of medical or other information about me to release to the Social Security Administration and Centers for Medicare & Medicaid Services or its intermediaries or carriers any information needed for this or a related Medicare claim. I permit a copy of this authorization to be used in place of the original, and request payment of medical insurance benefits either to myself or to the party who accepts assignment below.

Signature of patient *(See instructions on reverse where patient is unable to sign)*   Date signed

SIGN HERE ▶

PART II – AMBULANCE SUPPLIER TO FILL IN 7 THROUGH 25

7. Date of Service	☐ Emergency ☐ Admission ☐ Discharge ☐ Outpatient visit	8. Ordered By

9. Description of Illness or Injury *(Describe factors which made ambulance transportation necessary)*

10. Name of Treating Doctor	11. Address and Telephone Number of Doctor

12. Origin of Service	13. Destination of Service

14. Number of Miles	15. Cost per Mile	16. Mileage Charge	
22. Describe special service *(no none leave blank)*		17. Base Rate	
		18. Spec. Serv. Chg. *(Desc. Item 22)*	
23. Name and Address of Supplier *(Number and Street, City, State, ZIP Code)*	Supplier Code	19. Total Charges	
		20. Amount Paid	
	Telephone Number ( )	21. Any Unpaid Balance Due	

24. Assignment of Patient's Bill
☐ I accept assignment *(See reverse)*   ☐ I do not accept assignment

25. Signature of Supplier	Date Signed

CMS-1491 (SC) (01/89)

DEPARTMENT OF HEALTH AND HUMAN SERVICES
CENTERS FOR MEDICARE & MEDICAID SERVICES

ICD-10-PCS

KEY TERMS

Approach
Body part
Body system
Completeness
Device
Expandability
Multiaxial
Qualifier
Root operation term
Standardized terminology

LEARNING OUTCOMES

- Define the objectives that guided the development of ICD-10-PCS.
- Properly interpret the structure of ICD-10-PCS.
- Identify the differences between ICD-9-CM Volume 3 and ICD-10-PCS.
- Recognize the similarities between ICD-9-CM Volume 3 and ICD-10-PCS.
- Discern the circumstances that require CPT codes versus ICD-10-PCS.
- Determine the best, most accurate ICD-10-PCS code.

While not officially adopted yet, ICD-10-PCS is certainly going to be a part of your career. When ICD-9-CM is replaced by ICD-10-CM (a more precise and efficient diagnostic coding system), ICD-9-CM-Volume 3 Procedure Codes will be replaced by the new and improved ICD-10-PCS (International Classification of Diseases, 10th revision, Procedure Coding System).

ICD-10-PCS will be adopted in order to provide more specificity for different procedures, as well as making it easier to incorporate new procedures as they are developed and accepted by health care professionals.

This appendix identifies the distinct benefits of ICD-10-PCS. Then, step by step, the appendix differentiates the way the codes look and are constructed. The notations and explanations, exclusive to ICD-10-PCS, are all reviewed. Examples are provided to illustrate the concepts and elements throughout the chapter.

THE OBJECTIVES FOR ICD-10-PCS

One of the first tasks for the development of ICD-10-PCS was to establish its specific objectives. Four objectives were identified:

1. **Completeness**: A unique code for each procedure and for any possible procedure has been created.
2. **Expandability**: ICD-10-PCS has been developed so it can easily accept new procedures and incorporate them logically into the existing list. It acknowledges the incredible speed with which technology and science are working to develop new treatments and services.
3. **Multiaxial**: The characters used in creating the codes are used consistently within each section and, whenever possible, from section to section.
4. **Standardized terminology**: ICD-10-PCS uses only one meaning for each term, even if multiple meanings are accepted in the industry. In addition, ICD-10-PCS gives you the specific definition as it is intended for those terms.

The successful accomplishment of the four objectives will help ensure that ICD-10-PCS will make coding procedures more accurate, more efficient, and easier to assign.

ICD-10-PCS CODE DESCRIPTIONS

ICD-10-PCS has changed the way codes are described.

1. *Procedure descriptions will no longer include diagnostic information*: Previously, some of the procedure codes included diagnostic statements or categories in the description of the procedure code.

EXAMPLE

The repair of a *rupture* of an eyeball (16.82)
Correction of *cleft palate* (27.62).

The terms *rupture* and *cleft palate* are diagnoses, meaning this code can only be used for that specific type of repair or correction.

In ICD-10-PCS, the description of each procedure code is limited to the details of the procedure itself. The ICD-10-CM diagnostic codes will serve to explain the disease or condition.

EXAMPLE

Percutaneous needle core biopsy of right kidney 0TB03ZX

Open excision of tail of pancreas 0FBF0ZZ

2. *Not otherwise specified (NOS) options are omitted*: ICD-10-PCS requires you to have, at the very least, a minimum amount of detail

regarding each portion of the procedure. In those cases where the documentation has no additional specifics available and you cannot query the physician, ICD-10-PCS provides coding rules to guide you to the best, most appropriate code.

3. *Not elsewhere classified (NEC) options are reduced:* Due to the added levels of specificity throughout the ICD-10-PCS, the need for the NEC option is reduced. You will find the most common inclusion of NEC in procedure descriptions located in the sections on new devices and nuclear medicine, because such areas are more quickly affected by new technology and science.

THE STRUCTURE OF ICD-10-PCS CODES

Of course, the main purpose of creating ICD-10-PCS is to give you, the professional coder, an easier way to find the best, most accurate, and most specific code. That purpose has led to a new structure for the codes.

You may remember that ICD-9-CM Volume 3 procedure codes use a two-digit number to the left of a dot and up to two digits to the right of the dot.

EXAMPLE

18.09 Other incision of external ear (drainage, ear, external)

ICD-10-PCS codes have seven (7) characters. The codes are alphanumeric; the codes include both letters and numbers.

EXAMPLE

0990ZZZ Drainage, external ear, right, external approach

The first character in the seven-character sequence identifies the section of the ICD-10-PCS book to which the procedure belongs. The tabular (numeric) listing of ICD-10-PCS contains 17 sections, as identified in Box B-1.

EXAMPLE

An ankle x-ray is an imaging procedure—Section B

A breech extraction is an obstetrics procedure—Section 1

An amputation is a surgical procedure—Section 0

≪ CODING TIP

ICD-10-PCS codes may include any letter of the alphabet except the letters O and I. This is done to avoid any confusion between the letter O and the number 0, as well as any between the letter I and the number 1.

The 16 Sections of ICD-10-PCS

0 Medical and Surgical
1 Obstetrics
2 Placement
3 Administration
4 Measurement and Monitoring
5 Extracorporeal Assistance and Performance
6 Extracorporeal Therapies
7 Osteopathic
8 Other Procedures
9 Chiropractic
B Imaging

C Nuclear Medicine
D Radiation Oncology
F Physician Rehabilitation and Diagnostic Audiology
G Mental Health
H Substance Abuse Treatment

Note:

Until ICD-10-PCS has been approved and officially implemented, changes to the sections may still occur. This is the most recent at the time of this publication.

THE ICD-10-PCS BOOK

Just like the ICD-9-CM book and the CPT book, the ICD-10-PCS book is divided into two parts: the alphabetic index and the tabular (numerical) listing. The alphabetic index's entries are primarily sorted by **root operation terms**. Any root operation term identifies the specific service or type of treatment that is the basis of the entire procedure.

Root operation term

The exact procedure foundation.

CODING TIP »»

In ICD-10-PCS, the word operation has nothing to do with surgery.

Body system

The physiological system, or anatomical region, upon which the procedure was performed.

Body part

The anatomical site upon which the procedure was performed.

EXAMPLE

Root operation terms include bypass, drainage, excision, and insertion.

After you find the root operation term, as stated in the physician's notes, there are subentries listed by the following:

- **Body system**

EXAMPLE

Digestive system, musculoskeletal system

- **Body part**

EXAMPLE

Arm, leg, hand, foot

The alphabetic index also lists common terms for specific procedures.

EXAMPLE

Hysterectomy is listed and then cross-referenced to *resection* (a root operation term) and *female reproductive system* (body system).

A major difference between ICD-10-PCS, ICD-9-CM Volume 3, and CPT is the fact that the alphabetic index will only give you the first three or four characters of the actual seven-character procedure code. You will then *have* to go to the tabular (numeric) listing to find the additional characters.

Fragmentation

Of the Bladder OTF8-

You won't have to be reminded to *never code from the alphabetic index* once ICD-10-PCS comes into full effect. You won't be able to code from the alphabetic index alone anymore!

The tabular (numeric) list's entries are divided by body systems, similar to ICD-9-CM Volume 3. Of course, like all the other books, the section is in numerical order by the first character in the code.

Within each body system division of each section, the list continues in order by the root operation term for that procedure.

ICD-10-PCS CHARACTER ORDER AND PLACEHOLDERS

Each section of the tabular (numeric) list has a grid that specifies the assigned meaning to each letter or number along with its position in the seven-character code. (See Table B-1.)

Because the coding system is designed for future expansion, there will be cases where a specific procedure does not currently have the details to require all seven characters. In such cases, the letter Z is used to indicate that nothing in that position was applicable to the particular procedure.

«« CODING TIP

The sections are in order, as determined by the 16 sections listed in Box B-1—numbers 0 through 9 and then B through H— as indicated by the first character in the procedure code.

Table B-1 Sample from ICD-10-PCS Tabular Listing

0: Medical and Surgical (first character)

2: Heart and Great Vessels (second character)

7: Dilation: Expanding the orifice or the lumen of a tubular body part (third character)

Body Part Character 4	Approach Character 5	Device Character 6	Qualifier Character 7
0 Coronary Artery, One Site	0 Open	4 Drug-Eluting Intraluminal Device	6 Bifurcation
1 Coronary Artery, Two Sites	2 Open Endoscopic	D Intraluminal Device	Z No Qualifier
2 Coronary Artery, Three Sites	3 Percutaneous	Z No Device	
3 Coronary Artery, Four or More Sites	4 Percutaneous Endoscopic		

Approach

The specific technique used for the procedure.

Device

The identification of any materials or appliances that may remain in or on the body after the procedure is completed.

Qualifier

Any additional feature of the procedure, if applicable.

You will go through the grid and actually construct the correct code based on the physician's notes. As you have already learned, ICD-10-PCS codes are all seven characters. Therefore, you will build the code in this order, as directed by the grid (Table B-1).

First character: Section (e.g. Medicine, Mental Health, Imaging)
Second character: Body system
Third character: Root operation
Fourth character: Body part or region
Fifth character: **Approach**
Sixth character: **Device**
Seventh character: **Qualifier**

Therefore, when you review the information in Table B-1, you can see that the correct ICD-10-PCS code for the *Dilation of one site of a Coronary Artery, using an open approach with an Intraluminal device* is 02700DZ.

SUMMARY

Until the U.S. Congress approves an official start date for ICD-10-CM and ICD-10-PCS, you will have plenty of time to indoctrinate yourself to their proper usage. The purpose of this appendix is to provide an overview, giving you an idea of what to expect and establishing a comfort level so you are not apprehensive about the new system. It's going to be great!

1. In ICD-10-PCS, the initials PCS stands for

    a. Popular Coding System.

    b. Procedure Coding System.

    c. Possible Coding Solutions.

    d. Proper Coding System.

2. Of the four objectives for ICD-10-PCS, the one that relates to the meanings of the words and terms used is titled

    a. Completeness.

    b. Expandability.

    c. Multiaxial.

    d. Standardized terminology.

3. The descriptions for procedures identified in ICD-10-PCS

    a. Include diagnostic information.

    b. Define the disease or condition that caused the procedure.

    c. Do not include diagnostic information.

    d. Match those used in the CPT book exactly.

4. The structure of ICD-10-PCS codes includes

    a. Three numbers.

    b. Five numbers.

    c. Seven characters.

    d. Up to nine characters.

5. ICD-10-PCS codes include

    a. Only numbers.

    b. Only letters.

    c. One letter followed by numbers.

    d. Letters and numbers.

6. An example of a root operation term is

    a. Bypass.

    b. X-ray.

    c. Obstetrics.

    d. Hysterectomy.

7. Digestive system is an example of a

    a. Body part.

    b. Root operation term.

    c. Medical procedure.

    d. Body system.

8. The sections of ICD-10-PCS are identified by

    a. Numbers 1–17.

    b. Numbers 0–9 then Letters B–H.

    c. Letters A–Z.

    d. Alphabetical order by the name of the section.

9. Placeholders are used by ICD-10-PCS using

    a. The number 0.

    b. The letter X.

    c. The letter Z.

    d. The number 9.

10. ICD-10-PCS is designed to replace

    a. CPT.

    b. ICD-9-CM Volume 3.

    c. ICD-10-CM.

    d. ICD-9-CM.

11. An example of an approach is

    a. Anterior.

    b. Ileostomy.

    c. Pacemaker.

    d. Ventricular.

12. An example of a device, for purposes of ICD-10-PCS coding, is

    a. Ablation.

    b. Laparoscopy.

    c. Indwelling ureteral stent.

    d. Allotransplantation.

13. ICD-10-PCS uses characters consistently within the sections, and when possible, from section to section. This is called

    a. Expandability.

    b. Standardized Terminology.

    c. Completeness.

    d. Multiaxial.

14. The ICD-10-PCS code for the provision of a cesarean section would be found in

    a. Section 2 Placement.

    b. Section 1 Obstetrics.

    c. Section B Imaging.

    d. Section 6 Extracorporeal Therapies.

15. Coding a chiropractic manipulative treatment would begin in

    a. Section 0 Medical and Surgical.

    b. Section 4 Measurement and Monitoring.

    c. Section 7 Osteopathic.

    d. Section 9 Chiropractic.

Glossary

Ablation   Destruction or eradication of tissue.

Abstracting   The process of identifying the relevant words or phrases in health care documentation in order to determine the best, most appropriate code(s).

Adjunct code   The equivalent of a CPT add-on code. The code may not be reported alone or as a first-listed code.

Advanced life support (ALS)   Life-sustaining, emergency care is provided, such as airway management, defibrillation, and/or the administration of drugs.

Allotransplantation   The relocation of tissue from one individual to another (both of the same species) without an identical genetic match.

Alphanumeric   Expression containing both letters and numbers.

Ambulatory surgery center (ASC)   A facility specially designed to provide surgical treatments without an overnight stay; also known as same-day surgery center.

Anesthesia   The loss of sensation, with or without consciousness, generally induced by the administration of a particular drug.

Anesthesiologists   Physicians specializing in the administration of anesthesia.

Angiography   The imaging of blood vessels after the injection of contrast material.

Approach   The specific technique used for the procedure.

Anticipatory guidance   Recommendations for behavior modification and/or other preventive measures.

Arrhythmia   An irregular heartbeat.

Arthrodesis   The immobilization of a joint using a surgical technique.

Arthrography   The recording of a picture of an anatomical joint after the administration of contrast material into the joint capsule.

Basic life support (BLS)   The provision of emergency CPR, stabilization of the patient, first aid, control of bleeding, and/or the treatment of shock.

Basic personal services   Services that include washing/bathing, dressing and undressing, assistance in taking medications, and getting in and out of bed.

Bilateral   Both sides.

Body part   The anatomical site upon which the procedure was performed.

Body system   The physiological system, or anatomical region, upon which the procedure was performed.

Cannula   A tube that is inserted into the body to either deliver, or extract, fluid, such as a nasogastric tube.

Care plan oversight services   Evaluation and management of a patient, reported in 30-day periods, including infrequent supervision along with pre-encounter and postencounter work, such as reading test results and assessment of notes.

Category I codes   The codes listed in the main text of the CPT book; also known as *CPT codes*.

Category II codes   Performance measurement and tracking codes.

Category III codes   Emerging technology codes.

Catheter A thin flexible tube that is inserted into a body part and used to inject fluid, empty fluid, or to keep a passage open.

Caudal Near the hind part or tail of the body; the sacrum and coccyx areas.

Certified registered nurse anesthetist (CRNA) A registered nurse (RN) who has taken additional, specialized training in the administration of anesthesia.

Chelation therapy The use of a chemical compound that binds with metal in the body so that it will lose its toxic effect. It might be done when a metal disc or prosthetic is implanted in a patient, so there are no adverse reactions to the metal itself as a foreign body.

Class A finding Nontraumatic amputation of a foot or an integral skeletal portion.

Class B finding Absence of a posterior tibial pulse; absence or decrease of hair growth; thickening of the nail, discoloration of the skin, thinning of the skin texture; and/or absence of a posterior pedal pulse.

Class C finding Edema; burning sensation; temperature change (cold feet); abnormal spontaneous sensations in the feet; and/or limping.

Clinical Laboratory Improvement Amendment (CLIA) Federal legislation created for the monitoring and regulation of clinical laboratory procedures.

Closed treatment Fracture that is treated without surgically opening the affected area.

Code for coverage To choose a code by the insurance company's rules of what it will pay for, rather than a code that accurately reflects the truth about the encounter.

Completeness Structure that allows all procedures, services, and treatments to be represented by a code.

Complex closure (repair) A method of sealing an opening in skin involving a multilayered closure as well as reconstructive procedure, such as scar revision, debridement, or retention sutures.

Computerized tomography (CT) A specialized computer scanner with very fine detail that records images of internal anatomical sites.

Confirmatory consultation An encounter for purposes of a second physician's opinion or advice, requested by the patient, or a member of the patient's family, regarding the management of the patient's specific health concern.

Conscious sedation The use of a drug to reduce stress and/or anxiety.

Consultation An encounter for purposes of a second physician's opinion or advice, requested by another physician, regarding the management of a patient's specific health concern. A consultation is planned to be a short-term relationship between a health care professional and a patient.

Covered entities Businesses that have access to the personal health information of patients (health care providers, health plans, and health care clearinghouses).

CPT code modifier A two-character code that may be appended to a code from the main portion of the CPT book to provide additional information.

Critical care services Services for a patient who has a life-threatening condition expected to worsen.

Customary clinical documentation The usual contents of the notes and reports written after a health care encounter.

Cytology The investigation and identification of cells.

D

Decubitus ulcer Bedsore, or wound, created by lying in the same position on the same irritant without relief.

Diagnosis Physician's determination of a patient's condition, illness, or injury.

Device The identification of any materials or appliances that may remain in or on the body after the procedure is completed.

Disclosure The sharing of information between health care professionals working in separate entities, or facilities, in the course of caring for the patient.

DMEPOS An acronym for durable medical equipment, prosthetic, and orthotic supplies.

Donor area (site) The area or part of the body from which skin or tissue is removed with the intention of placing that skin or tissue in another area to help it heal.

Duplex scan Ultrasonic scanning procedure to determine blood flow and pattern.

Durable medical equipment (DME) Apparatus and tools that will last for a long time and/or be used to assist multiple patients over time.

Durable medical equipment regional carrier (DMERC) Companies that are contracted with Medicare to manage the day-to-day claims processing for durable medical equipment in a particular part of the country.

Early and periodic screening, diagnostic, and treatment (EPSDT) Medicaid preventive health program for children under 21.

End-stage renal disease (ESRD) Chronic, irreversible kidney disease requiring chronic dialysis.

Enteral Within, or by way of, the gastrointestinal tract.

Established patient A person who has received professional services within the last three years from the provider, or another provider of the same specialty belonging to the same group practice.

Etiology The study of the causes of disease.

Evaluation and management (E/M) Specific characteristics of a face-to-face meeting between a health care professional and a patient.

Excision The full-thickness removal of a lesion.

Expandability Structure that includes room for future growth.

Experimental A procedure or treatment that has not yet been accepted by the health care industry as the standard of care.

Fascia lata graft The transplantation of a connective tissue that encases the thigh muscles.

Fiscal intermediary A company that administers the day-to-day operation of reviewing and reimbursement of claims for state Medicare programs.

Fluoroscope A piece of equipment that emits x-rays through a part of the patient's body onto a fluorescent screen, causing the image to identify various aspects of the anatomy by density.

Full-thickness A measure that extends from the epidermis to the connective tissue layer of the skin.

General anesthesia The administration of a drug in order to induce a loss of consciousness; the condition by which a patient is unable to be aroused even by painful stimulation.

Global period The length of time allotted for postoperative care included in the surgical package; generally accepted to be 90 days for major surgical procedures and up to 10 days for minor procedures.

Global surgery package A group of services already included in the code for the operation and not reported separately.

Gross examination The study of a specimen by visual study (with the naked eye).

Harvesting The process of taking skin or tissue from one site (on the same body or another).

HCPCS Level II modifier A two-character alphabetic or alphanumeric code that may be appended to a code from the main portion of the CPT book or a code from the HCPCS Level II book.

HIPAA's Privacy Rule A portion of HIPAA ensuring that patient information is available to those who should see it while protecting that information from people who should not.

Hospice An organization that provides services to terminally ill patients and their families.

Hospital A facility that provides diagnostic, therapeutic (both surgical and nonsurgical), and rehabilitation services by, or under, the supervision of physicians to a patient admitted for a variety of medical conditions.

Immunization The process of making someone resistant to a particular disease by vaccination.

Incontinence The inability to control urination or fecal expulsion.

Infusion Introduction of a fluid into a blood vessel.

Injection The process of compelling a fluid into tissue or cavity.

Inpatient A patient staying overnight or longer in a hospital.

Intermediate closure (repair) A multilevel method of sealing an opening in the skin involving one or more of the deeper layers of the skin. *Note:* Single-layer closure of heavily contaminated wounds that require extensive cleaning or removal of particulate matter also constitutes intermediate repair.

Interval The time measured between one point and another, such as between physician visits.

Intervention   Action taken to change or prevent something that is happening, most often to stop or prevent something undesirable.

Invalid   An unacceptable code for reporting any procedure, service, or treatment.

Laboratory   A location with scientific equipment designed to perform experiments and tests.

Laminectomy   The surgical removal of a vertebral posterior arch.

Laterality   Relating to the side or sides of the body; *unilateral* meaning one side and *bilateral* meaning both sides.

Level of patient history   The amount of detail involved in the documentation of patient history.

Level of physical examination   The extent involved in the clinical assessment and inspection of the patient performed by the physician.

Liters per minute (LPM)   The measurement of how many liters of a drug or chemical is provided to the patient in 60 seconds.

Local anesthesia   The injection of a drug to prevent sensation in a specific portion of the body. Includes local infiltration anesthesia, digital blocks, and pudendal blocks.

Locum tenens physician   A physician that fills in, temporarily, for another physician.

Magnetic resonance arthrography (MRA)   MR imaging of an anatomical joint after the administration of contrast material into the joint capsule.

Magnetic resonance imaging (MRI)   A three-dimensional radiologic technique that uses nuclear technology to record pictures of internal anatomical sites.

Manipulation   The attempted return of a fracture or dislocation to its normal alignment manually by the physician.

Medical decision-making (MDM)   The description of how much knowledge and experience was needed by the provider for him or her to determine the diagnosis or to decide what to do next.

Medical exclusion criteria   A medical reason why a patient's data cannot be reported with a certain code.

Medical necessity   The assessment that the provider was acting according to standard practices in providing a procedure or service for an individual with a specific diagnosis.

Medicare code edit (MCE)   A computerized system to identify coding errors and/or concerns regarding medical necessity; a part of the Correct Coding Initiative.

Microscopic examination   The study of a specimen by using a microscope (under magnification).

Modifier   A two-character code that affects the meaning of another code; a code addendum that provides more to the meaning of the original code.

Multiaxial   Consistent use of characters and elements throughout a book.

Monitored anesthesia care (MAC)   The administration of sedatives, anesthetic agents, or other medications to relax but not render the patient unconscious while the patient is under constant observation of a trained anesthesiologist. Also known as "twilight" sedation.

Mutually exclusive codes   Codes that are not permitted to be used on the same claim form with each other.

New patient   A person who has not received any professional services within the past three years from the provider, or another provider of the same specialty who belongs to the same group practice.

Not otherwise specified (NOS)   The absence of more detailed information from the health care professional creating the documentation.

Nuclear medicine   Treatment that includes the injection or digestion of isotopes.

Nursing home   A facility that provides skilled nursing treatment and attention along with limited medical care for its residents, usually long-term, for individuals who do not require acute care services (hospitalization).

Open treatment   Surgically opening the fracture site, or another site in the body nearby, in order to treat a fractured bone.

Ophthalmologist   A physician qualified to diagnose and treat eye disease and conditions with drugs, surgery, and corrective measures.

Optional At your discretion; not required.

Optometrist A professional qualified to carry out eye examinations and to prescribe and supply eyeglasses and contact lenses.

Orthotic The making and fitting of orthopedic therapeutic devices.

Ostomy An artificial opening made surgically.

Otorhinolaryngology The study of the human ears, nose, and throat systems.

Outpatient A patient treated without being hospitalized.

P

Parenteral By way of anything other than the gastrointestinal tract, such as intravenous, intramuscular, intramedullary or subcutaneous.

Parenteral enteral nutrition (PEN) Nourishment delivered using a combination of means other than the gastrointestinal tract (e.g., IV), in addition to via the gastrointestinal tract.

Pathology The study of the nature, etiology, development, and outcomes of disease.

Patient population Common traits among patients using the same health care facility or health care provider.

Percutaneous skeletal fixation The insertion of fixation instruments (e.g., pins) placed across the fracture site. It may be done under x-ray imaging for guidance purposes.

Performance measure Criteria for gathering specific data to study.

Personnel modifiers A modifier providing additional information about the professionals attending to the treatment of the patient.

PFSH An acronym that stands for past, family, and social history.

Physical status modifier A two-character alphanumeric code used to describe the condition of the patient at the time anesthesia services were administered.

Preventive To stop something from happening or from getting worse.

Procedure A treatment or service provided by a health care professional.

Prosthetic Fabricated artificial replacement for a damaged or missing part of the body.

Protected health information (PHI) Any patient identifiable health information regardless of the form in which it is stored (paper, computer file, etc.).

Q

Qualifier: Any additional feature of the procedure, if applicable.

Qualitative The determination of a character or essential element(s).

Quantitative The counting or measurement of something.

Query To ask.

R

Radiation The high-speed discharge and projection of energy waves or particles.

Recipient area (site) The area or site of the body receiving a graft of skin or tissue.

Regional anesthesia The administration of a drug in order to interrupt the nerve impulses in a limited area without loss of consciousness. Includes epidural, caudal, spinal, axillary, stellate ganglion blocks, regional blocks, and brachial anesthesia.

Regional blocks Types of regional anesthesia applications that include axillary, bier, retrobulbar, peribulbar, interscalene, subarachnoid, supraclavicular, and infraclavicular blocks.

Reimbursement Payment for services provided.

Relationship The degree of familiarity between provider and patient.

Risk factor intervention Action taken by the attending physician to stop or reduce an impending health care concern.

Root operation term The exact procedure foundation. Root operation terms include bypass, drainage, excision, and insertion.

S

Saphenous vein Either of the two major veins in the leg that run from the foot to the thigh near the surface of the skin.

Self-administer To give medication to oneself, such as a diabetic giving herself an insulin injection.

Service-related modifier A modifier relating to a change or adjustment of a procedure or service provided.

Simple closure (repair) A method of sealing an opening in the skin (epidermis or dermis), involving only one layer.

Sonogram The use of sound waves to record images of internal organs and tissues. Also called an *ultrasound*.

Specialty care transport (SCT) A transportation vehicle that includes continuous care provided by one or more health professionals in an appropriate specialty area, such as respiratory care, cardiovascular care, or a paramedic with additional training.

Specimen A small part or sample of any substance or tissue obtained for analysis and diagnosis.

Standard of care The accepted principles of conduct, services, or treatments that are established as the expected behavior.

Standardized terminology One established meaning for each term.

Superbill A form preprinted with the diagnosis codes and procedure codes most frequently used in a particular facility.

Supplemental report A letter or report written by the attending physician or other health care professional to provide additional clarification or explanation.

Supporting documentation The paperwork in the patient's file that corroborates the codes presented on the claim form for a particular encounter; the written reports that provide evidence of what was provided to the patient and why.

Surgical pathology The study of tissues removed from a living patient during a surgical procedure.

Synchronous Simultaneous; occurring at the same time.

Topical anesthesia The application of a drug to the skin to reduce or prevent sensation in a specific area temporarily.

Transcutaneous electrical nerve stimulators (TENS) The use of electricity to agitate the skin to relieve pain.

Transplantation The transfer of tissue from one site to another.

Unbundling Coding individual parts of a specific procedure rather than one combination code that includes all the components.

Unlisted codes Codes that are shown at the end of each subsection of the CPT used as a catchall for any procedure not represented by an existing code.

Upcoding Using a code that indicates a higher level of service than that which was actually performed.

Urea reduction ratio (URR) A formula to determine the effectiveness of hemodialysis treatment.

Use The sharing of information between people working in the same health care facility for purposes of caring for the patient.

Venography The imaging of a vein after the injection of contrast material.

Credits

Chapter 13

p. 309: © Dynamic Graphics/JuperImages

p. 315: © Stockdisc/PunchStock

p. 318: © OS54 PhotoDisc/Getty

Chapter 14

p. 339: © Vol. 1 PhotoDisc/Getty Images

p. 346: © Ingram Publishing RF/Alamy

p. 353: © Vol. 40 PhotoDisc/Getty Images

Chapter 15

p. 383: © The McGraw-Hill Companies, Inc./Photo by JW Ramsey

Chapter 16

p. 395: © BrandX/Getty Images

Chapter 17

p. 417: © BrandX/Getty Images

Index

Note: Page numbers followed by f designate figures; b, boxes; and t, tables. A page number in **boldface** indicates the definition of the term on that page.

Symbols

A, 322
BI (dark grey box with a BI), 402
} (brace), 399
[ ] (brackets), 398
• (bullet symbol), 40, 77, 321
⊙ (bull's eye symbol), 40, 133, 278
☑ (check mark inside square box), 321, 352
○ (circle), 321
⮎ (circle with arrow), 40–41
⊘ (circle with slash), 40, 321
: (colon), 399
►◄, 40
EXCLUDES note, 400
♀, 322
INCLUDES note, 399
LC (blue-green box with an LC), 402–403
Line through code (Z1111), 322
M, 322
♂, 322
NC, 402
( ) (parentheses), 399
+ (plus symbol), 39–40
☑3ʳᵈ (red box with check mark and 3), 402
☑4ᵗʰ (red box with check mark and 4), 402
; (semicolon), 38
[ ] (slanted brackets), 398
▲ (triangle symbol), 40, 321

A

A codes (HCPCS), 314–315, 339–345
AAPC; *see* American Academy of Professional Coders (AAPC)
Abbreviations
    HCPCS, 328
    ICD-9-CM Volume 3 codes, 398–399
    laboratory tests, 242, 243t
    neurology, 271
Abdominal aortic aneurysm, 188, 318
Ablation, **269**
ABN; *see* Advance beneficiary notice (ABN)
Abstracting, **30**

Acronyms; *see* Abbreviations
Acupuncture, 274–275
Add-on codes, 39–40; *see also specific code*
    anesthesia services, 132–133
    immunizations, 258
Adjunct code, **401**
Administrative operations, information disclosure for, 8
Administrative services, 314
Administrative supplies, 344
Advance beneficiary notice (ABN), 376
Advanced life support (ALS), **314**, **354**
After-hours care, special rates for, 385
Age factors
    anesthesia services, 133, 278
    dialysis, 262
    symbol for, 322
AHIMA; *see* American Health Information Management Association (AHIMA)
Alcohol abuse treatment services, 317, 380–381
Allergy, 271
Allotransplantation, **181**; *see also* Recipient allotransplantation
Alphabetic lists
    differences between, 403
    format of, 38–39
    HCPCS codes, 312–313, 344, 350
    ICD-9-CM codes, 403–404
    ICD-10-PCS codes, 472
    verification with numerical list, 31, 107, 130, 266, 312, 404, 406, 472–473
Alphanumeric codes, **53**
Alphanumeric listing, HCPCS codes, 314–321
ALS; *see* Advanced life support (ALS)
Always report concurrent to the xxx procedure notation, 323
Alzheimer's facility, 105
Ambulance billing indicators, 357–358, 358b
Ambulance services, 314, 353–358
    CM-1491 claim form, 468
    modifiers, 356, 357b, 380
    waiting times, 354, 357, 357t
Ambulatory surgery center (ASC), **53**
    modifiers, 53, 58–59, 383
AMCC test; *see* Automated Multi-Channel Chemistry (AMCC) test
Amended claims, 15
American Academy of Professional Coders (AAPC), Code of Ethical Standards, 15–16, 18b
American Dental Association, 315